DENTAL SCIENCE, MATERIALS AND TECHNOLOGY

IMPLANT DENTISTRY

THEORY AND PRACTICE

DENTAL SCIENCE, MATERIALS AND TECHNOLOGY

DENTAL SCIENCE, MATERIALS AND TECHNOLOGY

IMPLANT DENTISTRY

THEORY AND PRACTICE

TIBOR KAROLY FABIAN
AND
HANS CHRISTIAN HIDALGO WULFF

NOVA BIOMEDICAL

New York

For permission to use material from this book please contact us:
Telephone 631-231-7269; Fax 631-231-8175
Web Site: http://www.novapublishers.com

Library of Congress Cataloging-in-Publication Data

ISBN: 978-63117-700-2

Library of Congress Control Number: 2014941040

Published by Nova Science Publishers, Inc. † New York

CONTENTS

PREFACE

Implant dentistry is a complex and rising field of dentistry and presents many intricate problems, which are being tackled by various disciplines for both basic and clinical research. There has been a great amount of scientific information gathered so far; however data are rather divergent, sometimes even contradictory. Therefore, there is an increasing need to integrate reviews about this highly important field of dentistry.

This work presents an integration of several prosthetic, surgical, and oral biological considerations of implant dentistry on a scientific level, with special respect to the problem of clinical decision-making. Further, this book also includes some chapters dedicated to rarely reviewed research areas like the use of physiotherapy and psychosomatic considerations for implant dentistry, which also satisfy a great want.

Relevant subject areas of this book include: applied anatomy and bone biology for implant dentistry; mechanisms of osseointegration and peri-implant soft tissue healing; biomaterials for implant surgery; medical and dental evaluation of patients; diagnostic imaging for implant dentistry and other diagnostic tools; several prosthodontic and surgical considerations for treatment planning; implant surgery; management of pain, inflammation, peri-implantitis and other complications; immediate and delayed loading of implants; implant maintenance and after care; physiotherapy and psychosomatic considerations for implant dentistry, and future perspectives on implant dentistry.

The book gathers and presents data on the leading edge of implant dentistry. However, there are many inadequacies in terms of study design and methodology present in the leading scientific literature. It is no wonder that there are numerous skeptic authors who are waiting for further data from well-designed studies before they will make any scientific conclusions. The authors of present work do not share such skeptical opinions and have intended this book to introduce the reader to what scientific research can tell us about implant dentistry today.

The anticipated principal audience for the present work is made up primarily of dental professionals having advanced knowledge related to implant dentistry (including university teachers and students of postgraduate and/or Ph.D. courses in dental schools). However, general dental practitioners, interested dental graduate students, and other professionals working in the orofacial region may also find the book serviceable.

The authors hope that this collection of data helps the reader be at home with implant dentistry related research and that the text will be used for professional reference. The authors also hope that the reader will be inspired to intensify efforts to discover this highly interesting field more deeply and to form a personal opinion by reading the cited references and other available literature.

INTRODUCTION

Knowing the applied anatomy of orofacial tissues is highly important for dentists practicing implant dentistry. Applied anatomy differs from classical descriptive anatomy significantly. Classical descriptive anatomy presents relevant details about an anatomical region, but the description is primarily about what the most typical variation looks like and details are discussed without (or with only moderate) respect to clinical significance. In contrast, applied anatomy is engaged in presenting those details that are of great clinical importance, including unusual and less frequently occurring variations of clinically important structures. From a surgical point of view, applied anatomy is crucial to understanding those practical morphological details that may help in avoiding unsuccessful surgical interventions because of laceration or damage done to highly important anatomical structures or because of misunderstanding clinically important anatomical situations. From a prosthodontic point of view, applied anatomy is highly important for planning, especially if a prosthodontic-driven implant-planning approach is used.

The success of implant dentistry strongly depends on proper diagnosis, optimal planning, and the degree of precision when implants are placed in the jaws. Therefore radiography plays a vital role in implant dentistry. Although a radiological diagnosis of the jaws and orofacial tissues may also include techniques like magnetic resonance imaging (MRI) and positron emission tomography (PET) in certain cases, in general, X-ray diagnostics is the most efficient tool for the analysis of orofacial hard tissues including bone and teeth and other related pathological conditions. Similarly, X-ray diagnostics is a major diagnostic tool for treatment planning and is needed to reach a proper level of surgical precision.

Titanium and its alloys are considered the most biocompatible and corrosion-resistant metals and are widely used as implant fixture materials today. Despite the high biocompatibility of titanium surfaces, certain materials (especially those used as bone substitutes as well) are frequently used as coatings for titanium fixtures. Therefore without having proper knowledge of bone substitutes and other biomaterials used for titanium coating, it would be difficult to understand certain aspects of current trends within implant fixture surface development.

Osseointegration is the stable and clinically asymptomatic rigid anchorage of an implant fixture achieved by direct bone-to-implant contact. The physiological cascade of osseointegration may be deconvoluted both phenomenologically and experimentally into three distinct phases: *osteoinduction*, *osteoconduction*, and *de novo bone formation*, which, in time, will be followed by the remodeling of the peri-implant bone tissue. The three premised peri-implant healing phases include the recruitment, maturation, and migration of osteogenic cells, followed by the bone formation of these cells on the implant surface result in a specific type of osteogenesis termed *contact osteogenesis*. Although contact osteogenesis is currently considered an optimum process, osseointegration may also occur via *distance osteogenesis*. In this case, *osteoinduction* is followed by the laying down of bone on the old bone surface in the peri-implant site instead of on the implant surface itself. The newly produced matrix encroaches on the implant, and in this way, the fixture becomes surrounded by bone, although there is no bone formation on the implant itself. Although most of the important aspects of osseointegration were recognized in relation to the osseointegration of titanium implants, it should be emphasized that the mechanism of osteogenesis seems to be rather similar in the case of many candidate implant materials, including newly developed metal alloys and ceramics as well as in the case of implant-coating materials or bone substitutes.

Successful dental implant treatment depends on the attachment of three basic components of healing peri-implant tissues, including the peri-implant bone, the peri-implant connective tissue, and the peri-implant gingival epithelium, which is composed of the apically located junctional epithelium and the peri-implant epithelium located farther away toward the peri-implant gingival sulcus. In the microenvironment of the peri-implant healing area, mesenchymal stem cells are stimulated by specific factors to differentiate into the adequate cell lineage. Under the influence of these factors, mesenchymal stem cells switch to osteoblastic cells that are in contact with bone tissue while they differentiate into a fibroblastic lineage in the gingival tissue region. The migration, early attachment, and proliferation of gingival epithelial cells occur in the same timeframe. Although bone and soft tissue processes are interconnected, thus they cannot be isolated, in reality, a separate chapter will focus on the healing and attachment of peri-implant gingival tissues for the sake of easier surveying.

Bone formation in the alveolar socket is a naturally occurring event as long as the surrounding alveolar walls remain intact. However, the volumetric contraction and sequential reparative resorption of the alveolar ridge may impair the implant placement; therefore several surgical techniques have been proposed to reduce the loss of the alveolar bone to an acceptable level. The primary aim of all these techniques is to reduce the postextraction loss of the alveolar bone and thereby enable the installation, primary stability, and osseointegration of dental implants as well as to improve the esthetic outcome of the final prosthesis, to reduce the need of additional bone grafting procedures, and to enable faster bone regeneration, allowing earlier prosthetic restoration. Thus the preservation of the alveolar ridge may be crucial for successful implant placement in many cases. For the preservation of the alveolar bone following tooth extraction, the use of common preservation techniques like "socket grafting," guided bone regeneration (GBR), immediate implant placement, and (in certain cases) forced eruption of compromised teeth may be considered.

There are various physiotherapeutic modalities that may be used in certain stages of implant-related treatments, including ultrasound, low-intensity pulsed ultrasound (LIPU), electric fields, light-emitting diode photomodulation therapy (LPT), and others. Some of them may be used before implant placement only (i.e. to promote bone augmentation before implant placement) but should not be used thereafter. Others may have compromised efficiency in deeper-located healing bone areas. Two major tools, namely, pulsed electromagnetic field (PEMF) therapy and low level laser therapy (LLLT), seem to be highly applicable in relation to implant dentistry; therefore, the related chapter will focus on these two modalities only.

It is obvious that the surgical aspects of implant dentistry are of primary importance; therefore the primary aim of the relevant chapter is to present a whole and comprehensive overview of several surgical techniques used in implant dentistry. Besides this, a few other closely related topics like the assessment of bone quality and primary stability as well as the complex problem of timing and the type of loading (i.e. functional, nonfunctional, and progressive loading) are also discussed in this chapter. This is because bone quality and primary stability can be evaluated best by a surgeon during surgery, and the surgeon's concrete observations in this regard should influence surgical techniques and surgical decision making as well as decision making related to the timing of, and the type of loading used for, the implants.

The abutment is a very important part of most implant systems. It is positioned between the fixture and the denture, and this "mesostructure" position (i.e. between the fixture as an "infrastructure" and the denture as a "suprastructure") makes it possible to connect dentures to fixtures and to modify the long axis of the implant-abutment-denture complex using an angled abutment that fits with a corresponding prosthetic emergence profile. Abutments may be classified as healing abutments or definitive abutments. If a healing abutment is used, it should be replaced with a definitive abutment after the healing phase. Healing abutments may be used right after the insertion of implant fixtures in cases of one-stage surgery or after the establishment of a mini-flap access during the uncovering stage of two-stage surgery. Accordingly, definitive abutments may be used either in all premised healing phases if no healing abutment was used or after the healing phase following the removal of the healing abutments. Abutments may also be classified based on the major fabrication technique, such as industrially manufactured straight/angled stock abutments (slightly modifiable chair-side), individually casted metal abutments, or CAD-CAM-milled (computer-aided design/computer-aided manufacturing) individual metal/zirconia abutments.

The survival rate of intraoral implants in *non*complex cases can be considered as rather high, being usually between 96%–100% in both the short-run (6–12 months) and the long-run (3 years or more). Although the documented results are rather satisfactory, patients who have undergone implant therapy should receive individualized, systematic, and continuous maintenance care for their peri-implant tissues to achieve favorable outcomes. Regular recall, proper personal and professional oral hygiene, and immediate adequate therapeutic interventions (if needed) are considered the cornerstones of well-founded maintenance care.

Implant dentistry may also utilize several specially sized implant systems, like short implants, narrow implants, and mini-implants. Short implants are manufactured for use in atrophic regions of the jaws and may be considered possible alternatives to bone augmentation, sinus floor elevation, or other advanced surgical procedures. Narrow diameter implants are potential solutions for specific clinical situations, such as reduced interradicular bone, thin alveolar crest (AC), and the replacement of teeth with small cervical diameters. Mini-implants are manufactured primarily for orthodontic purposes. The temporary placement of orthodontic mini-implants is widely employed to maximize anchorage during orthodontic treatment.

The orofacial region is an area of human privacy and is of special relevance to individual personality, with overproportional cortical representation that appears to be particularly predisposed for a large number of different functional and somatoform psychosomatic disorders. Oral psychogenic manifestations are based on unique psychological and depth psychological functions of the mouth and teeth during infancy (breasting), sexuality, aggressiveness, and communication. There is also great importance placed on the symbolic values of the mouth, teeth, tongue, and face. The mouth (including the teeth and tongue) also serves as a primary zone of interaction with the environment, and as such can have far-reaching emotional significance. It is surely tremendously important in a baby's life as an organ through which to receive nourishment; as an organ of pleasure; as an organ of contact with the mother; as an organ of testing, learning, and understanding; and as an organ of social signaling. The mouth should also be considered a highly charged erotogenic region right from childhood. Tooth loss may profoundly affect the psychosocial well-being of patients, even those who are apparently coping well with dentures and complete edentulousness can be a serious life event.

Medicamentous therapy is an important supplementary modality of implant dentistry. Medication is primarily utilized for the management of pain and inflammation, including antibiotic treatment if needed. Antibiotics may also be administered for preventative purposes in case of cardiac conditions associated with the highest risk of adverse outcomes from infective endocarditis and in the case of patients with total joint replacement. Besides these instances, medicamentous therapy may also be used for the management of fear of surgical intervention, for the management of muscle spasms, and for the management of allergic reactions in certain cases. In the related chapter, the most important aspects of medicamentous therapy from the viewpoint of implant dentistry will be introduced.

Implant failure can be considered a status of the implant performance that falls below an acceptable level. Despite the high success rate of oral implants, implant failure may sometimes occur. The distinction between the failed implant and a failing implant is clinically important because the failure process might be slow even if it is continual. In general, there are three major etiologic factors behind implant failure, such as bacterial infection, impaired healing, and overload. Besides implant failure, several other complications should also be considered. Complications are all the locally appearing conditions that materialize postoperatively; thus, complications may or may not lead to implant failure. Complications should be distinguished from surgical accidents, which may occur during surgery. Complications may be divided into two subclasses, such as early stage and late stage complications. Although various mechanisms are expected, not all the mechanisms responsible for the appearance of complications are known and the causative mechanisms often remain obscure. The most common causes are poor surgical technique (and/or an excessively traumatic surgical approach), bacterial contamination of the host site, decreased bone density, the presence of a bone dehiscence, a thin alveolar crest, wound dehiscence during healing, postoperative infection, excessive loading, the fabrication of an inadequate denture, and bad oral hygiene. Aside from the premised implant failure and other complications, adverse effects should also be considered. Adverse effects are conditions of general health significance that appear in relation to oral implant treatment. The appearance of adverse effects in relation to oral implants is rare.

There are only a few conditions that can be considered absolute contraindications in respect to dental implant rehabilitation, such as disease processes like recent myocardial infarction, recent cerebrovascular stroke, recent heart surgery, immune suppression, blood dyscrasias, *active* neoplastic disease undergoing treatment, drug abuse, certain psychiatric disorders, and more recently, intravenous bisphosphonate treatment. Accordingly, data suggest that patients with osteoporosis, cardiovascular diseases, and hypothyroidism are not at greater risk of implant failure. On the other hand, there are certain conditions that may negatively influence or jeopardize implant treatment outcomes. The most important conditions will be discussed in detail in the relevant chapter.

Future implant dentistry will utilize the body's own healing and reconstructive mechanisms by means of materials and concepts that are not available for regular use now but are readily envisioned by extrapolating information from current research efforts. Based on current developments, it is presumed that future implants will spontaneously heal and reconstruct surrounding tissues, which will revolutionize implant dentistry in the near future. Dental tissue engineering will provide an attractive alternative to traditional implantation therapies, with the hope that tissue-engineered teeth can be used to functionally replace missing teeth. However, tissue-engineering-based therapies are in their early phase of development and many issues need to be addressed before any clinical application occurs. Therefore the generation and clinical use of tissue-engineered teeth seems like it will be postponed for many years.

List of Abbreviations

2D	two-dimensional
3D	three-dimensional
AAOS	American Academy/Association of Orthopaedic Surgeons
ABH	available bone height
AC	alveolar crest
ADA	American Dental Association
AHA	American Heart Association
AMF	additional mental foramen
APF	apically positioned flap
BIC	bone-to-implant contact
BMPs	bone morphogenetic proteins
BPPV	benign paroxysmal positional vertigo
BRONJ	bisphosphonate-related osteonecrosis of the jaws
CAD/CAM	computer-aided design/computer-aided manufacturing
CAF	coronally advanced flap
CBCT	cone-beam CT, cone-beam computed tomography
CEJ	cementoenamel junction
CHD	congenital heart disease
C/I ratio	"crown-to-implant" ratio
CPC	calcium phosphate cement
cpTi	commercially obtainable pure titanium
CT	computed tomography
DD	dentine dysplasia
DGI	dentinogenesis imperfecta
DICOM	digital imaging and communications in medicine
DPCs	dental progenitor cells
DPR	digital panoramic radiography
DPT	definitive psychosomatic therapy
dPTFE	high-density polytetrafluoroethylene
DSI	distant site infection
EMD	enamel matrix derivative
ePTFE	expanded polytetrafluoroethylene
FA	fluoroapatite

FGF	fibroblast growth factor
FGG	free gingival graft
fMRI	see MRI
FOV	field of view
GBR	guided bone regeneration
GTR	guided tissue regeneration
HA	hydroxyapatite
HCA	carbonated apatite
HDPE	high density polyethylene
HIP	hot isostatic pressing
HLL	high level laser
HLLT	high level laser therapy
HU	Hounsfield unit(s)
IAN	inferior alveolar nerve
IE	infective endocarditis
IGF	insulin-like growth factor
IL-1β	interleukin-1-beta
IPT	initial psychosomatic therapy
ISQ	implant stability quotient
JE	junctional epithelium
LED	light-emitting diode
LF	lingual foramen
LIPU	low-intensity pulsed ultrasound
LLL	low level laser (soft laser)
LLLT	low level laser therapy
LPT	light-emitting diode photomodulation therapy
LT	linear tomography
MF	mental foramen
MIP	maximum intensity projection
MPR	multiplanar reconstruction
MR	see MRI
MRI	magnetic resonance imaging (MRI, fMRI, MR)
NDI	narrow diameter implant
NSAID	non-steroidal anti-inflammatory drug
OMI	orthodontic mini-implant
OP	orthopantomography (OP, PR)
OPG	osteoprotegerin
PDGF	platelet-derived growth factor
PDL	periodontal ligament
PDT	photodynamic therapy
PEMF	pulsed electromagnetic field
PET	positron emission tomography
PGA	polyglycolic acid
PHEMA	poly-hydroxyethyl methacrylate
PIE	peri-implant epithelium
PLA	polylactic acid

PLGA	poly-lactic-co-glycolic acid (copolymer of PLA and PGA)
PMMA	poly-methyl methacrylate
PPE	porous polyethylene
PR	panoramic radiography
PRP	platelet-rich plasma
PSAA	posterior superior alveolar artery
PSAN	posterior superior alveolar nerve
PTFE	polytetrafluoroethylene
PTH	parathyroid hormone
RANKL	receptor activator of nuclear factor-κβ ligand
RCC	right circular cylinder
RDI	regular diameter implant
RFA	resonance frequency analysis
ROI	region(s) of interest
RPD	removable partial denture
SCTG	subepithelial connective tissue graft
SIS	sinus implant stabilizer
SR	surface rendering
TENS	transcutaneous electric nerve stimulation
TGF-β	transforming growth factor beta
Ti	titanium (see also cpTi)
TMD	temporomandibular disorder
TMJ	temporomandibular joint
TNF-α	tumor necrosis factor alpha
TSAD	temporary skeletal anchorage devices
VIP	virtual implant placement
VR	volume rendering
Y-TZP	yttria-stabilized tetragonal zirconia polycrystals

CHAPTER 1

APPLIED ANATOMY FOR IMPLANT DENTISTRY

Abstract

The applied anatomy of the orofacial tissues is highly important for dentists practicing implant dentistry. Applied anatomy is engaged to present those details that are of high clinical importance, including unusual and less frequently occurring variations of clinically important structures. From a surgical point of view, applied anatomy is crucial in understanding those practical morphological details that may help to avoid unsuccessful surgical interventions. From a prosthodontic point of view, applied anatomy is highly important for planning, especially if a prosthodontic-driven implant-planning approach is used. In this chapter, the "hottest topics" from applied maxillary and mandibular anatomy are discussed. The text includes detailed applied anatomical descriptions of the maxillary sinus, frontal and zygomatic processes, and tuberal region and palatine processes of the maxillae as well as anatomical variations of the mandibular canal and other canals like the mental canal, lingual canal, and the incisive canal of the mandible. Anatomical variations of the mental foramen (MF), lingual foramen (LF), mental spinal foramen, and buccal foramen are also discussed in the text. Further, mandibular concavities as well as the applied anatomy of the alveolar bone of both jaws in dentate and edentulous, including an introduction of alveolar dehiscences and fenestrations, are also presented.

1.1. Introduction

The applied anatomy of the orofacial tissues is highly important for dentists practicing implant dentistry. Applied anatomy differs from classical descriptive anatomy significantly. Classical descriptive anatomy presents relevant details about an anatomical region, but the description is primarily about what the most typical variation looks like, and details are discussed without (or with moderate) respect to their clinical significance. In contrast, applied anatomy is engaged to present only those details that are of high clinical importance, including unusual and less frequently occurring variations of clinically important structures. From a surgical point of view, applied anatomy is crucial to understanding those practical morphological details that may help to avoid unsuccessful surgical interventions because of laceration or damage done to very important anatomical structures or because of misunderstandings about clinically important anatomical situations. From a prosthodontic point of view, applied anatomy is highly important for planning, especially if a prosthodontic-driven implant-planning approach is used.

1.2. The Applied Anatomy of Maxilla

1.2.1. The Applied Anatomy of Maxillary Sinus

The maxillary sinus is a large pyramidal-shaped cavity in the body of the maxilla (Williams and Warwick 1980; Pignataro et al. 2008). Its size shows great interindividual differences, and there are differences between the two sides within the same patient as well (Williams and Warwick 1980; Pignataro et al. 2008). Its size is also related to age and the presence or absence of upper teeth (Pignataro et al. 2008). The maxillary sinus is largely pyramidal-shaped (Williams and Warwick 1980). The base of this pyramidal cavity is the lateral wall of the nasal cavity, which presents the natural ostium to the middle meatus of the nose, generally through two small apertures, one of which is usually closed by a mucous membrane in living human body (Williams and Warwick 1980; Pignataro et al. 2008). The apex of the pyramid is laterally directed and extends into the zygomatic process (Williams and Warwick 1980), and in certain cases, it may reach the zygomatic bone itself (Williams and Warwick 1980). With the exception of the alveolar wall (also termed "floor"), which is formed from the alveolar process of the maxilla, all other walls of the maxillary sinus are rather thin and correspond to the orbital, anterior, and infratemporal aspects of the maxillary body and the lateral wall of the nasal cavity (Williams and Warwick 1980).

The lowest level of the alveolar wall (floor of sinus) is usually about 1.25 cm below the level of the floor of the nasal cavity (Williams and Warwick 1980). In many cases, radiating septa spring from the floor in the intervals between the adjacent teeth (Williams and Warwick 1980), especially at the border region between the premolars and molars and between the second and third molars (Underwood 1910; Krennmair et al. 1997; Beretta et al. 2012). The so-called secondary septa may also arise from the irregular pneumatization of the sinus floor following tooth loss (Krennmair et al. 1997; Beretta et al. 2012). All these septa should be considered carefully, because they can complicate sinus elevation by hampering the inversion of the bone plate and the lifting of the sinus membrane (Pignataro et al. 2008; Beretta et al. 2012). Besides premised septa, sinus floor extensions (alveolar recesses) may also appear between the roots of teeth in roughly 52% of cases (Nimigean et al. 2008), a fact that should also be considered because it may facilitate the violation of the sinus membrane through surgical procedures (Nimigean et al. 2008).

The bony lamella separating the maxillary sinus and the teeth decreases in thickness from the upper canine region (ca. 6.9 mm) to the second molar region (ca. 1.7 mm) and increases distal from this region, reaching a thickness of ca. 2.8 mm at the third molar region (Nimigean et al. 2008). Consequently, there is a very thin bony lamella in roughly 6% of teeth (primarily premolars and molars), and roughly 14% of teeth perforating the floor are covered by the sinus mucosa only (Nimigean et al. 2008). Perforations most frequently occur in the case of molars (Williams and Warwick 1980), but premolars (especially second premolars) may also penetrate the sinus floor (Nimigean et al. 2008).

The posterior wall of the maxillary sinus contains alveolar canals that may project as ridges into the sinus and transmit the posterior superior alveolar artery (PSAA) and nerve (PSAN) to the molar teeth (Williams and Warwick 1980; Sato et al. 2010). Similarly, the infraorbital canal also projects an extending ridge from the orbital wall (also termed "roof") to the anterior wall (Williams and Warwick 1980; Sato et al. 2010) and transmits the infraorbital artery and nerve (Sato et al. 2010). Importantly, the posterior superior alveolar artery anastomoses with the infraorbital artery at the anterolateral region (Solar et al. 1999; Traxler et al. 1999), forming the extended and contiguous bony canal structure of the anterior and lateral wall of the maxillary sinus (Solar et al. 1999; Traxler et al. 1999; Sato et al. 2010; Yoshida et al. 2010). The location of these bony canal structures can be evaluated via CBCT (cone-beam computed tomography) (Sato et al. 2010; Yoshida et al. 2010) and should be considered before sinus surgery to avoid laceration or damage of the PSAA and PSAN and consequent bleeding, vascular impairment, ischemia, or pain (Sato et al. 2010; Yoshida et al. 2010). This is especially true because in many cases (ca. 53%), these bony canals run in the deeper regions of the lateral wall, and in some cases (ca 23.5%), they run rather near to the sinus floor (Yoshida et al. 2010).

1.2.2. Frontal and Zygomatic Processes

The frontal and zygomatic processes are important bony structures around the maxillary sinus. In certain cases these bony structures may allow the insertion of angulated/tilted implants (Sorni et al. 2005). Although the insertion of such angulated/tilted implants into the premised maxillary processes is clearly not easy, the surgical technique itself has undergone considerable development in recent years (Sorni et al. 2005). Insertion of the implants into the premised bony structures may be of importance in the rehabilitation of patients with larger bony defects and/or with an extremely resorbed alveolar process. There is usually a rather compact cortical layer and a rather dense medullary bone from the *lower part of the frontal process* positioned between the nasal cavity and the maxillary sinus (Sorni et al. 2005), which may be used for the insertion of tilted/angulated implants in certain cases (Mattsson et al. 1999; Krekmanov et al. 2000; Sorni et al. 2005). Similarly, there is a rather compact bone structure for the zygomaticoalveolar crest along with the zygomatic process (Sorni et al. 2005) that may advantageously be utilized for the insertion of implants in certain cases (Krekmanov 2000; Balshi and Wolfinger 2001; Parel et al. 2001); however the extension of the maxillary sinus into the zygomatic process should be carefully evaluated before surgery.

1.2.3. The Tuberal Region

The tuberal region comprises three bony structures, including the maxillary tuberosity, the pyramidal process of the palatine bone, and the pterygoid process of the sphenoid bone (Williams and Warwick 1980; Sorni et al. 2005). The maxillary tuberosity is usually composed of a scantly dense medullary bone covered by a rather thin cortical layer (Sorni et al. 2005); therefore, it is usually not an ideal structure for implant placement (Sorni et al. 2005). In contrast, the pyramidal process of the palatine bone and the anterior portion of the pterygoid process are composed of cortical bone (Sorni et al. 2005); therefore, the junction-region of the above-mentioned three bony structures (i.e. the maxillary tuberosity, pyramidal process, and pterygoid process) may be used for implant placement in certain cases (Graves 1994; Balshi et al. 1995; Fernandez and Fernandez 1997; Balshi and Wolfinger 1999; Nocini et al. 2000). However, an extremely careful surgical technique is needed if an implant is placed into this region, because there is high risk of damaging branches of the maxillary artery (Fernandez and Fernandez 1997; Sorni et al. 2005) and the maxillary nerve. The fact that the pterygopalatine fossa is nearby should also be considered carefully since serious complications because of the dangerous spreading of the occasional infection through this fossa may also appear.

1.2.4. The Applied Anatomy of the Palatine Process

The thickness and quality of the bone from the maxillary palatine process are crucial factors for the planning and success of palatal implants used for orthodontic anchorage. Most orthodontic implants are placed either in the midline and 6–12 mm posterior to the incisive foramen or are placed into an ovoid area located on both sides of the midline, 3–9 mm lateral from the midline and 3–9 mm posterior from the papillary coronal plane (Lai et al. 2010). In general, bone height is lowest in the midline and increases gradually lateral to the midline. In contrast, bone mineral density is the highest in the midline (in the median-palatal suture) and decreases gradually lateral to the midline (Lai et al. 2010). Taking into consideration both factors (bone height and density), the median-palatal suture and at least 6 mm posterior to the incisive foramen appears to be the most suitable location for implantation even if very short implants are used (Lai et al. 2010). However, it should be considered that the median-palatal suture seems to be an important center of maxillary growth and development (Lai et al. 2010); therefore, in the case of children and adolescents, any real need for palatal implantation, especially into the median-palatal suture, should be evaluated carefully (Lai et al. 2010) to avoid affecting maxillary growth and development.

1.3. The Applied Anatomy of the Mandible

1.3.1. Anatomical Variations of the Mandibular Canal

The mandibular canal runs more or less horizontally in the mandibular body below the sockets of the teeth with which it communicates through small canals (Williams and Warwick 1980). It contains the inferior alveolar nerve and vessels from which branches enter the roots of the teeth (Williams and Warwick 1980). However it should be considered that there are certain variations of the mandibular canal. A double ("duplicated" or "bifid") mandibular canal is the most frequent such variation (Karamifar et al. 2009; Bogdan et al. 2006), but in certain cases, even a triple mandibular canal may be observed (Bogdan et al. 2006). The existence of such variations should certainly be recognized and carefully evaluated before implant surgery (Karamifar et al. 2009; Bogdan et al. 2006).

1.3.2. Anatomical Variations of the Mental Canal and Mental Foramen

Between (or below) the roots of the first and second premolars, the mandibular canal divides into incisive and mental canal (Williams and Warwick 1980). The mental canal typically swerves upward, backward, and laterally to reach the mental foramen (Williams and Warwick 1980). This typical swerve is referred to as an "*anterior loop*." The prevalence of a loop-shaped mental canal has been reported between 88% (Neiva et al. 2004) and 96% (Arzouman et al. 1993) of the time, and in most cases (76%), it was observed bilaterally (Neiva et al. 2004). The mean mesial extent of the anterior loop was reported to be between 4.3 mm (Neiva et al. 2004) and 6.95 mm (Arzouman et al. 1993), but even longer loops may also appear, indicating a need for the exact radiological determination of the course and location of the mental canal before implant placement into the interforaminal region occurs (Uchida et al. 2007). In rare cases, an accessory mental canal may also exist, especially distal to the mental foramen (Kulkarni et al. 2011).

Anatomical variations of the mental foramen have also been reported in many studies. In most cases, double or multiple mental foramina appear (Kaufman et al. 2000; Igarashi et al. 2004; Santos Jr. et al. 2013) as a result of the branching of the mental nerve before it passes through the MF. In contrast, the MF may be single but hypoplastic, or it may even not exist in rare cases (Silva Ramos Fernandes et al. 2011). The reported frequency of occurrence of additional mental foramen (AMF) is between 1.4% and 7% (Sawyer et al. 1998; Hanihara and Ishida 2001). In most cases the AMF is located rather near (1.3–1.5 mm) to the MF in an apico-coronal direction (in coronal plane); however, the distance between the MF and AMF may be up to 5–6 mm in the mesio-distal direction (Kulkarni et al. 2011; Santos Jr. et al. 2013), which should be considered when safety distance is being determined for implant surgery.

1.3.3. The Lingual Canal and Lingual Foramen

The lingual canal descends from the mandibular canal to the lingual side of the mandible and opens to the sublingual region through the lingual foramen (Yoshida et al. 2005). This canal contains branches of the inferior alveolar artery and nerve running in the mandibular canal. However, branches of the sublingual artery may also enter the mandible via this canal, leading to the risk of dangerous sublingual bleeding if any injury of larger branches occurs (Hofschneider et al. 1999; Gultekin et al. 2003). An auxiliary nerve, which supplies the teeth and alveolar bone, may also arrive from the sublingual area and its occurrence may cause difficulties in relation to the mandibular nerve block techniques (Williams and Warwick 1980).

The prevalence of the lingual canal and lingual foramen is rather high; reported values were 15% (Yoshida et al. 2005), 46% (Yoshida et al. 2005), 73% (Jaju and Jaju 2011), and 82% (Jacobs et al. 2002). Importantly, roughly 30%–40% of patients seem to have two or more lingual canals (Gultekin et al. 2003). The typical location of the lingual foramen is the premolar region on the inside surface of the mandible (Gultekin et al. 2003; Yoshida et al. 2005), somewhat basal and mesial to the location of the mental foramen (Yoshida et al. 2005). The mean diameter of the lingual canal(s) is 0.6 mm in the premolar region (Gultekin et al. 2003); however, somewhat larger canals may also appear, which should be considered before implant planning to avoid dangerous sublingual bleeding complications (Gultekin et al. 2003; Yoshida et al. 2005).

1.3.4. The Incisive Canal, Mental Spinal Foramen, and Buccal Foramen

The frequency of occurrence of the incisive canal of the mandible is roughly 93% (Jacobs et al. 2002). The diameter of incisive canals is roughly between 1–7 mm (mean 3.1 mm) at the origin and 0.5–5 mm (mean 1.7 mm) at 5 mm mesially (Uchida et al. 2007). The mean diameter of the incisive canal at the midline region is roughly 0.8 mm (Gultekin et al. 2003); however, there are certainly also much smaller and much larger canals.

The incisive canal continues below the incisor teeth (Williams and Warwick 1980) and may have an opening on the lingual side at the midline of the mandible (referred to as the "mental *spinal* foramen"). The prevalence of the mental spinal foramen is rather high; values have been reported to be between 13% (Yoshida et al. 2005), 53% (Tepper et al. 2001), and 99% (McDonnell et al. 1994). It is believed that arterial branches from the sublingual region may enter the mandible via the mental spinal foramina, which should be considered before implant placement because of the real risk of dangerous sublingual bleeding (Gultekin et al. 2003). In roughly 50% of cases, supplementary branches of the mylohyoid nerve enter the mandible via the mental spinal foramina, serving as supplementary innervation for the lower incisor region (Madeira et al. 1978), which may also be considered for implant surgery, especially in relation to the efficiency of local anesthesia (Sutton 1974).

The incisive canal may also have an opening(s) in the buccal side (referred to as "buccal foramen"), especially in the incisor, canine, or premolar region; in rare cases, they can also appear in the midline (Naitoh et al. 2009). The prevalence of foramina entering the buccal side of the mandible is rather high; roughly 44% of the patients have at least one, but in many cases, they have at least two such foramina (Naitoh et al. 2009). These foramina appear roughly 2%–3% of the time in the midline, 42% of the time in the incisor/canine region, 27% of the time in the premolar region, and 15% of the time posterior to the mental foramen (Naitoh et al. 2009); however not all of them belong to the incisive canal (Naitoh et al. 2009). It should be noted that some of these foramina (especially those located in the premolar region or behind the mental foramen) more likely belong to the mental canal (Naitoh et al. 2009) or to an accessory mental canal of the mandibular canal (Kulkarni et al. 2011) and therefore should be considered anatomical variations of the mental foramen. In the case of buccal foramina, it may also be the case that the auxiliary nerve supply or arterial branches may enter the mandible (Williams and Warwick 1980); however, their clinical significance is much less than those entering via the mental spinal foramen or via the lingual foramen (see above).

1.3.5. Mandibular Concavities

There are three major mandibular concavities (Williams and Warwick 1980), including the "*incisive fossa*" (below the incisor teeth, labial side), the "*sublingual fossa*" (at the location of the sublingual gland), and the "*submandibular fossa*" (at the location of the submandibular gland). These concavities should be considered carefully, especially if the placement of longer implants is planned (Madrigal et al. 2008). In certain cases, however, unusual concavities of the mandible may also appear (Williams and Warwick 1980; Aguiar et al. 2011). Therefore, detailed radiological examination of the mandibular surface is crucial before implant planning.

1.4. Applied Anatomy of the Alveolar Bone (Both Jaws)

1.4.1. Anterior Maxilla and Mandible in Dentate

A sufficient thickness of the residual cancellous and cortical bone is a primary factor in the initial fixation and osseointegration of implants placed following tooth extraction. In dentate, the thickness of the alveolar bone normally increases from the alveolar crest to the root apex and from the anterior region to the molar region (Kim et al. 2012). The thickness of the alveolar bone following extraction may be critical, especially in the anterior region, because of both anatomical and esthetic reasons (Kim et al. 2012). In dentate, the anterior region cortical bone thickness increases from the crestal side to the apical side in both the labial and lingual/palatal sides of both jaws (Kim et al. 2012). The labial cortical bone of maxilla is the thinnest compared to the other regions (Kim et al. 2012). The cancellous bone of anterior maxilla in dentate is thinnest at the crestal region and its thickness increases from the crestal side to the apical side in the maxilla (Kim et al. 2012). In contrast, the crestal bone of the anterior dentate mandible is thinnest around the middle of the root (Kim et al. 2012).

The amount of total (cancellous and cortical) bone thickness gradually increases from the crestal to the apical side in both the labial and palatal/lingual sides of both dentate jaws. The increase of the total amount of bone is rather pronounced in the palatal/lingual side of both jaws (Han and Jung 2011), whereas it is less pronounced in the labial side of both jaws (Han and Jung 2011) around the middle region of the roots in both the maxilla and the mandible (Han and Jung 2011). The distance between the alveolar crest and the cementoenamel junction (CEJ) is much longer in the labial than the palatal side of the maxilla (Han and Jung 2011). In contrast, the distance between the AC and CEJ is rather similar when comparing the labial and lingual sides of the mandible (Han and Jung 2011). Absolute values of mandibular AC-CEJ distances are somewhat higher than *palatal* maxillary values but are much lower than *labial* maxillary values (Han and Jung 2011). In general, a labial bone thickness of more than 1.91 mm following implant placement could prevent a failure of the implant resulting from severe labial bone resorption (Cho et al. 2011; Kim et al. 2012). However, the buccal wall of the frontal/premolar region may be thinner, averaging ca. 0.8 mm in the anterior and ca. 1.1 mm in the premolar sites (Pagni et al. 2012).

After tooth extraction, the alveolar bone undergoes sequential reparative resorption/remodeling and in particular the labial cortical bone and alveolar crest suffer strong dimensional changes (Kim et al. 2012; Pagni et al. 2012) that may compromise both implant stability and esthetics, especially in the case of the anterior maxilla. This initial reparative bone resorption/remodeling occurs in two phases. *During the first phase*, there is initially a blood clot; subsequently granulation tissue and then later a provisional matrix and woven bone fill up the alveolus (Pagni et al. 2012). These processes lead to the rapid resorption of the thin layer of alveolar bundle bone that lines the alveolar socket and extends coronally, forming the alveolar crest (and also makes part of the periodontal structure as it encloses the external terminations of Sharpey's fibers). Thus, a consequent and rather quick resorption of the thin alveolar crest occurs, especially if the alveolar wall is thin (Pagni et al. 2012). *During the second phase*, the outer surface of the alveolar bone is remodeled, which causes further overall horizontal and vertical bone tissue contraction (Pagni et al. 2012). Interestingly, the horizontal bone tissue contraction is greater in the molar region compared to the premolar area (Pagni et al. 2012).

To prevent the premised dimensional changes of the maxillary labial cortical bone from the crestal region following tooth extraction, immediate implant placement, "socket grafting," or guided bone regeneration may be used (Covani et al. 2003, 2007; Nevins et al. 2006; Yoo et al. 2006; Pagni et al. 2012). Reducing the extraction trauma and limiting flap elevation (if any) are essentials for each surgical procedure in this respect (Fickl et al. 2008; Pagni et al. 2012). Following the initial bone resorption/remodeling phase, the remaining parts of the alveolar bone are gradually absorbed throughout life (Williams and Warwick 1980; Pagni et al. 2012). The resorption rate of the alveolar ridges is faster during the first six months following the extraction and proceeds at an average of 0.5%–1.0% per year for the rest of an individual's lifetime (Williams and Warwick 1980; Pagni et al. 2012).

1.4.2. Alveolar Resorption in the Edentulous Mandible

In the case of the edentulous mandible, the alveolar ridge is strongly resorbed. The process of resorption affects primarily the thinner of the two alveolar walls, which is the labial wall in the anterior and the lingual wall in the molar regions (Williams and Warwick 1980). Therefore, the resorption process frequently results in a linear (sometimes "knife-edge-shaped") alveolar ridge that lies within the (previously existing) line of teeth in the anterior and outside that line in the molar region (Williams and Warwick 1980). In the case of the premised linear "knife-edge-shaped" alveolar bone, the height of the edentulous mandibular bone should be further reduced to reach a bucco-lingual diameter of a minimum of 5–6 mm, which is necessary for successful implant placement into edentulous arches (Madrigal et al. 2008). This means that the mandibular bone height may need to be reduced by up to roughly 3–5 mm, which corresponds to a rather significant reduction (roughly 14%–18%) of total bone height in certain cases (Madrigal et al. 2008).

In the case of edentulous maxilla, the process of resorption is rather similar to that of the mandible, although the contour of the resorbed alveolar ridge is more rounded (instead of "knife-edge-shaped") in this case (Williams and Warwick 1980). In the case of the maxilla, the labial alveolar wall is thinner everywhere (Williams and Warwick 1980); therefore, the rest of the alveolar ridge lies wholly within the curve of the previously existing line of teeth (Williams and Warwick 1980). Consequently, the maxillary line of the edentulous alveolar ridge nearly always lies within the mandibular line in the molar region, but in many cases it also lies in the premolar, canine, or incisor region. The significantly altered relation between the mandibular and maxillary alveolar aches should also be considered carefully from a prosthodontic point of view before implant surgery.

1.4.3. Alveolar Dehiscences and Fenestrations

Alveolar dehiscences (lack of cortical bone at the level of roots) and fenestrations (localized defect in the alveolar bone that exposes the root surface) are common findings (Williams and Warwick 1980), being present in roughly 54% and 70% of patients, respectively (Nimigean et al. 2009). The prevalence of dehiscences is higher (72%) in the mandible, whereas the prevalence of fenestrations is higher (75%) in the maxilla (Nimigean et al. 2009). Alveolar dehiscences and fenestrations are considered non-pathological conditions. However, their undiagnosed or unexpected appearance may unnecessarily complicate implant surgical procedures (Nimigean et al. 2009), especially in the case of fenestrations. Most fenestrations are located at the apical third of the roots (49%), whereas their prevalence at the middle of the root (28%) and at the coronal third of the root (19%) is somewhat lower (Nimigean et al. 2009). There are a few percentages (4%) of large fenestrations extending from the apical to the middle third of the root (Nimigean et al. 2009). Apical fenestrations typically appear in the maxilla, whereas coronal fenestrations appear mostly in the mandible (Nimigean et al. 2009). Although fenestrations appear primarily in the buccal side, lingual fenestrations of molar sockets may also appear (Williams and Warwick 1980). The prevalence of fenestrations is highest in the case of the first molar (43%), followed by the first premolar (14%) in the maxilla, whereas their prevalence is highest in the case of the first molar (16%), followed by the canine (5%), in the case of the mandible (Nimigean et al. 2009).

Conclusion

Applied anatomy of the orofacial tissues is of great significance for dentists practicing implant dentistry. In this chapter, the "hottest topics" of applied maxillary and mandibular anatomy were discussed to help the reader avoid unsuccessful surgical interventions arising from misunderstanding practical morphological details of clinical importance and to help implant planning from both a surgical and prosthodontic point of view.

References

Aguiar, LBV; Neves, FS; Bastos, LC; Crusoe-Rebello, I; Ambrosano, GMB; Campos, PSF. *ISRN Dentistry*, 2011, Article ID 792145. DOI: 10.5402/2011/792145.

Arzouman, MJ; Otis, L; Kipnis, V; Levine, D. Observations of the anterior loop of the inferior alveolar canal. *Int J Oral Maxillofac Implants*, 1993, 8, 295–300.

Balshi, TJ; Lee, HY; Hernandez, RE. The use of pterygomaxillary implants in the partially edentulous patient: a preliminary report. *Int J Oral Maxillofac Implants*, 1995, 10, 89–98.

Balshi, TJ; Wolfinger, GJ. Analysis of 356 pterygomaxillary implants in edentulous arches for fixed prosthesis anchorage. *Int J Oral Maxillofac Implants*, 1999, 14, 398–406.

Balshi TJ; Wolfinger, GJ. Treatment of congenital ectodermal dysplasia with zygomatic implants: a case report. *Int J Oral Maxillofac Implants*, 2002, 17, 277–281.

Beretta, M; Cicciu, M; Bramanti, E; Maiorana, C. Schneider membrane elevation in presence of sinus septa: anatomic features and surgical management. *Int J Dentistry*, 2012, Article ID 261905. DOI: 10.1155/2012/261905.

Bogdan, S; Pataky, L; Barabas, J; Nemeth, Z; Huszar, T; Szabo, G. Atypical courses of the mandibular canal: comparative examination of dry mandibles and x-rays. *J Craniofac Surg*, 2006, 17, 487–491.

Cho, YB; Moon, SJ; Chung, CH; Kim, HJ. Resorption of labial bone in maxillary anterior implant. *J Adv Prosthodont*, 2011, 3, 85–89.

Covani, U; Cornelini, R; Barone, A. Bucco-lingual bone remodeling around implants placed into immediate extraction sockets: a case series. *J Periodontol*, 2003, 74, 268–273.

Covani, U; Cornelini, R; Barone, A. Vertical crestal bone changes around implants placed into fresh extraction sockets. *J Periodontol*, 2007, 78, 810–815.

Fernandez, J; Fernandez L. Placement of screw type implants in the pterygo-maxillary-pyramidal region: a surgical procedure and preliminary results. *Int J Oral Maxillofac Implants*, 1997, 12, 814–819.

Fickl, S; Zuhr, O; Wachtel, H; Bolz, W; Huerzeler, M. Tissue alterations after tooth extraction with and without surgical trauma: a volumetric study in the beagle dog. *J Clin Periodontol*, 2008, 35, 356–363.

Graves, SL. The pterygoid plate implant: a solution for restoring the posterior maxilla. *Int J Periodontics Restorative Dent*, 1994, 14, 513–523.

Gultekin, S; Arac, M; Celik, H; Karaosmaoglu, AD; Isik, S. Assessment of mandibular vascular canals by dental CT. *Tani Girisim Radyol*, 2003, 9, 188–191.

Han, JY; Jung, GU. Labial and lingual/palatal bone thickness of maxillary and mandibular anteriors in human cadavers in Koreans. *J Periodontal Implant Sci*, 2011, 41, 60–66.

Hanihara, T; Ishida, H. Frequency variations of discrete cranial traits in major human populations. IV. Vessel and nerve related variations. *J Anat*, 2001, 199, 273–287.

Hofschneider, U; Tepper, G; Gahleitner, A; Ulm, C. Assessment of the blood supply to the mental region for reduction of bleeding complications during implant surgery in the interforaminal region. *Int J Oral Maxillofac Implants*, 1999, 14, 379–383.

Igarashi, C; Kobayashi, K; Yamamoto, A; Morita, Y; Tanaka, M. Double mental foramina of the mandible on computed tomography images: a case report. *Oral Radiol*, 2004, 20, 68–71.

Jaju, P; Jaju, S. Lingual vascular canal assessment by dental computed tomography: A retrospective study. *Ind J Dental Res*, 2011, 22, 232–236.

Jacobs, R; Mraiwa, N; van Steenberghe, D; Gijbels, F; Mirynen, M. Appearance, location, course, and morphology of the mandibular incisive canal: an assessment on spiral CT scan. *Dentomaxillofac Radiol*, 2002, 31, 322–327.

Karamifar, K; Shahidi, S; Tondari, A. Bilateral bifid mandibular canal: Report of two cases. *Ind J Dent Res*, 2009, 20, 235–237.

Kaufman, E; Serman, NJ; Wang, PD. Bilateral mandibular accessory foramina and canals: a case report and review of the literature. *Dentomaxillofac Radiol*, 2000, 29, 170–75.

Kim, HJ; Yu, SK; Lee, MH; Lee, HJ; Kim, HJ; Chung, CH. Cortical and cancellous bone thickness on the anterior region of alveolar bone in Korean: a study of dentate human cadavers. *J Adv Prosthodont*, 2012, 4, 146–152.

Kulkarni, S; Kumar, S; Kamath, S; Thakur, S. Accidental identification of accessory mental nerve and foramen during implant surgery. *J Indian Soc Periodontol*, 2011, 15, 70–73.

Krekmanov, L. Placement of posterior mandibular and maxillary implants in patients with severe bone deficiency: a clinical report of procedure. *Int J Oral Maxillofac Implants*, 2000, 15, 722–730.

Krekmanov, L; Kahn, M; Rangert, B; Lindstrom, H. Tilting of posterior mandibular and maxillary implants for improved prosthesis support. *Int J Oral Maxillofac Implants*, 2000, 15, 405–414.

Krennmair, G; Ulm, C; Lugmayr, H. Maxillary sinus septa: incidence, morphology and clinical implications. *J Cranio-Maxillo-Facial Surg*, 1997, 25, 261–265.

Lai, RF; Zou, H; Kong WD; Lin, W. Applied anatomic site study of palatal anchorage implants using cone beam computed tomography. *Int J Oral Sci*, 2010, 2, 98–104.

Madeira, MC; Percinoto, C; das Garcas, M; Silva, M. Clinical significance of supplementary innervation of the lower incisor teeth: a dissection study of the mylohyoid nerve. *Oral Surg Oral Med Oral Pathol*, 1978, 46, 608–614.

Madrigal, C; Ortega, R; Meniz, C; Lopez-Quiles, J. Study of available bone for interforaminal implant treatment using cone-beam computed tomography. *Med Oral Patol Oral Cir Bucal*, 2008, 13, E307–E312.

Mattsson, T; Kondell, PA; Gynther, GW; Fredholm, U; Bolin, A. Implant treatment without bone grafting in severely resorbed edentulous maxillae. *Int J Oral Maxillofac Surg*, 1999, 57, 281–287.

McDonnell, D; Reza, NM; Todd, ME. The mandibular lingual foramen: a consistent arterial foramen in the middle of the mandible. *J Anat*, 1994, 184, 363–369.

Naitoh, M; Nakahara, K; Hiraiwa, Y; Aimiya, H; Gotoh, K; Ariji, E. Observation of buccal foramen in mandibular body using cone-beam computed tomography. *Okajimas Folia Anat Jpn*, 2009, 86, 25–29.

Neiva, RF; Gapski, R; Wang, HL. Morphometric analysis of implant-related anatomy in Caucasian skulls. *J Periodontol*, 2004, 75, 1061–1067.

Nevins, M; Camelo, M; De Paoli, S; Friedland, B; Schenk, RK; Parma-Benfenati, S; Simion, M; Tinti, C; Wagenberg, B. A study of the fate of the buccal wall of extraction sockets of teeth with prominent roots. *Int J Periodontics Restorative Dent*, 2006, 26, 19–29.

Nimigean, V; Nimigean VR; Maru, N; Salavastru, DI; Badita, D; Tuculina, MJ. The maxillary sinus floor in the oral implantology. *Romanian J Morphol Embryol*, 2008, 49, 485–489.

Nimigean, VR; Nimigean, V; Bencze, MA; Dimcevici-Poesina, N; Cergan, R; Moraru, S. Alveolar bone dehiscences and fenestrations: an anatomical study and review. *Romanian J Morphol Embryol*, 2009 50, 391–397.

Nocini, PF; Albanese, M; Fior, A; De Santis, D. Implant placement in the maxillary tuberosity: the Summers' technique performed with modified osteotomes. *Clin Oral Impl Res*, 2000, 11, 273–278.

Pagni, G; Pellegrini, G; Giannobile, WV; Rasperini, G. Postextraction alveolar ridge preservation: Biological basis and treatments. *Int J Dentistry*, 2012, Article ID: 151030. DOI: 10.1155/2012/151030.

Parel, SM; Branemark, PI; Ohrnell, LO; Sensson, B. Remote implant anchorage for the rehabilitation of maxillary defects. *J Prosthet Dent*, 2001, 86, 377–381.

Pignataro, L; Mantovani, M; Torretta, S; Felisati, G; Sambataro, G. ENT assessment in the integrated management of candidate for (maxillary) sinus lift. *Acta Otorhinolaryngologica Italica*, 2008, 28, 110–119.

Santos Jr., O; Pinheiro, LR; Umetsubo, OS; Sales, MAO; Cavalcanti, MGP. Assessment of open source software for CBCT in detecting additional mental foramina. *Braz Oral Res (Sao Paulo)*, 2013, 27, 128–135.

Sato, I; Kawai, T; Yoshida, S; Miwa, Y; Imura, K; Asaumi, R; Sunohara, M; Yosue, T. Observing the bony canal structure of the human maxillary sinus in Japanese cadavers using cone beam CT. *Okajimas Folia Anat Jpn*, 2010, 87, 123–128.

Sawyer, DR; Kiely, ML; Pyle, MA. The frequency of accessory mental foramina in four ethnic groups. *Arch Oral Biol*, 1998, 43, 417–420.

Silva Ramos Fernandes, L; Capelozza, A; Rubira-Bullen, I. Absence and hypoplasia of the mental foramen detected in CBCT images: a case report. *Surg Radiol Anat*, 2011, 33, 731–734.

Solar, P; Geyerhofer, U; Traxler, H; Windisch, A; Ulm, C; Watzek, G. Blood supply to the maxillary sinus relevant to sinus floor elevation procedures. *Clin Oral Impl Res*, 1999, 10, 34–44.

Sorni, M; Guarinos, J; Penarrocha, M. Implants in anatomical buttresses of the upper jaw. *Med Oral Patol Oral Cir Bucal*, 2005, 10, 163–168.

Sutton, RN. The practical significance of mandibular accessory foramina. *Aust Dent J*, 1974, 19, 167–173.

Tepper, G; Hofschneider, UB; Gahleitner, A; Ulm, C; Computed tomographic diagnosis and localization of bone canals in the mandibular interforaminal region for prevention of bleeding complications during implant surgery. *Int J Oral Maxillofac Implants*, 2001, 16, 68–72.

Traxler, H; Windisch, A; Geyerhofer, U; Surd, R; Solar, P; Firbas, W. Arterial blood supply of the maxillary sinus. *Clin Anat*, 1999, 12, 417–421.

Uchida, Y; Yamashita, Y; Goto, M; Hanihara, T. Measurement of anterior loop length for the mandibular canal and diameter of the mandibular incisive canal to avoid nerve damage when installing endosseous implants in the interforaminal region. *J Oral Maxillofac Surg*, 2007, 65, 1772–1779.

Underwood, AS. An inquiry into the anatomy and pathology of the maxillary sinus. *Journal of Anatomy and Physiology*, 1910 44, 354–369.

Williams, PL; Warwick, R. (Ed-in-chiefs). *Gray's Anatomy*. Thirty-sixth edition. Edinburgh-London-Melbourne-New York: Churchill Livingstone; 1980. 316–319, 340, 342.

Yoo, RH; Chuang, SK; Erakat, MS; Weed, M; Dodson, TB. Changes in crestal bone levels for immediately loaded implants. *Int J Oral Maxillofac Implants*, 2006, 21, 253–261.

Yoshida, S; Kawai, T; Okutsu, K; Yosue, T; Takamori, H; Sunohara, M; Sato, I. The appearance of foramen in the internal aspect of the mental region of mandible from Japanese cadavers and dry skulls under macroscopic observation and three-dimensional CT images. *Okajimas Folia Anat Jpn*, 2005, 82, 83–88.

Yoshida, S; Kawai, T; Asaumi, R; Miwa, Y; Imura, K; Koseki, H; Sunohara, M; Yosue, T; Sato, I. Evaluation of the blood and nerve supply patterns in the molar region of the maxillary sinus in Japanese cadavers. *Okajimas Folia Anat Jpn*, 2010, 87, 129–133.

CHAPTER 2

RADIOGRAPHIC IMAGING FOR IMPLANT DENTISTRY

Abstract

The success of implant dentistry depends on proper diagnosis, optimal planning, and the degree of precision when implants are placed in the jaws. Therefore radiography plays a vital role in implant dentistry. X-ray diagnostics is the most efficient tool for the analysis of orofacial hard tissues, including bone and teeth, and related pathological conditions; therefore, this chapter focuses primarily on X-ray diagnostics although some other radiographic tools like MRI and PET are also briefly discussed. X-ray diagnostics for implant dentistry usually includes the evaluation of intraoral radiographs, images of orthopantomography, and images of cone-beam computed tomography. *Intraoral radiographs* are primarily used for follow up, including the examination of a bone-implant interface for signs of failure such as a radiolucent rim around the implant body and loss of crestal bone and augmented/grafted bone. In certain cases, intraoral radiographs may also be used for planning. *Orthopantomography* (OP) is one of the most frequently used modalities for presurgical planning, including both finding an appropriate location and measuring the available bone. Within certain limitations bone quality may also be evaluated. OP is generally also useful in ruling out gross pathosis within the jaws before implant surgery as well as for follow up with multiple implants and augmented/grafted bone. However, the reliability of panoramic radiography for presurgical implant planning in the anterior area is questionable. *Cone-beam computed tomography* (CBCT) was designed specifically for visualizing the maxillofacial region and offers both two- and three-dimensional images with high spatial resolution. CBCT can be used to rule out gross pathosis and other unexpected findings/conditions within the jaws and the orofacial region before implant surgery as well as to detect or rule out procedural errors following implant treatment. Further, CBCT is an important tool in the evaluation of those anatomical structures that may limit implant placement. The assessment of the quality of bone is also possible but it comes with certain limitations. For dental implant surgery, easily comprehensible volumetric maxillo-mandibular images of high spatial resolution and high dimensional accuracy are available in any plane. CBCT-based CAD/CAM surgical guide technology allows dentists to place implants using a surgical guide and place fixed prosthesis during the same dental visit.

2.1. Introduction

The success of implant dentistry mostly depends on proper diagnosis, optimal planning, and the degree of precision when implants are placed in the jaws. Therefore radiography plays a vital role in implant dentistry (Mupparapu and Singer 2004). Although radiological diagnosis of the jaws and orofacial tissues may also include techniques like magnetic resonance imaging and positron emission tomography in certain cases, in general, X-ray diagnostics is the most efficient tool for the analysis of orofacial hard tissues, including bones and teeth, and related pathological conditions (Scarfe et al. 2006; Nair and Nair 2007). Similarly, X-ray diagnostics is a major diagnostic tool for treatment planning and to reach a proper level of surgical precision, especially because those anatomical structures that may limit implant placement (Pompa et al. 2010) as well as the quantity and quality of the bone can be best evaluated with X-ray (de Carvalho Crusoe Silva 2012). As a consequence of the above considerations, this chapter focuses primarily on X-ray diagnostics, although some other radiographic tools like MRI and PET are also briefly discussed.

2.2. Radiological Diagnostic Tools

2.2.1. X-Ray

X-ray diagnostics is highly efficient in the analysis of orofacial hard tissues, including bones and teeth, and related pathological conditions (Scarfe et al. 2006; Nair and Nair 2007). Radiographic evidence of sialolithiasis and certain other pathological condition of the soft tissues, like mineralization in the stylohyoid or stylomandibular ligament (Eagle syndrome), may also be recognized (Correll and Wescott 1982); however, in such cases, the diagnostic value of X-ray images is limited. X-ray diagnostics is a major diagnostic tool for implant dentistry, especially because anatomical structures that may limit implant placement, such as the maxillary sinus, incisive foramen (Pompa et al. 2010), mandibular canal, mental canal, mental foramen, additional mental foramen (Naitoh et al. 2009; Georgescu et al. 2010; Santos Jr. et al. 2013), incisive canal of the mandible, mental spinal foramen, lingual foramen, and the lingual canal (Yoshida et al. 2005; Naitoh et al. 2009; Jaju and Jaju 2011) as well as the morphology of the maxillary vascular network and nerve supply (Sato et al. 2010; Yoshida et al. 2010) can be best evaluated with X-ray. Similarly, the quantity and quality of the bone can be best evaluated with X-ray (de Carvalho Crusoe Silva 2012).

X-ray diagnostics includes the evaluation of several two-dimensional (2D) images including *intraoral radiographs*, *extraoral radiographs*, and images of *orthopantomography*. X-ray diagnostics also includes evaluation of three-dimensional (3D) images from *computed tomography* (CT) (Hazey et al. 2009; Spin-Neto et al. 2013; Wenzel et al. in press). 3D imaging was developed to overcome the major drawbacks of 2D images, like inherent magnification, distortion, and the overlap of anatomical structures (Howerton Jr. and Mora 2008). In contrast to 2D imaging, 3D imaging was developed as a digital-imaging modality, but within the last few decades, digital radiological imaging has also been replacing the traditional film-based radiography in all 2D-imaging modalities, including periapical, bitewing, panoramic, and cephalometric imaging (Howerton Jr. and Mora 2008).

A number of technological advances in radiology have attempted to improve the standard of two-dimensional and computed tomographic (3D) images (Scarfe et al. 2006; Hazey et al. 2009). For the enhanced visualization of 2D images, *magnification*, *gamma adjustment*, and *enhanced two-dimensional imaging* (Parks 2008; Hazey et al. 2009) including *color enhancement*, *image reversal*, *histogram equalization* (accentuating a small area), *contrast enhancement*, and several *measurement tools* (Parks 2008; Hazey et al. 2009) are the most important techniques. In the case of 3D computed tomography, a new and highly efficient method called *cone-beam computed tomography* was developed roughly fifteen years ago (Mozzo et al. 1998). The CBCT method reaches higher diagnostic value in the orofacial region, like other medical CT methods (Scarfe et al. 2006; Hintze et al. 2007; Spin-Neto et al. 2013; Wenzel et al. in press), with the use of a lower X-ray dose and does so at lower costs (Berrington De Gonzalez and Darby 2004; Silva et al. 2008; Spin-Neto et al. 2013), but it requires careful interpretation to achieve optimum results (Howerton Jr. and Mora 2008; de Carvalho Crusoe Silva 2012).

2.2.2. MRI

*Magnetic resonance imaging (*including *fMRI)* uses the principle of nuclear magnetic resonance to produce cross-sectional images with high spatial resolution without the use of ionizing radiations (Pompa et al. 2010). All the data employed to create the final image comes from properly stimulated hydrogen atoms, which first absorb and then give out energy that is detected in the form of electrical signals (Pompa et al. 2010). MRI is a highly sensitive and noninvasive tool, especially suitable for the diagnosis of heterogeneous pathologies because soft tissues and bones as well as their changes during function (i.e. continuous moving images) may be analyzed (Ogasawara et al. 2001; Larheim 2005). In general, MRI is suitable to detect bone marrow and cortical bone abnormalities, osteoarthritis, sinovial proliferation, joint effusion (more fluid than seen in healthy individuals), TMJ (temporomandibular joint) disc displacement, disc morphology, and TMJ functioning (de Laat et al. 1993; Larheim 2005). MRI may also be used to evaluate the constriction or dilatation of blood vessels (Ogasawara et al. 2001), which could be important for the diagnosis of vascular orofacial pain symptoms. Recently, MRI was also considered for implant dentistry (Pompa et al. 2010). The relative biological safety of MRI and the fact that MRI makes it possible to create 3D images of both hard and soft tissues are key elements that led to the testing of its clinical applications. The first results were promising (Pompa et al. 2010), but the quality of the images of bony structures were not as high as those of X-ray CBCT images.

2.2.3. Positron Emission Tomography (PET)

Although *positron emission tomography* is not considered a usual diagnostic tool for implant dentistry, it may be mentioned for the sake of completeness. PET is primarily used as a highly sensitive tool for the diagnosis of primary or metastatic malign tumors in the orofacial region (Baek et al. 2008) because actively growing malignant tumor cells take up much higher amounts of nutrition (including positron-emitting diagnostic radioisotopes like ^{18}F, ^{11}C, ^{15}O, or ^{13}N) from the environment than normal cells (Rother 2001). This kind of tomography is rather expensive because of the use of a positron-camera and the need for administered radioisotopes. It may be used to verify or to exclude primary, metastatic, or recidival tumors (Rother 2001; Baek et al. 2008; White and Pharoah 2008) in connection with orofacial reconstructive implantology.

2.3. Conventional X-Ray Diagnostics

2.3.1. Intraoral Radiographs

Intraoral radiographs are primarily used for follow up, including the examination of a bone-implant interface for signs of failure, such as a radiolucent rim around the implant body or loss of crestal bone (Mupparapu and Singer 2004) and augmented/grafted bone (Jung et al. 2010; Cha et al. 2011). Using an individually fabricated bite-block with a film-holder (i.e. using hard body impression materials or other proper dental materials), a series of standardized periapical radiographs may be taken with a conventional paralleling technique before and after implant placement (Wakoh et al. 2006; Fernandez-Formoso et al. 2011).

The parallel technique is defined as parallelism between the object to be studied and the plane of the film, with a perpendicular central axis coming from the X-ray (Fernandez-Formoso et al. 2011). These radiographs may be used for longitudinal assessment in a routine follow-up regarding bone changes around implant fixtures (Grondahl et al. 1996; Wakoh et al. 2006; Fernandez-Formoso et al. 2011; Schropp et al. 2012). For the optimization of standard projections, a simple "RB-RB/LB-LB mnemonic rule" may be used as follows (Schropp et al. 2012): if implant threads are blurred at the right side of the implant (Right Blur or "RB"), the X-ray beam direction must be raised (Raise Beam or "RB"); whereas if implant threads are blurred at the left side (Left Blur or "LB"), the direction of the X-ray beam must be lowered (Lower Beam or "LB") to obtain sharp projections of the implant on both sides (Schropp et al. 2012). Importantly, the "RB-RB/LB-LB" rule applies irrespective of whether the implant was placed in the upper or lower jaw (Schropp et al. 2012).

When intraoral films are well angulated and applying the premised standardized projection, the periapical radiographs have minimal distortion (Fernandez-Formoso et al. 2011) that can be corrected with a software program (Wakoh et al. 2006). Therefore, these images are appropriate for application with a digital subtraction technique (Wakoh et al. 2006) and are well suited for longitudinal assessment of peri-implant bone change after implantation (Wakoh et al. 2006; Fernandez-Formoso et al. 2011).

Using certain software, the pose determination of implants with a shape (at least in part or in whole) of right circular cylinder (RCC) in three dimensions is also possible from a single two-dimensional radiograph (Schulze 2010).

In certain cases intraoral radiographs may also be used for planning (Lim et al. 2004; Mupparapu and Singer 2004). Periapical views may be used for the initial evaluation of available bone. Intraoral occlusal projections may be used for the determination of the width of a ridge (Lim et al. 2004; Desai et al. 2013). Making intraoral occlusal projections with a denture-shaped template (with radio-opaque markers like gutta-percha or the metal ball of a known diameter, etc.) placed in the mouth, possible differences (if any) between the prosthetic and radiological optimum positions of the implant placement may also be recognized at least in the case of the mandible (Desai et al. 2013).

2.3.2. Orthopantomography (OP, DPR)

Orthopantomography (also referred to as panoramic radiography "PR/" or digital panoramic radiography "DPR") is one of the most frequently used modalities for presurgical planning, including both finding an appropriate location and measuring the available bone (Rockenbach et al. 2003; Mupparapu and Singer 2004; Hu et al. 2012). Within certain limitations, bone quality may also be evaluated via panoramic radiography using the fractal dimension analysis method (Lee et al. 2010). Further, orthopantomography is generally useful in ruling out gross pathosis within the jaws before implant surgery (Mupparapu and Singer 2004) as well as for follow up with multiple implants and augmented/grafted bone (Hieu et al. 2010; Cha et al. 2011).

Panoramic radiographs display the body of the mandible and maxilla, including the maxillary sinus, on a single image (Hu et al. 2012). The length and mesiodistal angulation of an implant may be accurately determined, especially in the posterior area (Rockenbach et al. 2003; Hu et al. 2012). In this area, bifid mandibular canals are also rather recognizable (Langlais et al. 1985; Karamifar et al. 2009). However the accuracy is not as high as that of CBCT; the vestibulo-oral angulation of an implant placement cannot be obtained (Rockenbach et al. 2003; Hu et al. 2012), and the evaluation of smaller bone defects (Aguiar et al. 2011; Penarrocha et al. 2012) or concavities of bone contour (Madrigal et al. 2008) are not possible (Madrigal et al. 2008; Aguiar et al. 2011; Penarrocha et al. 2012).

Further, a roughly 20%–30% overestimation of the available bone height (ABH) frequently occurs in both jaws even in the posterior region (Park 2010). Mandible overestimation may occur especially if there is resorption of the buccal aspect of the ridge and the alveolar crest has moved to the lingual side (Lee et al. 2012). The above-mentioned high risk of overestimation should be considered and calculated when safety distances are determined based on panoramic radiography in the posterior region.

In the anterior area, where more distortions may appear (Park 2010; Hu et al. 2012), the height of available bone may be greatly overestimated (Hu et al. 2012, Georgescu et al. 2010), the distortion of one side compared to the contralateral side may also appear (Park 2010), and the evaluation of the morphology of the incisive and mental canal (both considered the extension of the mandibular canal) and/or additional mental foramen (if any) is also severely compromised (Georgescu et al. 2010; Santos Jr. et al. 2013). The evaluation of the presence or absence of an anterior loop (typical swerve of the mental canal, which rises from the mandibular canal and runs outward, upward, and backward again to open at the mental foramen) is also rather compromised (Kuzmanovic et al. 2003; Ngeow et al. 2009). The evaluation of the presence or absence of the mental spinal foramen, lingual canal, and lingual foramen is also nearly impossible to verify with any certainty. Therefore the reliability of panoramic radiography for presurgical implant planning is questionable in this region (Ngeow et al. 2009; Hu et al. 2012; Georgescu et al. 2010).

In recent years, several software programs for implant planning have been developed, but the manual methods still seem to be more accurate than the software (de Freitas and Montebello Filho 2004). However, planning software may be used advantageously to improve a patient's understanding of the implant placement process by making communication between the patient and dentist easier (de Freitas and Montebello Filho 2004). Certain software programs may also be used advantageously to compare a series of OP images and in this way they will evaluate in the long run changes of graft height utilizing a software-based superimposition technique (Riachi et al. 2012).

2.3.3. Linear Tomography and Complex Motion Tomography

Linear tomography (LT) is the simplest conventional tomographic technique based on the linear movement of the X-ray tube and the detector cassette (Mupparapu and Singer 2004). Linear tomography is frequently available as an additional function in equipment used for panoramic radiography. This technique allows the obtainment of a transversal image of the alveolar bone. Linear tomography has the advantage of low cost, low radiation dose, and speed and ease of execution (Rockenbach et al. 2003; Mupparapu and Singer 2004). However its exactness and validity are questionable, especially because of non-uniform magnification and decreased sharpness (Rockenbach et al. 2003). The accuracy of LT is not as good as that of CBCT. Values of available bone may be significantly overestimated using this technique (Rockenbach et al. 2003).

To overcome the weaknesses of linear tomography, more complex computer-controlled motions (i.e. circular, trispiral, elliptical, and hypocycloidal) for an X-ray tube and detector cassette were introduced. This more developed type of conventional tomography is referred to as complex motion tomography or computer-*assisted* tomography (Mupparapu and Singer 2004). Although images of complex motion tomography are of higher quality than those of LT (Mupparapu and Singer 2004), their quality does not match those of CBCT images (Mupparapu and Singer 2004).

2.4. X-Ray Diagnostics with CBCT

2.4.1. About CBCT in General

Cone-beam CT (CBCT) systems belong to the highest level of computed tomography systems. These CT systems were designed specifically for the visualization of the maxillofacial region. The major advantage of CBCT compared to the medical CT is that it can collect volume data by means of a *single* rotation (taking between ca. 9–40 sec.) due to the use of a *cone*-shaped X-ray beam and two-dimensional detectors (Yajima et al. 2006; Howerton Jr. and Mora 2008). In this way, CBCT overcomes the major drawback of medical CT methods in which the scanner acquires *sliced*-image data with a *fan*-shaped X-ray beam and captures portions (slices) of anatomy as the source and receptor rotate and move along the long axis of the section of anatomy being examined (Yajima et al. 2006; Howerton Jr. and Mora 2008). Therefore medical CT images are reconstructed based on numerous projection data from several slices (Yajima et al. 2006; Howerton Jr. and Mora 2008). Consequently, resolution is sometimes compromised (i.e. there are "blind spaces" between slices), and the details of anatomical structures in the maxillofacial region are insufficient to allow adequate visualization (Yajima et al. 2006).

CBCT offers a great advantage in comparison to medical CT in terms of accuracy, scan time reduction, dose reduction, and its lower number of artifacts (Yajima et al. 2006; de Carvalho Crusoe Silva 2012; Spin-Neto et al. 2013; Wenzel et al. in press). In certain cases the advantage of dose reduction may be further enhanced, because the dose may be further reduced (sometimes to approximately ⅛ of the standard exposure) based on the careful individual evaluation of patients (Dawood et al. 2012).

CBCT offers both two- and three-dimensional images with high spatial resolution through the employment of an isotropic voxel matrix, and it has the potential to offer additional benefits in hard-tissue visualization and the evaluation of the morphology of the maxillofacial region (Yajima et al. 2006; Howerton Jr. and Mora 2008), because CBCT reformats the raw data of radiation detectors into "Digital Imaging and Communications in Medicine" (DICOM) data (Yajima et al. 2006; Howerton Jr. and Mora 2008), which are imported into viewing software that enables the manipulation of multiplanar reconstructed slices.

Importantly, using the DICOM data format, a dentist can make *precise* measurements in *any plane* within the viewing software (Yajima et al. 2006; Howerton Jr. and Mora 2008). Based on the above possibilities, CBCT can be used to rule out gross pathosis and other unexpected findings/conditions within the jaws and the orofacial region before implant surgery (Caglayan and Tozoglu 2012; Silva et al. 2012) as well as to detect or rule out procedural errors following implant treatment (Silva et al. 2012). CBCT is also very important in the evaluation of those anatomical structures that may limit implant placement. Assessing the quality of hard tissue is also possible (Howerton Jr. and Mora 2008) but comes with certain limitations (de Carvalho Crusoe Silva 2012).

DICOM data may also be used in additional software. Using several available dental software programs, CBCT is capable of displaying various processed images (Yajima et al. 2006; Howerton Jr. and Mora 2008), such as a multiplanar reconstruction (MPR), volume rendering (VR), surface rendering (SR), maximum intensity projection (MIP), or cross-sectional views of various planes. CBCT also provides simulation tools to bridge the gap between 2D and 3D image types via lateral and posteroanterior cephalometric views (Cevidanes et al. 2006) as well as panoramic ("OP-like") or partial panoramic views (the latter is a smaller field within the panoramic view).

In most cases, there are possibilities for a detailed (0.1 mm voxel sizes) and a less detailed (0.2 mm voxel sizes) projection with a smaller or a larger field of view (FOV), respectively (Yajima et al. 2006). For dental implant surgery, easily comprehensible volumetric maxillo-mandibular images of high spatial resolution and high dimensional accuracy are also available in any plane (Yajima et al. 2006). Moreover, there is software available to aid in the placement of implants and/or grafting, as well as to aid orthodontic assessment and orthognathic surgery (Yajima et al. 2006; Howerton Jr. and Mora 2008).

2.4.2. CBCT and the Evaluation of Anatomical Structures

CBCT is crucial in the evaluation of those anatomical structures that may limit implant placement. Aside from in the evaluation of the morphology of the maxillary sinus, incisive foramen, mandibular canal, and mental foramen, CBCT is also very useful in evaluating the presence or absence of an additional mental foramen, mental spinal foramen, lingual canal, and lingual foramen as well as in the evaluation of the detailed morphology of the mental canal and incisive canal (Naitoh et al. 2009; Georgescu et al. 2010; Santos Jr. et al. 2013). Incisive canals are detectable in the CBCT sagittal section view of the anterior mandible, whereas they were detectable only in 6% of cases in the central incisor region and 32% of cases in the lateral incisor and canine region with the aid of orthopantomography (Georgescu et al. 2010); this indicates the clear superiority of CBCT compared with OP in this situation.

In the case of CBCT evaluation of *section views* from various planes and/or in 3D-MPR mode and 3D reconstruction, the tool should be used to localize incisive/mental canals because the panoramic view of CBCT (even though it is much better than OP) does not reach the same diagnostic value in this case (Naitoh et al. 2009; Georgescu et al. 2010). Similarly, for the detection of additional mental foramen, the use of section views (Naitoh et al. 2009) and/or 3D-MPR mode and 3D reconstruction seems to be the most efficient method and is superior to that of the panoramic view of CBCT (Naitoh et al. 2009; Santos Jr. et al. 2013). Accordingly, the presence or absence of a mental spinal foramen (the lingual opening of incisive canal at the midline of mandible) as well as a lingual canal (extends internally from mandibular canal) and lingual foramen (the opening of lingual canal) may also be evaluated most advantageously when section views as well as 3D-MPR and 3D reconstruction modes are used (Yoshida et al. 2005; Naitoh et al. 2009; Jaju and Jaju 2011).

Importantly, the morphology of the maxillary vascular network and nerve supply should also be studied (Sato et al. 2010; Yoshida et al. 2010), because the most important arteries and nerves have bony canals clearly appearing on CBCT images of the sinus wall (Sato et al. 2010; Yoshida et al. 2010). Special attention should be paid to the morphology of the lateral sinus wall because of the posterior superior alveolar artery and nerve as well as their distributed arteries/nerves (Sato et al. 2010; Yoshida et al. 2010). The evaluation of the anastomoses of PSAA with the infraorbital artery in the anterolateral wall of the sinus may also be important (Sato et al. 2010; Yoshida et al. 2010). The location of the bony canals of the PSAA/PSAN can be detected using CBCT frontal section views and a 3D reconstruction of the lateral sinus wall (Sato et al. 2010; Yoshida et al. 2010). The detected locations of the premised canals should be considered in relation to the sinus floor elevation procedures (especially in the molar region) to avoid laceration of the premised arteries/nerves and consequent bleeding, vascular impairment, ischemia, pain, etc. (Sato et al. 2010; Yoshida et al. 2010).

2.4.3. CBCT and Bone Density

CBCT may also be used for the evaluation of bone density expressed in Hounsfield units (HU). Hounsfield units are standard numbers originating from medical CT images and represent the relative density of tissues according to a calibrated gray-level scale (de Carvalho Crusoe Silva 2012) that ranges from -1000 (air) to 3000 (enamel) (Turkyilmaz and McGlumphy 2008). When compared with the Misch classification (Misch 1990), < 150 HU refers to D5, 150–350 HU refers to D4, 350–850 HU refers to D3, 850–1250 HU refers to D2, and > 1250 refers to the D1 Misch class (Turkyilmaz and McGlumphy 2008; de Carvalho Crusoe Silva 2012). The HU values correlate well with the real bone quality (Homolka et al.

2002; Turkyilmaz and McGlumphy 2008; Farre-Pages et al. 2011) and may predict implant insertion torque and implant stability (Homolka et al. 2002; Turkyilmaz and McGlumphy 2008; Farre-Pages et al. 2011). However, in the case of CBCT images, the accuracy of bone density measurements has certain limitations because HU values may be overestimated (de Carvalho Crusoe Silva 2012). In general, the accuracy of the D2 and D3 classifications seems to be relatively good but D4 is compromised (de Carvalho Crusoe Silva 2012), which demands attention during surgery and indicates a need for the development of more suitable software (de Carvalho Crusoe Silva 2012).

2.4.4. CBCT, Virtual Implant Placement, and Navigational Surgery

With the aid of CBCT images, a dentist can place implants virtually (VIP: virtual implant placement) into the surgical region of interest (ROI) from the images. Thereafter, the data can be sent to a CAD/CAM manufacturing facility, which creates (through a process termed "stereolithography") a surgical guide including metal cylinders that direct the osteotomy drills into precise locations of the jaws as planned by the dentist (Howerton Jr. and Mora 2008; Pozzi et al. 2008; De Vico et al. 2012; Svensson et al. 2014).

However, the weak points of surgical template-based methods should also be considered (Frisardi et al. 2011). The weak point of such surgical template-based procedures relies on the accuracy in transferring information derived from CBCT based on VIP data into surgery, because deviations between the virtually planned and real post-insertion positions of the implants could cause irreversible damage to important anatomical structures such as sensory nerves or the maxillary sinus floor (Frisardi et al. 2011).

Even if the surgical template may be considered accurate (Huh et al. 2012) and may be supported/anchored on teeth or stabilized by placing anchor pins through the template into the bone (Serrano et al. 2008; De Vico et al. 2011, 2012), it may still be difficult sometimes to guarantee a close fit with the hard and/or soft tissue surfaces in a proper and stable position in order to accurately transfer the preoperative VIP treatment plan into the real surgical implant placement (Frisardi et al. 2011).

To overcome the premised problem of inaccuracy, real-time computer-assisted navigational surgery allowing virtual direct vision of the drill tip in relation to the bone and other surrounding tissues (i.e. the sinus floor or alveolar nerve) during surgery is available (Ng et al. 2005). In this case, navigation is made possible through a series of sensors attached to the rotary instruments, to the surgical template, and to a cap fixed on the patient's head, all of which are coupled with the same data-analyzing system (Serrano et al. 2008). The surgical template can be supported/anchored by the teeth, the teeth and mucosa, the mucosa, or by the bone itself (by raising a flap) and may be stabilized by placing anchor pins through the template into the bone (Serrano et al. 2008; De Vico et al. 2011, 2012). Data obtained are transferred immediately to the computer and enable the dental surgeon to see the real situation on CBCT images that are then used as a map and provide the dental surgeon with a real-time representation of the surgical instruments in relation to the anatomical structures of the patient (Serrano et al. 2008).

2.4.5. CBCT and Prosthodontic-Driven Implant Planning

In the frame of prosthodontic-driven implant planning, fixed prostheses may also be planned virtually and manufactured in connection with the above-mentioned CAD/CAM surgical guide technology that allows a dentist to place implants using a surgical guide and place a fixed prosthesis during the same dental visit (Howerton Jr. and Mora 2008; Pozzi et al. 2008; De Vico et al. 2012; Svensson et al. 2014). Recently, 3D CBCT images of the cranium, mandible, and dental surfaces can also be combined with computed three-dimensional movement recording, performing dynamic and precise simulation of condyle to fossa distances, and occlusal contacts during mandibular function (Palla et al. 2003; Terajima et al. 2008) to evaluate chewing-functional and occlusal aspects of VIP-planned implant-supported dentures. Nowadays, a full digital prosthodontic-driven pre-operative planning workflow, including VIP as well as the virtual planning of reconstructive bone surgery, is also available for oral/maxillofacial surgeons who are working in the field of oral/maxillofacial oncology or traumatology (Essig et al. 2011; Pedersen et al. 2014).

In the absence of available CAD/CAM manufacturing technologies, a diagnostic wax-up of the planned prosthodontic restoration is made in the dental laboratory for the patient (based on previously made impressions, bite registration, and study casts) and the optimal locations for implants (from a prosthodontic view) are determined (Serrano et al. 2008; Talwar et al. 2010). Thereafter a special denture-shaped radio-opaque (barium sulfate coated) radiographic template or a denture-shaped template with radio-opaque position markers (gutta-percha, metal ball of known diameter, etc.) is manufactured (Lim et al. 2004; Serrano et al. 2008; Talwar et al. 2010). A CBCT image with this template placed in the mouth is made and VIP is carried out using this kind of image (Lim et al. 2004; Serrano et al. 2008; Talwar et al. 2010). Finally, the radiographic template can be modified (or a new template can be manufactured) and used as a surgical template based on the results of the VIP-planning procedure (Lim et al. 2004; Serrano et al. 2008; Talwar et al. 1010).

In certain cases, a patient's existing denture may also be used as a "radiographic and surgical template." In this case, light-activated radio-opaque calcium-hydroxide liner may be placed as a marker on the denture's surface chair-side for CBCT imaging (Huynh-Ba et al. 2013); whereas bore-holes for surgical guidance (optimally with metal guide tubes) may be prepared later in the dental laboratory.

Alternatively, the above-mentioned traditional and CAD/CAM-based VIP methods may also be combined. In this case, a denture-shaped template with radio-opaque position markers (i.e. gutta-percha, metal ball, barium sulfate coated) should be manufactured based on a traditional diagnostic wax-up in a dental technical laboratory and placed in the mouth during the diagnostic CBCT scanning (De Vico et al. 2012). Thereafter the surgical template and fixed denture may be manufactured via the VIP and CAD/CAM methodology as mentioned above (De Vico et al. 2012).

2.4.6. Other Related CBCT Applications

An important additional application of CBCT is its use in the planning of the shape of membranes if there is a need for guided bone/tissue regeneration because of bone defects with complex morphology (Takane et al. 2010). Using CBCT images, the membrane can be pre-cut into an optimal shape to cover the bone defect and to fit the roots and/or implants present in the treatment area (Takane et al. 2010), leading to a decrease in the amount of time used for surgery and improvement of clinical outcome (Takane et al. 2010).

Another important application that should be mentioned is the fact that CBCT may also be used efficiently to determine optimal sites to place palatal and/or approximal anchorage implants for orthodontic purposes (Lai et al. 2010; Miyazawa et al. 2010). In the case of the palatal bone, both bone height and bone mineral density can be evaluated, and an optimum implant position considering both safety and stability can be determined (Lai et al. 2010). Similarly, cortical thickness as well as the quality and quantity of the bone in the alveolar process may also be determined accurately for optimal placement of the orthodontic mini-implants (Miyazawa et al. 2010). CBCT- and VIP-based surgical guides (similar to that of implant placement for prosthodontic purposes, see above) are also available for the safe insertion of orthodontic miniscrews (Miyazawa et al. 2010).

Conclusion

The major diagnostic tool for implant dentistry is X-ray diagnostics. X-ray diagnostics for implant dentistry usually includes the evaluation of several two-dimensional images like *intraoral radiographs* and images of *orthopantomography* as well as three-dimensional images such as those obtained from *cone-beam computed tomography* (Hazey et al. 2009).

Intraoral radiographs are primarily used for follow up, including the examination of a bone-implant interface for signs of failure such as a radiolucent rim around the implant body and loss of crestal bone (Mupparapu and Singer 2004) and augmented/grafted bone (Jung et al. 2010; Cha et al. 2011). In certain cases intraoral radiographs may also be used for planning (Lim et al. 2004; Mupparapu and Singer 2004).

Orthopantomography (also referred to as *panoramic radiography*) is one of the most frequently used modalities for presurgical planning, including both finding an appropriate location and measuring the available bone (Rockenbach et al. 2003; Mupparapu and Singer 2004; Hu et al. 2012). Within certain limitations, bone quality may also be evaluated via panoramic radiography using the fractal dimension analysis method (Lee et al. 2010). Further, orthopantomography is generally useful in ruling out gross pathosis within the jaws before implant surgery (Mupparapu and Singer 2004) as well as for follow up on multiple implants and augmented/grafted bone (Hieu et al. 2010; Cha et al. 2011). However, the reliability of panoramic radiography for presurgical implant planning in the anterior area is questionable (Ngeow et al. 2009; Hu et al. 2012; Georgescu et al. 2010).

Cone-beam computed tomography systems belong to the highest level computed tomography systems. These CT systems were designed specifically for the visualization of the maxillofacial region and offer both two- and three-dimensional images with high spatial resolution. CBCT offers a great advantage in comparison to the medical CT in terms of accuracy, scan time reduction, dose reduction, and its lower number of artifacts (Yajima et al. 2006; de Carvalho Crusoe Silva 2012). CBCT can be used to rule out gross pathosis and other unexpected findings/conditions within the jaws and the orofacial region before implant surgery (Caglayan and Tozoglu 2012; Silva et al. 2012) as well as to detect or rule out procedural errors following implant treatment (Silva et al. 2012). CBCT is also important in evaluating most anatomical structures that might be limiting implant placement, such as the maxillary sinus, the incisive foramen, the mandibular canal, the mental canal, the mental foramen, additional mental foramen (Naitoh et al. 2009; Georgescu et al. 2010; Santos Jr. et al. 2012), the incisive canal of the mandible, the mental spinal foramen, the lingual canal and lingual foramen (Yoshida et al. 2005; Naitoh et al. 2009; Jaju and Jaju 2011), and the morphology of the maxillary vascular network and nerve supply (Sato et al. 2010; Yoshida et al. 2010). Assessing the quality of hard tissue is also possible (Howerton Jr. and Mora 2008) but only within certain limitations (de Carvalho Crusoe Silva 2012), which indicates a need for the development of more suitable software for this purpose.

For dental implant surgery, easily comprehensible volumetric maxillo-mandibular CBCT images with high spatial resolution and high dimensional accuracy are also available in any plane (Yajima et al. 2006). A dentist can place implants virtually into the surgical region of interest within the images and data can be sent to a CAD/CAM manufacturing facility, which creates (through a process termed "stereolithography") a surgical guide including metal cylinders that direct osteotomy drills into precise locations within the jaws as planned by the dentist (Howerton Jr. and Mora 2008; Pozzi et al. 2008; De Vico et al. 2012). In the frame of prosthodontic-driven implant planning, fixed prostheses may also be planned virtually and manufactured in connection with the aforementioned CAD/CAM surgical guide technology that allows a dentist to place implants using a surgical guide and to place a fixed prosthesis during the same single dental visit (Howerton Jr. and Mora 2008; Pozzi et al. 2008; De Vico et al. 2012). Planning of the shape and pre-cut of membranes is also possible with the use of CBCT images if there is a need for GBR/GTR (guided tissue regeneration) of bone defects with complex morphology (Takane et al. 2010).

References

Aguiar, LBV; Neves, FS; Bastos, LC; Crusoe-Rebello, I; Ambrosono, GMB; Campos, PSF. Multiple Stafne Bone Defects: A rare entity. *ISRN Dentistry*, 2011, ID792145. DOI: 10.5402/2011/792145.

Baek, CH; Chung, MK; Son, YI; Choi, JY; Kim, HJ; Yim, YJ; Ko, YH; Choi, J; Cho, JK; Jeong, HS. Tumor volume assessment by ^{18}F-FDG PET/CT in patients with oral cavity cancer with dental artifacts on CT or MR images. *J Nucl Med*, 2008, 49, 1422–1428.

Berrington De Gonzalez, A; Darby, S. Risk of cancer from diagnostic X-rays: Estimates for the UK and 14 other countries. *Lancet*, 2004, 363, 345–351.

Caglayan, F; Tozoglu, Ü. Incidental findings in the maxillofacial region detected by cone beam CT. *Diagn Interv Radiol*, 2012, 18, 159–163.

Cevidanes, LHS; Styner, MA; Proffit, WR. Image analysis and superimposition of 3-dimensional cone-beam computed tomography models. *Am J Orthod Dentofacial Orthop*, 2006, 129, 611–618.

Cha, JK; Park, JC; Jung, UW; Kim, CS; Cho, KS; Choi, SH. Case series of maxillary sinus augmentation with biphasic calcium phosphate: a clinical and radiographic study. *J Periodontal Implant Sci*, 2011, 41, 98–104.

Correll, RW; Wescott, WB. Eagle's syndrome diagnosed after history of headache, dysphagia, otalgia, and limited neck movement. *J Am Dent Assoc*, 1982 104, 491–492.

Dawood, A; Brown, J; Sauret-Jackson, V; Purkayastha, S. Optimization of cone beam CT exposure for pre-surgical evaluation of the implant site. *Dentomaxillofac Radiol*, 2012, 41, 70–74.

de Carvalho Crusoe Silva, IM; de Feritas, DQ; Ambrosano, GMB; Boscolo, FN; Almeida, SM. Bone density: comparative evaluation of Hounsfield units in multislice and cone-beam computed tomography. *Braz Oral Res (Sao Paulo)*, 2012, 26, 550–556.

de Freitas, DQ; Montebello Filho, A. Evaluation of two methods of tracing for implants in panoramic radiographs. *J Appl Oral Sci*, 2004, 12, 84–88.

Desai, SR; Karthikeyan, I; Singh, R. An in-office, cost effective technique for measuring width of bone using intra-oral periapical radiographs in occlusal projections. *J Indian Soc Periodontol*, 2013, 17, 82–86.

De Vico, G; Bonino, M; Spinelli, D; Schiavetti, R; Sannino, G; Pozzi, A; Ottria, L. Rationale for tilted implants: FEA considerations and clinical reports. *ORAL & Implantology*, 2011, 4, 23–33.

De Vico, G; Spinelli, D; Bonino, M; Schiavetti, R; Pozzi, A; Ottria, L. Computer-assisted virtual treatment planning combined with flapless surgery and immediate loading in the rehabilitation of partial edentulism. *ORAL & Implantology*, 2012, 5, 3–10.

de Laat, A; Horvath, M; Bossuyt, M; Fossion, E; Baert, AL. Myogenous or arthrogenous limitation of mouth opening: Correlations between clinical findings, MRI, and clinical outcome. *J Orofac Pain*, 1993, 7, 150–155.

Essig, H; Rana, M; Kokemueller, H; von See, C; Ruecker, M; Tavassol, F; Gellrich, NC. Pre-operative planning for mandibular reconstruction – A full digital planning workflow resulting in a patient specific reconstruction. *BMC Head & Neck Oncology*, 2011, 3, 45.

Farre-Pages, N; Augé-Castro, ML; Alaejos-Algarra, F; Mareque-Bueno, J; Ferres-Padro, E; Hernández-Alfaro, F. Relation between bone density and primary implant stability. *Med Oral Patol Oral Cir Bucal*, 2011, 16, e62–e67.

Fernandez-Formoso, N; Rilo, B; Mora, MJ; Martinez-Silva, I; Santana, U. A paralleling technique modification to determine the bone crest level around dental implants. *Dentomaxillofac Radiol*, 2011, 40, 385–389.

Frisardi, G; Chessa, G; Barone, S; Paoli, A; Razionale, A; Frisardi, F. Integration of 3D anatomical data obtained by CT imaging and 3D optical scanning for computer aided implant surgery. *BMC Medical Imaging*, 2011, 11, 5.

Georgescu, CE; Mihai, A; Didilescu, AC; Moraru, R; Nimigean, V; Nimigean, VR; Tanase, G. Cone beam computed tomography as a method of quantitative and qualitative analysis of alveolar crest in the frontal mandibular area. *Romanian J Morphol Embriol*, 2010, 51, 713–717.

Grondahl, K; Ekestubbe, A; Grondahl, HG. Postoperative radiographic examinations. In: Grondahl K, Ekestubbe A, Grondahl HG editors. *Radiography in oral endosseous prosthetics*. Goteborg: Nobel Biocare AB; 1996. 111–126.

Hazey III, MA; Ngan, P; Reed, H; Razmus, T; Crout, R; Kao, E. Comparison of computer-generated, enhanced and conventional 2-dimensional radiographic imaging. *Am J Orthod Dentofacial Orthop*, 2009, 135, 463–467.

Hieu, PD; Chung, JH; Yim, SB; Hong, KS. A radiographical study on the changes in height of grafting materials after sinus lift: a comparison between two types of xenogenic materials. *J Periodontal Implant Sci*, 2010, 40, 25–32.

Hintze, H; Wiese, M; Wenzel, A. Cone beam CT and conventional tomography for the detection of morphological temporomandibular joint changes. *Dentomaxillofacial Radiol*, 2007, 36, 192–197.

Homolka, P; Beer, A; Birkfellner, W; Nowotny, R; Gahleitner, A; Tschabitscher, M; Bergmann, H. Bone mineral density measurement with dental quantitative CT prior to dental implant placement. *Radiology*, 2002, 224, 247–252.

Howerton, Jr. WB; Mora, MA. Advancements in digital imaging: What is new and on the horizon? *Am J Dent Assoc*, 2008, 139(suppl 3), 20S–24S.

Hu, KS; Choi, DY; Lee, WJ; Kim, HJ; Jung, UW; Kim, S. Reliability of two different presurgical preparation methods for implant dentistry based on panoramic radiography and cone-beam computed tomography in cadavers. *J Periodontal Implant Sci*, 2012, 42, 39–44.

Huh, YJ; Choi, BR; Huh, KH; Yi, WJ; Heo, MS; Lee, SS; Choi, SC. In-vitro study on the accuracy of a simple-design CT-guided stent for dental implants. *Imaging Sci Dent*, 2012, 42, 139–146.

Huynh-Ba, P; Alexander, P; Vargas, A; Vierra, M; Oates, TW. A radiographic template for a two-implant mandibular overdenture using the patient's existing denture. *J Prosthet Dent*, 2013, 109, 53–56.

Jaju, P; Jaju, S. Lingual vascular canal assessment by dental computed tomography: A retrospective study. *Indian J Dent Res*, 2011, 22, 232–236.

Jung, JH; Choi, SH; Cho, KS; Kim, CS. Bone-added osteotome sinus floor elevation with simultaneous placement of non-submerged sand blasted with large grit and acid etched implants: a 5-year radiographic evaluation. *J Periodontol Implant Sci*, 2010, 40, 69–75.

Karamifar, K; Shahidi, S; Tondari, A. Bilateral bifid mandibular canal: Report of two cases. *Indian J Dent Res*, 2009, 20, 235–237.

Kuzmanovic, DV; Payne, AG; Kieser, JA; Dias, GJ. Anterior loop of the mental nerve: a morphological and radiological study. *Clin Oral Implant Res*, 2003, 14, 464–471.

Lai, RF; Zou, H; Kong, WD; Lin W. Applied anatomic site study of palatal anchorage implants using cone beam computed tomography. *Int J Oral Sci*, 2010, 2, 98–104.

Langlais, RP; Broadus, R; Glass, BJ. Bifid mandibular canals in panoramic radiographs. *J Am Dent Assoc*, 1985, 110, 923–926.

Larheim, TA. Role of magnetic resonance imaging in the clinical diagnosis of the temporomandibular joint. *Cells Tissues Organs*, 2005, 180, 6–21.

Lee, DH; Ku, Y; Rhyu, IC; Hong, JU; Lee, CW; Heo, MS; Huh, KH. A clinical study of alveolar bone quality using the fractal dimension and the implant stability quotient. *J Periodontal Implant Sci*, 2010, 40, 19–24.

Lee, SM; Lee, SS; Huh, KH; Yi, WJ; Heo, MS; Choi, SC. The effects of location of alveolar crest on the vertical bone heights on panoramic radiographs. *Dentomaxillofac Radiol*, 2012, 41, 117–121.

Lim, TJ; Csillag, A; Irinakis, T; Nokiani, A; Wiebe, CB. Intentional angulation of an implant to avoid a pneumatized maxillary sinus: A case report. *J Can Dent Assoc*, 2004, 70, 164–168.

Madrigal, C; Ortega, R; Meniz, C; Lopez-Quiles, J. Study of available bone for interforaminal implant treatment using cone-beam computed tomography. *Med Oral Patol Oral Cir Bucal*, 2008, 13, E307–E312.

Misch, CE. Density of bone: effect on treatment plans, surgical approach, healing, and progressive bone loading. *Int J Oral Implantol*, 1990, 6, 23–31.

Miyazawa, K; Kawaguchi, M; Tabuchi, M; Goto, S. Accurate pre-surgical determination for self-drilling miniscrew implant placement using surgical guides and cone-beam computed tomography. *Eur J Orthodontics*, 2010, 32, 735–740.

Mozzo, P; Procacci, C; Tacconi, A; Tinazzi Martini, P; Bergamo Andreis, IA. A new volumetric CT machine for dental imaging based on the cone-beam technique: preliminary results. *Eur Radiol*, 1998, 8, 1558–1564.

Mupparapu, M; Singer, SR. Implant imaging for the dentist. *J Can Dent Assoc*, 2004, 70, 32 (a–g).

Nair, MK; Nair, UP. Digital and advanced imaging in endodontics: A review. *J Endod*, 2007, 33, 1–6.

Naitoh, M; Nakahara, K; Hiraiwa, Y; Aimiya, H; Gotoh, K; Ariji, E. Observation of buccal foramen in mandibular body using cone-beam computed tomography. *Okajimas Folia Anat Jpn*, 2009, 86, 25–29.

Ng, FC; Ho, KH; Wexler, A. Computer-assisted navigational surgery enhances safety in dental implantology. *Ann Acad Med Singapore*, 2005 34, 383–388.

Ngeow, WC; Dionysius, DD; Ishak, H; Nambiar, P. A radiographic study on the visualization of the anterior loop in dentate subjects of different age groups. *J Oral Sci*, 2009, 51, 231–237.

Ogasawara, T; Kitagawa, Y; Ogawa, T; Yamada, T; Kawamura, Y; Sano, K. MR imaging and thermography of facial angiooedema: A case report. *Oral Surg Oral Med Oral Pathol Oral Radiol Endod*, 2001, 92, 473–476.

Palla, S; Gallo, LM; Gossi, D. Dynamic stereometry of the temporomandibular joint. *Orthod Craniofac Res*, 2003, 6 (suppl.1), 37–47.

Park, JB. The evaluation of digital panoramic radiographs taken for implant dentistry in the daily practice. *Med Oral Patol Oral Cir Bucal*, 2010, 15, e663–e666.

Parks, ET. Digital radiographic imaging. Is the dental practice ready? *J Am Dent Assoc*, 2008, 139, 477–481.

Pedersen, TK; Dalstra, M; Cattaneo, P; Blomlof, J; Buhl, J; Norholt, SE. Use of digital dental cast and 3D models in orthodontics, orthognathic and reconstructive surgery. *Danish Dent J*; 2014, 118, 14–19

Penarrocha, M; Vina, J; Maestre, L; Penarrocha, D; Balaguer, J. Guided implant surgery with modification of the technique involving the raising of a semicircular miniflap: A preliminary study. *Med Oral Patol Oral Cir Bucal*, 2012, 17, e775–780.

Pompa, V; Galasso, S; Cassetta, M; Pompa, G; De Angelis, F; Di Carlo, S. A comparative study of Magnetic Resonance (MR) and Computed Tomography (CT) in the pre-implant evaluation. *Annali di Stomatologia*, 2010, 1, 33–38.

Pozzi, A; Gargari, M; Barlattani, A. CAD/CAM technologies in the surgical and prosthetic treatment of the edentulous patient with biomymetic individualized approach. *ORAL & Implantology*, 2008, 1, 2–14.

Riachi, F; Naaman, N; Tabarani, C; Aboelsaad, N; Aboushelib, MN; Berberi, A; Salameh, Z. Influence of material properties on rate of resorption of two bone graft materials after sinus lift using radiographic assessment. *Int J Dentistry*, 2012, ID 737262.

Rockenbach, MIB; Sampaio, MCC; da Costa, LJ; da Costa, NP. Evaluation of mandibular implant sites: Correlation between panoramic and linear tomography. *Braz Dent J*, 2003, 14, 209–213.

Rother, UJ. *Moderne bildgebende Diagnostic in der Zahn-, Mund-, und Kieferheilkunde*. Munchen: Urban & Fisher, 2001, 171.

Santos Jr., O; Pinheiro, LR; Umetsubo, OS; Sales, MAO; Cavalcanti, MGP. Assessment of open source software for CBCT in detecting additional mental foramina. *Braz Oral Res (Sao Paulo)*, 2013, 27, 128–135.

Sato, I; Kawai, T; Yoshida, S; Miwa, Y; Imura, K; Asaumi, R; Sunohara, M; Yosue, T. Observing the bony canal structure of the human maxillary sinus in Japanese cadavers using cone beam CT. *Okajimas Folia Anat Jpn*, 2010, 87, 123–128.

Scarfe, WC; Farman, AG; Sukovic, P. Clinical applications of cone-beam computed tomography in dental practice. *J Can Dent Assoc*, 2006, 72, 75–80.

Schropp, L; Stavropoulos, A; Spin-Neto, R; Wenzel, A. Evaluation of the RB-RB/LB-LB mnemonic rule for recording optimally projected intraoral images of dental implants: an in-vitro study. *Dentomaxillofac Radiol*, 2012, 41, 298–304.

Schulze, RKW. Pose determination of a cylindrical (dental) implant in three dimensions from a single two-dimensional radiograph. *Dentomaxillofac Radiol.*, 2010, 39, 33–41.

Serrano, MR; Estela, SA; Diago, MP; Diago, MP. Software applied to oral implantology: Update. *Med Oral Patol Cir Bucal*, 2008, 13, E661–E665.

Silva, MAG; Wolf, U; Heincke, F; Bumann, A; Visser, H; Hirsch, E. Cone-beam computed tomography for routine orthodontic treatment planning: A radiation dose evaluation. *Am J Orthod Dentofac Orthop*, 2008, 133, 640.e1–640.e5.

Silva, JA; de Alencar, AHG; da Rocha, SS; Lopes, LG; Estrela, C. Three-dimensional image contribution for evaluation of operative procedural errors in endodontic therapy and dental implants. *Braz Dent J*, 2012, 23, 127–134.

Spin-Neto, R; Stavropoulos, A; Pereira, LAVD; Marcantonio Jr., E; Wenzel, A. Fate of autologous and fresh-frozen allogenic block bone grafts used for ridge augmentation. A CBCT-based analysis. *Clin Oral Implant Res*, 2013, 24, 167–173.

Svensson, KG; Trulsson, M; Hultin, M. Computer aided implant treatment. *Danish Dent J*, 2014, 118, 22–29.

Takane, M; Sato, S; Suzuki, K; Fukuda, T; Asano, Y; Honda, K; Arai, Y; Ito, K. Clinical application of cone beam computed tomography for ideal absorbable membrane placement in interproximal bone defects. *J Oral Sci*, 2010, 52, 63–69.

Talwar, N; Singh, BP; Chand, P; Pal, US. Use of diagnostic and surgical stent: A simplified approach for implant placement. *J Indian Prosthodont Soc*, 2010, 10, 234–239.

Terajima, M; Endo, M; Aoki, Y; Yuuda, K; Hayasaki, H; Goto, TK; Tokumori, K; Nakasima, A. Four-dimensional analysis of stomatognathic function. *Am J Orthod Dentofacial Orthop*, 2008, 134, 276–287.

Turkyilmaz, I; McGlumphy, EA. Influence of bone density on implant stability parameters and implant success: a retrospective clinical study. *BMC Oral Health*, 2008, 8, 32.

Wakoh, M; Nishikawa, K; Otonari, T; Yamamoto, M; Harada, T; Sano, T; Yajima, Y; Ooguro, T. Digital subtraction technique for evaluation of peri-implant bone change in digital dental imaging. *Bull Tokyo Dent Coll*, 2006, 47, 57–64.

Wenzel, A; Hirsch, E; Christensen, J; Matzen, LH; Scaf, G; Frydenberg, M. Detection of cavitated approximal surfaces using cone beam CT and intraoral receptors. *Dentomaxillofac Radiol*, in press DOI: 10.1259/dmfr/39458105.

White, SC.; Pharoah, MJ. The evolution and application of dental maxillofacial imaging modalities. *Dent Clin North Am*, 2008, 52, 689–705.

Yajima, A; Otonari-Yamamoto, M; Sano, T; Hayakawa, Y; Otonari, T; Tanabe, K; Wakoh, M; Mizuta, S; Yonezu, H; Nakagawa, K; Yajima, Y. Cone-beam CT (CB Throne) applied to dentomaxillofacial region. *Bull Tokyo Dent Coll*, 2006, 47, 133–141.

Yoshida, S; Kawai, T; Okutsu, K; Yosue, T; Takamori, H; Sunohara, M; Sato, I. The appearance of foramen in the internal aspect of the mental region of mandible from Japanese cadavers and dry skulls under macroscopic observation and three-dimensional CT images. *Okajimas Folia Anat Jpn*, 2005, 82, 83–88.

Yoshida, S; Kawai, T; Asaumi, R; Miwa, Y; Imura, K; Koseki, H; Sunohara, M; Yosue, T; Sato, I. Evaluation of the blood and nerve supply patterns in the molar region of the maxillary sinus in Japanese cadavers. *Okajimas Folia Anat Jpn*, 2010, 87, 129–133.

CHAPTER 3

BIOMATERIALS FOR IMPLANT SURGERY

Abstract

In this chapter, the most important current knowledge related to biomaterials used for implant surgery is summarized. Only the materials used for implant surgery are included, while other dental materials used for making impressions and dentures are not discussed. Bone substitutes are introduced in detail because these materials are also frequently used as coatings for fixtures. Consequently, without having proper knowledge of these materials it would be difficult to understand the current trends of implant fixture surface development. Titanium and its alloys, considered the most biocompatible and corrosion-resistant metals and widely used as implant fixture materials nowadays, are also discussed in detail. Besides the premised materials of primary importance, several other materials currently used in implant surgery, like membranes and sutures, as well as materials that may be of historical importance or of use to future perspectives are also briefly introduced. A high number of various biomaterials may be used for implant surgery, and the number of such biomaterials is increasing continuously. Consequently, it is rather difficult for both researchers and clinicians to keep abreast of the developments in this field. Therefore, there is a need for general reviews on the available current scientific data to keep related knowledge up-to-date and functional. In this chapter the most important data are summarized.

3.1. Introduction

In this chapter the most important current knowledge related to biomaterials used for implant surgery is summarized. Only materials used for implant surgery are included, while other dental materials used for making impressions and dentures are not discussed. Bone substitutes are introduced in detail because these materials are also frequently used as coatings for fixtures (Mano et al. 2011; Kuwabara et al. 2012; Bose and Tarafder 2012). Consequently, without having proper knowledge of these materials, it would be difficult to understand the current trends in implant fixture surface development. Titanium and its alloys, considered the most biocompatible and corrosion-resistant metals (Letic-Gavrilovic et al. 2000; Neumann and Kevenhoerster 2009; Hanawa 2011) and widely used as implant fixture materials nowadays (Letic-Gavrilovic et al. 2000; Neumann and Kevenhoerster 2009;

Yamashita et al. 2009; Saulacic et al. 2012), are also discussed in detail. Besides the premised materials of primary importance, numerous other materials currently used in implant surgery as well as materials that may be of historical importance or of use to future perspectives are also briefly introduced.

3.2. Bone Substitutes

3.2.1. General Considerations

The ability of bone to regenerate depends on the size of the bone defect (Neumann and Kevenhoerster 2009; Liu et al. 2010), and above a critical size (i.e. congenital, traumatic, cystic, or tumorous defects), the defect will not heal properly without intervention (Neumann and Kevenhoerster 2009; Liu et al. 2010). In such cases (referred to as "critical size defects"), an application of bone substitutes is required (Neumann and Kevenhoerster 2009; Liu et al. 2010). The use of bone substitutes may also be considered for other indications like reinforced bearing for dental implants (i.e. sinus elevation, alveolar ridge augmentation) or bone augmentation because of periodontal or esthetic reasons (Neumann and Kevenhoerster 2009).

Bone substitutes may be divided into four major subtypes: "*autologous*" derived from the same individual, "*allogenic*" derived from the same species, "*xenogenic*" derived from another species, or "*alloplastic*" derived from non-biologic material like metal, ceramic, or plastic. The autologous, allogenic, or xenogenic bone substitutes may also be termed "*grafts*," meaning that these substitutes may be considered "tissues" that have been moved from their original place and inserted into a new one without bringing their own blood supply with them.

The biological interaction between bone and bone substitute may be divided into four major subtypes as follows (Neumann and Kevenhoerster 2009): (1) *Substitution*: complete resorption and replacement of the bone substitute through the healing/new development of surrounding bone. Although this process is considered the optimum choice, in cases where resorption occurs too quickly, a disadvantageous fibrous interlayer may appear (between the newly formed bone and the resorbed bone substitute) that may compromise healing (Neumann and Kevenhoerster 2009). (2) *Osteoconduction*: directed growth of bone tissue on a surface due to the geometric form of the bone substitute. In this case, the bone substitute serves as a scaffold along which osteoblasts can migrate into the defect. Evidence suggests that interconnecting pores of roughly 150–450 μm (inside of and/or among the substitute particles) are likely to be optimum for osteoconduction (Tsuruga et al. 1997; Albrektsson and Johansson 2001; Neumann and Kevenhoerster 2009). (3) *Osteoinduction*: recruitment and differentiation of mesenchymal precursor cells into osteoprogenitor cells by means of the interaction of the bone substitute and the bone, and the subsequent endochondral ossification (Letic-Gavrilovic et al. 2000; Albrektsson and Johansson 2001; Neumann and Kevenhoerster 2009). (4) *Osteostimulation*: activation of differentiated bone cells and the stimulation of bone metabolism through the bone substitute (Neumann and Kevenhoerster 2009). (Please note that the premised categories are also used to describe interactions between the bone and implant fixtures.)

Autologous bone (exerting optimal properties for all major types of a substitute—bone interaction) is the gold standard of bone substitutes (Neumann and Kevenhoerster 2009; Liu et al. 2010; Spin-Neto et al. 2013). The demand for other bone substitutes is generally justified by certain disadvantages of autologous bone, including the morbidity/scarring of the donor site, the prolongation of operation time, highly complex operative procedures, the limited individual shape modulation, and the limited availability in cases of large defects (Neumann and Kevenhoerster 2009; Liu et al. 2010; Carlsen et al. 2013; Andersen et al. in press). This is in opposition to the problems of non-autologous bone substitutes, including expenses, storage, biocompatibility, rejection, and product safety with regard to infectious diseases in the case of non-autologous bone products (Neumann and Kevenhoerster 2009).

3.2.2. Autologous Bone Grafts

Autologous bone has been used as a bone substitute since the 19th century (Macewen 1885; Neumann and Kevenhoerster 2009) and is considered a gold standard among biomaterials (Nuss and von Rechenberg 2008; Neumann and Kevenhoerster 2009; Spin-Neto et al. 2013). The autologous bone is clearly biocompatible and can be either resorbed or integrated during osteogenesis. Further, even if not a cortical bone (pore size ca. 1–100 µm), cancellous bone has a pore size of 200–400 µm, which is optimum for osteoconduction (Neumann and Kevenhoerster 2009). The presence of various growth/morphogenetic factors and other promoters ensuring the osteoinductive and osteostimulative effect of autologous bone may also be considered.

Different donor sites (i.e. calvaria, rib, iliac ala, tibia, scapula, and sternum) were already described in the early 20th century and the procedure was referred to as “spongioplasty” (Neumann and Kevenhoerster 2009). Intraoral donor sites were also available (Akintoye et al. 2008; Carlsen et al. 2013; Andersen et al. in press), and it is notable that autologous bone grafts originating from intraoral (maxillary or mandibular) sources seem to exert superior osteogenic properties around oral implants when compared to autologous bone grafts of other origins (Akintoye et al. 2008).

Although the transplanted bone graft may be considered largely necrotic, it acts as a scaffold for the ingrowth of granulation tissue containing osteoprogenitor cells (Nuss and von Rechenberg 2008); and under the influence of local factors, these osteoprogenitor cells differentiate into osteoblasts that are responsible for new bone formation (Nuss and von Rechenberg 2008). At the same time, the graft matrix is resorbed through osteoclasts (Nuss and von Rechenberg 2008). This kind of graft resorption occurring parallel to bone formation was historically referred to as “creeping substitution” (Phemister 1914; Nuss and von Rechenberg 2008). Autologous bone grafts are osteoconductive, osteoinductive, and osteostimulative, and can be easily resorbed/substituted (or reintegrated) (Liu et al. 2010). The essential disadvantage of an autologous bone graft is the limited possibility of transplant forming and modeling (Neumann and Kevenhoerster 2009), along with the risk that bone grafts may partially be resorbed (Neumann and Kevenhoerster 2009; Liu et al. 2010; Maiorana et al. 2011).

3.2.3. Anorganic Bone Allografts

Anorganic allograft (also termed "homograft") bone is harvested from human donors. All the organic components are industrially removed or denaturated/inactivated by means of ultrasound baths and a denaturating ethanol lavage, and the product is sterilized thereafter by means of antimicrobial lavage and/or gamma radiation. These implants may be characterized as an anorganic bone matrix having a normal bone structure (Neumann and Kevenhoerster 2009). These grafts may advantageously be supplemented with autologous bone marrow (Neumann and Kevenhoerster 2009) and/or with autologous bone and/or autologous platelet-rich plasma (PRP) in order to support their transformation into a more "vital" bone substitute (Neumann and Kevenhoerster 2009; Saini et al. 2011).

Anorganic bone allograft can also be substituted with a recombinant human bone morphogenetic protein (Sasikumar et al. 2012) or with a recombinant human platelet-derived growth factor (Kaigler et al. 2011); these possibilities are likely to further improve new bone formation around the grafts as well as the implant fixtures (Kaigler et al. 2011; Sasikumar et al. 2012). Anorganic bone allografts may also be coupled with the human bone morphogenetic protein (BMP) gene in the future (Song et al. 2008).

Although anorganic bone allografts may be considered osteoconductive, osteoinductive, and osteostimulative, their resorption and substitution can be rather slow. Although manufacturers attest high safety, there still remains some concern regarding the safety of allograft bone substitutes (Neumann and Kevenhoerster 2009; Liu et al. 2010).

3.2.4. Demineralized Bone Allografts

Demineralized allograft (homograft) bone is harvested from human donors in a manner similar to anorganic allograft bone (Neumann and Kevenhoerster 2009). The demineralization is usually performed through acidification, resulting in a matrix containing type-I-collagen and osteoinductive growth factors (Neumann and Kevenhoerster 2009). Lyophilization makes the material storable. The demineralized allograft is porous and can be easily formed and remodeled intraoperatively but it is not load resistant until fully ossified (Neumann and Kevenhoerster 2009). The demineralized bone allografts are considered osteoconductive, osteoinductive, and osteostimulative. They can also be resorbed and substituted. These grafts may also be advantageously supplemented with autologous platelet-rich plasma (Piemontese et al. 2008) as well as with several growth factors like bone morphogenetic proteins (Ho et al. 2010). Although manufacturers attest high safety, there still remains some concern regarding the safety of demineralized allograft bone substitutes (Liu et al. 2010).

3.2.5. Anorganic Bone Xenografts

The xenogenic (also termed "heterogenic") bone is usually of bovine origin. The deproteinization process is similar to that of the allogenic bone. Anorganic bone xenografts may be considered osteoconductive, osteoinductive, and osteostimulative, but their resorption and substitution is rather slow. Although there may be concern about the safety of xenografts, both manufacturers and many publications attest the high safety of these products. Similar to anorganic bone allografts, these grafts may also be advantageously supplemented with a recombinant human bone morphogenetic protein (Sasikumar et al. 2012), with a recombinant human platelet-derived growth factor (Kaigler et al. 2011), with autologous bone marrow (Neumann and Kevenhoerster 2009), with autologous platelet-rich plasma, and/or with autologous bone (Dori et al. 2007/b; Neumann and Kevenhoerster 2009; Saini et al. 2011; Jensen et al. 2012/a, b, c).

3.2.6. Calcium Phosphate Ceramics

Besides bone-based grafts, calcium phosphates may be considered the most biocompatible synthetic bone-substitutes (Letic-Gavrilovic et al. 2000; Bose and Tarafder 2012). They do not cause inflammatory reactions or a foreign body response, and the surrounding tissue may chemically bond to their surface (Tomsia et al. 2011). Although calcium phosphates may be used in their "biomimetic" simple crystal forms or cement forms for bone substituting (Nuss and von Rechenberg 2008; Moreau et al. 2009; Rajesh et al. 2009; Sugawara et al. 2010; Zhao et al. 2010), in dentistry, calcium phosphates are primarily used in their *ceramic form* for these purposes (Neumann and Kevenhoerster 2009; Bose and Tarafder 2012). (This means they are used in a form that develops after sintering, heating, or firing at a very high temperature but somewhat below the melting point.)

Although calcium phosphate ceramics are primarily manufactured synthetically, hydroxyapatite (HA) ceramics may also be manufactured using alloplastic materials, or they may have xenogenic sources like xenogenic cancellous bone or a hard skeleton of corals (Neumann and Kevenhoerster 2009). The most important calcium phosphates used in their *ceramic form* for bone substitution are *hydroxyapatite* and *β-tricalcium phosphate* and their compound termed *biphasic calcium phosphate* (Letic-Gavrilovic et al. 2000; Neumann and Kevenhoerster 2009; Bose and Tarafder 2012). Basically all calcium phosphate ceramics are osteoconductive (Letic-Gavrilovic et al. 2000; Neumann and Kevenhoerster 2009; Bose and Tarafder 2012) but they are neither osteoinductive nor osteostimulative (Letic-Gavrilovic et al. 2000). Some of them, like β-tricalcium phosphate ceramics, may be resorbed and substituted, whereas hydroxyapatite ceramics will be poorly resorbed and substituted (Letic-Gavrilovic et al. 2000; Masago et al. 2007; Neumann and Kevenhoerster 2009).

Calcium phosphate ceramics may be coated with various molecules like allogenic collagen, an allogenic demineralized bone matrix, a xenogenic non-collagen protein, or biodegradable synthetic polymers (etc.), which may improve their biological properties (Takahashi 2009) and/or may act as carriers being impregnated with several growth/morphogenetic factors like bone morphogenetic proteins, a platelet-derived growth factor (PDGF) of several cytokines, or other promoters, including several drugs (Letic-Gavrilovic et al. 2000; Kaigler et al. 2011; Tamazawa et al. 2011; Bose and Tarafder 2012; Sasikumar et al. 2012). More recently, synthetic calcium phosphate was engineered with stem/progenitor cells that also significantly improved osteogenesis in an animal study (Barboni et al. 2013). Calcium phosphate ceramics may also be supplemented with autologous platelet-rich plasma (Saini et al. 2011), with autologous bone (Shigeishi et al. 2012), or with autologous bone marrow (Neumann and Kevenhoerster 2009).

3.2.7. Calcium Phosphate Cements

In contrast to calcium phosphate *ceramics*, which are widely used for dental applications, calcium phosphate *cements* (CPC) are not frequently used in implant dentistry, perhaps because of their brittleness and low strength (Moreau et al. 2009; Zhao et al. 2010). However, they are more frequently used as bone substitutes in craniofacial surgery for non-load-bearing bone repair (Nuss and von Rechenberg 2008; Zhao et al. 2010), and it should be mentioned that they will be used in dental applications more frequently in the future (Fujikawa et al. 2002; Moreau et al. 2009; Rajesh et al. 2009; Sugawara et al. 2010; Zhao et al. 2010). Their use in periodontal surgery especially seems to be promising (Sugawara et al. 2010), because they seem to induce new cement (and also perhaps periodontal ligament) formation in animal studies (Sugawara et al. 2010).

Similar to calcium phosphate ceramics, the cement form of calcium phosphates is also highly biocompatible (Sugawara et al. 2010); they induce no (or negligible) inflammatory reactions and also exert osteoconductive properties (Sugawara et al. 2010). The advantage of this form of calcium phosphate is that it can be administered very easily in paste form that is injected into bone defects (Nuss and von Rechenberg 2008; Moreau et al. 2009; Rajesh et al. 2009; Sugawara et al. 2010). In certain cases it may even be administered (injected) through the soft tissues without the need of open approaches (Nuss and von Rechenberg 2008). Calcium phosphate cements set in situ to form bioresorbable hydroxyapatite (Nuss and von Rechenberg 2008; Moreau et al. 2009; Sugawara et al. 2010; Zhao et al. 2010), although in certain cases (if $pH < 4.2$), the setting may also partially result in brushite (Nuss and von Rechenberg 2008).

Recent data indicate that the addition of fluoride (up to 3.1 mass %) into the mass of CPCs may result in the formation of large amounts of fluoroapatite (FA, up to 87 mass %) during the in situ setting (Takagi et al. 2010). Increased formation of fluoroapatite leads to a significant decrease (or absence) of bioresorbability (Takagi et al. 2010), which may be useful for applications where slow or no resorption of CPC is required (Takagi et al. 2010). The incorporation of other inorganic materials like strontium, zinc, magnesium, sodium, silver, yttrium, etc., may also be useful in improving biological and/or physical properties (Fu et al. 2012).

Collagen molecules may also be incorporated into CPCs, which further improves their physical properties (i.e. toughness) as well as their biological properties by increasing osteoblast cell attachment onto their surface (Moreau et al. 2009). CPCs may also be substituted with human recombinant BMPs or PDGF as well (Kaigler et al. 2011; Sasikumar et al. 2012). Calcium phosphate cements can also be used advantageously as constituents of composites (Davies et al. 2010; Zhao et al. 2010).

3.2.8. Glass-Ceramics

Glass-ceramic bone substitutes (also termed "bioactive" glass-ceramics) are composed of the ceramic form of four major ingredients (Neumann and Kevenhoerster 2009), including: silicon dioxide (ca. 45%), sodium dioxide (ca. 45%), calcium oxide (ca. 5%), and phosphorus oxide (ca. 5%). Their physical and biological properties can be significantly altered by changing the ratio of calcium oxide and phosphorus oxide (Neumann and Kevenhoerster

2009). Glass-ceramics are not osteoinductive and instead exert significant osteostimulative and osteoconductive properties (Letic-Gavrilovic et al. 2000; Neumann and Kevenhoerster 2009). Glass-ceramics show only minimal fibrous encapsulation (Neumann and Kevenhoerster 2009), which may be degraded and replaced by bone (Tomsia et al. 2011); whereas the resorption and substitution of these materials does not occur (Neumann and Kevenhoerster 2009). The surrounding tissue may chemically bond to their surface (Tomsia et al. 2011).

They may be coated by biologically active molecules like platelet-derived growth factor, bone morphogenetic proteins, and/or other growth/morphogenetic factors, cytokines, or other promoters or drugs (Letic-Gavrilovic et al. 2000; Kaigler et al. 2011; Tamazawa et al. 2011; Sasikumar et al. 2012) following a coating with bioactive carrier molecules like allogenic collagen, an allogenic demineralized bone matrix, a xenogenic non-collagen protein, biodegradable synthetic polymers (Tamazawa et al. 2011), or others. Glass-ceramics may advantageously be supplemented with autologous bone marrow (Neumann and Kevenhoerster 2009) or with autologous bone and autologous platelet-rich plasma (Saini et al. 2011).

3.2.9. Resorbable Polymers

Resorbable (biodegradable) polymers are primarily used for resorbable sutures (Aderriotis and Sandor 1999; Zhao et al. 2010), for resorbable osteosynthesis systems (Neumann and Kevenhoerster 2009), and for resorbable membranes in guided tissue regeneration techniques (Letic-Gavrilovic et al. 2000). However they may also be used as bone substitute, especially in the form of composites (Zhao et al. 2010; Pamula et al. 2011; Tamazawa et al. 2011; Takechi et al. 2012). They may also be used as bioactive carriers of antibiotics (Tamazawa et al. 2011; Thomas et al. 2011) and/or other antimicrobial agents like chlorhexidine or halogenated furanone (Thomas et al. 2011; Cheng et al. 2012) as well as several growth factors (Yu et al. 2010; Sasikumar et al. 2012).

The most promising materials nowadays may be polyglycolic acid (PGA) and polylactic acid (PLA), including their copolymer called poly-lactic-co-glycolic acid (PLGA); but numerous other polyesters like polytrimetylcarbonate polyurethane, polycaprolactone, polyhydroxibutirate, polyhydroxialkanoate, or polyglactin (as well as their mixture) may also be mentioned (Aderriotis and Sandor 1999; Neumann and Kevenhoerster 2009; Yu et al. 2010; Tamazawa et al. 2011; Takechi et al. 2012). Experimental results with chitosan, a natural biocompatible osteoconductive and biodegradable biopolymer used as a constituent for composites, are also rather promising (Zhao et al. 2010), especially because chitosan also exerts certain antibacterial properties (Renoud et al. 2012).

3.2.10. Composites and Nanocomposites

The aim of composite materials is a synthesis of the advantageous properties of several biomaterials (Letic-Gavrilovic et al. 2000; Neumann and Kevenhoerster 2009; Bose and Tarafder 2012). Although there are composites that are simple mixtures of several particles, most composites consist of a molecular matrix (i.e. degradable polymers, collagen sponge, alginate, calcium phosphate cements, gypsum, etc.) mixed with variously sized particles from various biomaterials (Matsuno et al. 2008; Takahashi 2009; Moreau et al. 2009; Zhao et al. 2010; Liu and Webster 2010; Pamula et al. 2011; Takechi et al. 2012). Recently, the *nanosized* particles of several ceramics like titanium oxide ceramics (also called "titania") or calcium phosphate ceramics as well as antibacterial silver nanoparticles (etc.) have become available for such purposes (Liu and Webster 2010; Cabal et al. 2012; Wu et al. 2012).

The size of the premised nanoparticles ranges between roughly 10–100 nm (Liu and Webster 2010; Cabal et al. 2012; Wu et al. 2012); although sometimes their size is up to few hundred nanometers (Liu and Webster 2010; Wu et al. 2012). Composites that consist of this type of nanosized particle are referred to as "*nanocomposites*" (Liu and Webster 2010; Wu et al. 2012). Data indicate that the addition of nanosized particles (also called "*nanophase*") to composites may significantly improve both their biological and physical properties (Lavenus et al. 2010; Liu and Webster 2010; Wu et al. 2012) as opposed to conventional composites consisting of micron-scale particles (Lavenus et al. 2010; Liu and Webster 2010; Wu et al. 2012).

Composite particles may also be coated with various bioactive molecules like allogenic collagen, an allogenic demineralized bone matrix, a xenogenic non-collagen protein, or biodegradable synthetic polymers (etc.), which can be followed by impregnation with more specific promoters like bone morphogenetic proteins and/or other growth/morphogenetic factors, cytokines, or other promoters, including several drugs (Letic-Gavrilovic et al. 2000; Yu et al. 2010; Tamazawa et al. 2011; Bose and Tarafder 2012). They may also be supplemented with autologous bone marrow (Neumann and Kevenhoerster 2009) and/or with autologous bone and/or autologous platelet-rich plasma (Saini et al. 2011). The combination of composites with stem/progenitor cells also seems to be rather promising according to an experimental study (Zhao et al. 2010).

A large number of various composites and nanocomposites are already available in the market or are under development now. A "classical" example may be a calcium phosphate ceramic composite consisting of a mixture of hydroxyapatite and beta-tricalcium phosphate (60:40) interconnected by a silicon dioxide matrix; the composite is available for mandibular defects or for a sinus elevation procedures as a granule (Neumann and Kevenhoerster 2009). Other promising examples may be: an injectable composite of beta-tricalcium phosphate ceramic beads and alginate, which shows rather promising results under experimental conditions (Matsuno et al. 2008); a biphasic composite of beta-tricalcium phosphate ceramics and calcium sulfate (Smeets et al. 2009); a composite of beta-tricalcium phosphate ceramics and an antibiotic-loaded degradable polymer (copolymer of lactic acid and glycolic acid) for bone substitution in infected osseous lesions (Tamazawa et al. 2011); and a composite of beta-tricalcium phosphate ceramics and collagen for bone substitution purposes (Brkovic et al. 2008; Takahashi 2009), and particularly for the prevention of alveolar crest resorption following tooth extraction (Brkovic et al. 2008).

3.2.11. Autologous Platelet-Rich Plasma (PRP)

Autologous platelet-rich plasma is a concentrated suspension of platelets containing growth factors like platelet-derived growth factor, transforming growth factor-β (TGF-β), and others in their granules (Saini et al. 2011; Forni et al. 2013). The use of autologous platelet-rich plasma along with bone-substituting procedures was shown to significantly increase bone formation and maturation as well as soft tissue healing in numerous studies (Marx et al. 1998; Dori et al. 2007/a, b; Piemontese et al. 2008; Saini et al. 2011). PRP may advantageously be combined with all kinds of available bone grafts and/or bone substitutes (Marx et al. 1998; Dori et al. 2007/a, b; Piemontese et al. 2008; Saini et al. 2011; Forni et al. 2013). Autologous platelet-rich plasma is prepared from a patient's whole blood (collected by means of venipuncture of the (median) cubital vein).

3.3. Titanium

3.3.1. General Considerations

Metals are probably the oldest forms of materials used for dental implants, and because of their superior fracture and fatigue resistance they have been the most common material used so far (Letic-Gavrilovic et al. 2000; Neumann and Kevenhoerster 2009). A large spectrum of metals and alloys have been used as subperiosteal and endosseus implants, including gold-based alloys, stainless steel, and especially cobalt-chromium alloys (Letic-Gavrilovic et al. 2000; Neumann and Kevenhoerster 2009); however the fundamental problem with these metals/alloys was the fibrous response (fibrous interface) that they promoted with the bone (Letic-Gavrilovic et al. 2000; Neumann and Kevenhoerster 2009). By today's standards, none of these metals/alloys can achieve osseointegration; therefore they have largely been replaced by titanium and titanium alloys (Letic-Gavrilovic et al. 2000).

Although in the next paragraph issues related to the use of titanium as an implant fixture are discussed, it should be mentioned that titanium implants in the form of a web of titanium fibers (Masago et al. 2007) or in the form of porous titanium granules (Thor 2013) mixed with PRP/blood (Masago et al. 2007; Thor 2013) may also be used as bone substitute for alveolar ridge augmentation (Masago et al. 2007) and for the regeneration of bone defects around dental implants (Thor 2013). Similarly, porous granules made of titanium oxide (TiO_2) *ceramics* may also be used to prevent alveolar ridge resorption following the removal of a tooth (Tiainen et al. 2012).

3.3.2. Major Properties of Titanium

Titanium (Ti) is characterized by high stability at a light mass, and it is the most biocompatible and corrosion-resistant metal (Letic-Gavrilovic et al. 2000; Neumann and Kevenhoerster 2009; Hanawa 2011). Although its elasticity modulus is well above that of human bone (105 kN/mm^2 and ca. 20 kN/mm^2, respectively), it corresponds to the elasticity modulus of the bone more than other more or less biocompatible metals like stainless steel or cobalt-chrome alloys (Neumann and Kevenhoerster 2009). Titanium also has a light weight and a uniquely high strength to weight ratio (Letic-Gavrilovic et al. 2000; Hanawa 2011). Moreover, titanium exerts osteoconductive properties, although alternatives concerning the type of Ti alloy being used and its surface properties generate diverse osseointegration results (Letic-Gavrilovic et al. 2000). Although titanium implants provide a physical matrix that is suitable for the deposition of new bone and may guide both the growth and extension of the bone (Letic-Gavrilovic et al. 2000), they do not exert osteoinductive or osteostimulative properties (Letic-Gavrilovic et al. 2000).

Importantly, an approx. 5–10 nm thick, strong, and tightly-bound superficial layer of titanium oxide develops spontaneously and instantaneously (in 30 ms, Hanawa 2011) on the surface of titanium when it comes into contact with air (Letic-Gavrilovic et al. 2000; Neumann and Kevenhoerster 2009; Hanawa 2011). The premised oxide layer has a tendency to grow spontaneously up to 200 nm, leading to a "matured" titanium-oxide layer (Letic-Gavrilovic et al. 2000). The appearance of a matured Ti-oxide layer could lead to improved biological properties but unfortunately, the premised "maturation" is coupled with a certain "aging" (also referred to as "biological aging") that may occur because of the progressive accumulation of hydrocarbons and the time-related disappearance of hydrophilic properties and/or the electrostatic positivity occurring within a few weeks (Iwasa et al. 2011; Yoneyama et al. 2013). Despite the premised "biological aging" (which may somewhat compromise the biological properties of the Ti surface), the titanium-oxide layer is very important for the biocompatibility of titanium, because it is responsible for both the corrosion-resistance and surface adhesion of the glycoproteins that play a crucial role in the osseointegration processes (Letic-Gavrilovic et al. 2000; Neumann and Kevenhoerster 2009; Hanawa 2011).

Although titanium is commonly found in the crust of lithosphere, the industrial production of pure titanium is complex and therefore expensive. Commercially obtainable pure titanium (cpTi) is classified into four quality grades as specified in ISO 5832-2:2000-08 (Letic-Gavrilovic et al. 2000; Neumann and Kevenhoerster 2009). "Pure titanium" refers to an amount containing less than 1% of additives like nitrate, carbon, hydrogen, oxygen, or iron (Letic-Gavrilovic et al. 2000; Neumann and Kevenhoerster 2009). Although commercially pure titanium is also commonly used as dental implant material (Yamashita et al. 2009; Saulacic et al. 2012), titanium-based implant materials regularly consist of alloys, e.g. Ti-6Al-4V (6% aluminum, 4% vanadium), Ti-6Al-7Nb (6% aluminum, 7% niobium), Ti-5Nb-5Zr (5% niobium 5% zirconium), and others as standardized in ISO 5832-3 (Letic-Gavrilovic et al. 2000; Neumann and Kevenhoerster 2009). It should be noted that the composition of a Ti alloy may determine not only its physical, but also certain biological properties.

3.3.3. Surface Modification of Titanium Fixtures

Although the "original" root-form implant fixtures were made of pure titanium (cpTi) with a turned surface (Branemark et al. 1969; Branemark 1972; Branemark et al. 1977; Albrektsson et al. 1981; Branemark 1983; Palmquist et al. 2012), later manufacturers created various Ti alloys with different surface roughness properties to achieve better bone healing, osseointegration, and osteoconduction (Letic-Gavrilovic et al. 2000; Yamashita et al. 2009; Tomsia et al. 2011). Titanium by itself does exert osteoconductive properties (Letic-Gavrilovic et al. 2000); however, alternatives concerning the type of Ti alloy as well as its surface roughness definitely influence its osteoconductivity (Letic-Gavrilovic et al. 2000; Yamashita et al. 2009; Bose and Tarafder 2012). It is generally accepted that rough surfaces promote cell differentiation (Ramaglia et al. 2011), cell proliferation, and the spread of the cells (Osathanon et al. 2011) as well as the attachment of osteoblasts (Koh et al. 2009) and the increased formation of an extracellular matrix and bone apposition (Yamashita et al. 2009; Ramaglia et al. 2011; Tomsia et al. 2011; Palmquist et al. 2012; Teng et al. 2012). Rough surfaces also favor mechanical interlocking with the surrounding tissue (Palmquist et al. 2012).

The most important techniques that can be used to increase the surface roughness of titanium fixtures (without coating) are sandblasting, grinding, Ti-plasma spraying, laser texturing (Tomsia et al. 2011), and acid etching (Kimura et al. 2009; Ramaglia et al. 2011). Hydrothermal treatment of Ti surfaces with 3% H_2O_2 using an autoclave (Yoneyama et al. 2013) as well as the treatment of Ti surfaces with UV light (referred to as "UV-photofunctionalization," Iwasa et al. 2011) are used to recover the biological activity of aged ("biologically aged") Ti implant surfaces (Iwasa et al. 2011; Yoneyama et al. 2012). Recently, anodic oxidation (also referred to as "anodization") has also been used to modify the surface of Ti-based alloys by creating an adherent Ti-oxide layer with a wide range of available morphology and micro-/nano-porosities on the implant surface (Kim and Ramaswamy 2009; Tomsia et al. 2011; Ma et al. 2012; Kang et al. 2012; Min et al. 2013). Through anodization it is possible to create a *nanotubular structure* (ca. 120 nm pore size) in the Ti-oxide layer that can advantageously affect the adhesion, orientation, proliferation, and gene expression of various types of cells (Ma et al. 2012). Similarly, a nanostructured Ti-oxide layer may also be manufactured by means of TiO_2 sputtering (Iwasa et al. 2011).

Besides improving surface roughness properties, certain surface treatments (i.e. chemical etching) are also used to create more hydrophilic implant surfaces (Tomsia et al. 2011) that may also promote protein adhesion and subsequently cell attachment (Ishizaki et al. 2011; Tomsia et al. 2011; Jung et al. 2012).

3.3.4. Coating of Titanium Fixtures

The classical protocol of osseointegration was based on the success of uncoated root-form pure titanium (cpTi) implants (Branemark et al. 1969; Branemark 1972; Branemark et al. 1977; Albrektsson et al. 1981; Branemark 1983; Palmquist et al. 2012). In the case of the earliest (turned) forms of cpTi implants, distance osteogenesis occurred; thus the fixtures are coated with an interfacial layer immediately after implantation that degrades and is replaced ideally by bone (Tomsia et al. 2011). In the case of cpTi implants with increased surface roughness contact, osteogenesis can occur (Davies 2003; Palmquist et al. 2012), leading to an intimate bone-implant contact at a nanoscale level (Davies 2003; Palmquist et al. 2012).

Although long-term clinical data supports the use of cpTi-based protocols even today, current data substantiate the use of implant surface modifications by means of various coatings to further improve osseointegration (Letic-Gavrilovic et al. 2000; Hanawa 2011; Mano et al. 2011; Tomsia et al. 2011). Coatings may have significant clinical importance especially in the following cases: where there are big defects and poorly supported bone (Letic-Gavrilovic et al. 2000; Davies 2003), very small or very big implants (Letic-Gavrilovic et al. 2000), repeated surgical procedures or re-implantation (Letic-Gavrilovic et al. 2000), type III or type IV bone quality (Letic-Gavrilovic et al. 2000; Davies 2003), and at implantation into fresh extraction sites (Letic-Gavrilovic et al. 2000).

The idea is to apply a thin coating layer (usually a ceramic layer) that will improve *de novo* bone apposition (Dziedzich et al. 1996; Davies 2003) and will also chemically bond to both the implant and the surrounding bone (Hench and Wilson 1984; Letic-Gavrilovic et al. 2000; Tomsia et al. 2011; Bose and Tarafder 2012; Fu et al. 2012). While this layer is aimed to optimize the closure between the *de novo* synthesized bone and the osseointegrating implant by means of optimal micromechanical interdigitation (Dziedzich et al. 1996; Davies 2003) and chemical binding, its additional important function is to optimize *de novo* bone apposition (Davies 2003) as a scaffold and by means of gaining osteoinductive and/or osteostimulating properties (Letic-Gavrilovic et al. 2000; Davies 2003; Tomsia et al. 2011; Bose and Tarafder 2012).

Over the years, various coating methods were developed to manufacture the coatings themselves (i.e. plasma spraying, flame spraying, chemical vapor deposition, physical vapor deposition, slip casting/sintering, electrophoretic deposition/sintering, electrochemical deposition, sputtering, pulsed-laser deposition, blast coating, etc.) and a large number of implant systems consisting of many different biomaterials have been introduced (Letic-Gavrilovic et al. 2000; Kim and Ramaswamy 2009; Hanawa 2011; Mano et al. 2011; Roy et al. 2011; Tomsia et al. 2011; Kuwabara et al. 2012; Bressan et al. 2013).

The most frequently used coatings are of the ceramic type, like calcium phosphate ceramics, glass-ceramics, titanium nitride ceramics (TiN), titanium carbide ceramics (TiC), titanium oxide ceramics, diamond-like carbon ceramics, silicon carbide ceramics (SiC), or aluminum-calcium-phosphate (AlCaP) ceramics (Letic-Gavrilovic et al. 2000; Mano et al. 2011; Kuwabara et al. 2012; Bose and Tarafder 2012); the most prevalently used are calcium phosphate ceramics (i.e. hydroxyapatite and tricalcium phosphate) or glass-ceramics (Mano et al. 2011; Tomsia et al. 2011). Ceramic coatings appear to have better biological properties than cpTi or Ti alloys alone, even if the clinical results are somewhat controversial (Letic-Gavrilovic et al. 2000; Tomsia et al. 2011; Bose and Tarafder 2012). When implanted, certain ceramic coatings form a carbonated apatite (HCA) layer on their surfaces. HCA agglomerates are rather similar in composition and structure to the mineral phase of osseous tissue (Tomsia et al. 2011) and at the same time they can incorporate collagen fibrils from the environment (Tomsia et al. 2011). Today, coatings may also be made of *nanosized particles* (within roughly 10–100 nm in size), which may further improve their biological and physical properties (Lavenus et al. 2010; Roy et al. 2011; Variola et al. 2011; Yamada et al. 2012) since the data indicate that physicochemical features in the nanometer range are likely to ultimately control the adsorption of proteins as well as the adhesion and differentiation of cells (Lavenus et al. 2010; Lavenus et al. 2011; Bueno et al. 2011; Variola et al. 2011).

The addition of biologically active molecules to the implant surface was also widely investigated and may lead to a breakthrough in maximizing the osseointegration of titanium implant fixtures (Letic-Gavrilovic et al. 2000; Simon and Watson 2002; Hanawa 2011; Tomsia et al. 2011; Bose and Tarafder 2012; Cabal et al. 2012; Bressan et al. 2013; Min et al. 2013). These molecules may be bonded directly to Ti surfaces via certain carrier molecules (Petrie et al. 2008; Liu et al. 2010; Min et al. 2013), for example, by means of silanation (Kammerer et al. 2011; Renoud et al. 2012,) and tresyl chloride activation (Yamamichi et al. 2008). Biologically active molecules may also be bonded directly onto Ti via the formation of a *nanotubular structure* (ca. 120 nm pore size) on the Ti oxide layer by means of anodization, followed by repeated lyophilization of the biologically active molecule on the Ti oxide layer's surface (Ma et al. 2012). *Non*-ceramic crystalline calcium phosphates (primarily carbonated apatite) that crystallize in the presence of biologically active molecules directly onto titanium surfaces by means of supersaturated calcium phosphate solutions may also be used; this is referred to as "biomimetic calcium phosphate coating" (Liu et al. 2006; Lavenus et al. 2010; Liu et al. 2010; Kang et al. 2012).

However, in most cases, the main carrier of the premised biologically active molecules is the ceramic coating (primarily calcium phosphate ceramics) of the implant surfaces (Barros et al. 2009; Cabal et al. 2012), which is often combined with a second bioactive carrier (i.e. allogenic collagen, allogenic demineralized bone matrix, xenogenic non-collagen protein, biodegradable synthetic polymers, etc.) prior to impregnation with bone morphogenetic proteins, platelet-derived growth factor, and/or other growth/morphogenetic factors and cytokines as well as other promoters including several anti-inflammatory drugs, antimicrobial agents, or antibiotics (Letic-Gavrilovic et al. 2000; Simon and Watson 2002; Tamazawa et al. 2011; Kaigler et al. 2011; Tomsia et al. 2011; Bose and Tarafder 2012; Cheng et al. 2012). Recently, it has also been possible to bond synthetic functional domains (bioactive motif oligopeptides) of extracellular matrix proteins (i.e. fibronectin, vitronectin, laminin, etc.) to coatings of implant surfaces (Petrie et al. 2008; Yamamichi et al. 2008; Barros et al. 2009; Tomsia et al. 2011; Min et al. 2013), which may improve cell adhesion and osseointegration. The surface density of these motifs is adjustable during manufacturing and this seems to be rather important in relation to the biological effect (Barros et al. 2009; Tomsia et al. 2011). Similarly, the *nanopattern* (i.e. ordered distribution vs. random distribution) of the premised oligopeptides may be adjusted using functionalized gold nanoparticles (Tomsia et al. 2011) to match the corresponding receptors on the osteogenic cell surfaces (Tomsia et al. 2011), which may further enhance overall functionality.

3.3.5. Carcinogenicity, Allergic Reactions, and Toxicity

Animal tests do not show any indication of tumorigenicity of titanium or titanium alloys (Neumann and Kevenhoerster 2009). Although there are a few reports of individual cases of malignant tumors in the tissue surrounding titanium alloys (Friedman and Vernon 1983), pathogenically these cases remain speculations (Neumann and Kevenhoerster 2009). Regarding the great amount of titanium-alloy dental implants used throughout the world, tumorigenicity has been practically ruled out (Neumann and Kevenhoerster 2009). Similarly, allergic reactions do not seem to play any significant role concerning the dental applications of titanium alloys (Neumann and Kevenhoerster 2009). Sensitization through titanium is rare. Although a few individual cases have been described for orthopedic or cardiologic (pacemaker implant) applications, no type IV allergic reactions have been described for the oral applications of titanium alloys to date (Neumann and Kevenhoerster 2009).

Overall, both titanium oxide and pure titanium (both ionic or particle) show very low toxicity (Neumann and Kevenhoerster 2009); there was no local toxic effect found in the bone or skeletal muscle neither in animal experiments nor in clinical experiences (Neumann and Kevenhoerster 2009). However, both titanium oxide and titanium itself may cause certain toxic effect and disorders like yellow nail syndrome (Berglund and Carlmark 2011) in rare cases, especially if a larger amount is released through galvanic action or other physico-chemical corrosion. As indicated above, titanium is a highly corrosion-resistant metal (Letic-Gavrilovic et al. 2000; Neumann and Kevenhoerster 2009) due to its spontaneously developing titanium-oxide surface layer (Neumann and Kevenhoerster 2009). However, despite the titanium-oxide layer, a slight amount of corrosion may occur as a result of flexure under mechanical stress as well as because of the friction between the implant fixture and the abutment (Neumann and Kevenhoerster 2009). This corrosion phenomenon may be intensified in the presence of macrophages through the production of H_2O_2 (Neumann and Kevenhoerster 2009). Corrosion may also occur through galvanic action (Berglund and Carlmark 2011) and/or through the oxidative action of fluorides (Roselino Ribeiro et al. 2007; Yamazoe et al. 2007; Berglund and Carlmark 2011; Lelli et al. 2013).

Somewhat higher toxicity potential may also arise from titanium-alloy additives like aluminum and vanadium, as well as from several titanium corrosion products (Letic-Gavrilovic et al. 2000; Neumann and Kevenhoerster 2009; Tomsia et al. 2011); however, it should be emphasized that there is currently no indication for clinically relevant systemic toxicity caused by oral titanium-alloy implants (Neumann and Kevenhoerster 2009). There are a few reports about localized reactions of mucosa caused by screws protruding into the maxillary sinuses (Neumann and Kevenhoerster 2009), and localized oral soft tissue reactions around titanium dental implants have also been extensively described (Letic-Gavrilovic et al. 2000; Myshin and Wiens 2005). However, in these cases, it is not exclusively the local toxic effect of the titanium alloys but also the accumulation of bacteria (and their interactions with the surroundings) that play a pivotal role.

Importantly, an addition of 0.5% platinum (Pt) to cpTi or Ti alloys seems to improve both mechanical strength and corrosion resistance, including fluoride corrosion (Yamazoe et al. 2007). This may be significant in preventing various types of corrosion phenomena, including the premised galvanic corrosion, flexure/friction related corrosions, and fluoride corrosion in relation to the maintenance of oral health (i.e. natural teeth) using fluoride-containing mouthwash and toothpaste (Yamazoe et al. 2007).

3.4. Zirconium Dioxide Ceramics

The ceramic form of zirconium dioxide (ZrO_2, also referred to as "zirconia") has the potential for use as a dental implant fixture material (Yamashita et al. 2009; Hashimoto et al. 2011; Borgonovo et al. 2012). Early clinical results in humans have been promising (Borgonovo et al. 2012), and the use of zirconia may resolve esthetic problems appearing in connection with titanium (Yamashita et al. 2009; Borgonovo et al. 2012), such as the grayish color of titanium fixtures shining through thin peri-implant mucosa (if any) and the appearance of exposed metal due to recession (if any). The biocompatibility of zirconium dioxide ceramics is superior to that of titanium (Hashimoto et al. 2011) and especially to those of titanium alloys, which may also be considered advantageous (Yamashita et al. 2009; Hashimoto et al. 2011).

Although there may be certain differences in relation to the early cellular response of osteoblastic cells (Depprich et al. 2008/a), in general, the osseointegration of zirconia is rather similar to that of titanium on the histological level (Depprich et al. 2008/c), resulting in intimate bone contact without the interposition of any interfacial layer at the ultrastructural level (Depprich et al. 2008/b). Importantly, the surface properties of zirconia are just as significant as those of titanium implants, and rough surfaces also show improved initial cell responses in this case (Yamashita et al. 2009; Hashimoto et al. 2011; Ito et al. 2013).

The most important method to increase the surface roughness of zirconia may be sandblasting followed by heating to recover the crystal phase of the zirconia surface (Yamashita et al. 2009; Hashimoto et al. 2011); but acid etching has also been studied

(Depprich et al. 2008/a, b, c; Hashimoto et al. 2011; Ito et al. 2013). For the chemical modification of zirconia surfaces, acid treatment, cold plasma, oxygen plasma, and UV light treatment may be used (Hashimoto et al. 2011; Watanabe et al. 2012). Acid etching, oxygen plasma treatment, and UV light treatment were reported to increase the hydrofilicity properties of zirconia significantly (Watanabe et al. 2012), which advantageously increases the initial surface attachment of osteoblast-like cells (Watanabe et al. 2012). Recently, the biomimetic coating of zirconia with highly affine zirconia-bonding peptide motives capable of attaching a targeted protein to zirconia surfaces has also become available (Hashimoto et al. 2011).

The major problem with zirconium dioxide ceramics is their low fracture resistance compared to titanium; therefore efforts are now being made to develop zirconium dioxide ceramics of higher flexural strength and fracture toughness (Yamashita et al. 2009). Recently, yttria-stabilized tetragonal zirconia polycrystals (Y-TZP) have exerted rather good physical characteristics (Yamashita et al. 2009; Hashimoto et al. 2011; Borgonovo et al. 2012), especially in their hot isostatic-pressing processed (HIP Y-TZP) form (Koyama et al. 2012; Iijama et al. 2013). Similarly, the physical properties of a zirconia/alumina nanocomposite (30 vol% Al_2O_3) stabilized with 10 mol% ceria (CeO_2) have also been very promising (Yamashita et al. 2009).

3.5. Membranes

3.5.1. Non-Resorbable Membranes

These kinds of membranes are primarily made of expanded polytetrafluoroethylene (ePTFE). Since these membranes are not resorbable, they require a second procedure to be removed (Letic-Gavrilovic et al. 2000; Irinakis 2006; Kim et al. 2011). These membranes can be combined with carrier materials for the delivery of several growth/morphogenetic substances to promote bone regeneration under both the guided bone regeneration and guided tissue regeneration techniques (Letic-Gavrilovic et al. 2000; Irinakis 2006; Parrish et al. 2009; Kim et al. 2011). Clinical results have demonstrated that this technique allows the bone to grow directly around the implant (Letic-Gavrilovic et al. 2000).

3.5.2. Resorbable Membranes

The major synthetic materials for biologically resorbable membranes are primarily polyglycolic acid and polylactic acid or their combination (Letic-Gavrilovic et al. 2000; Kim et al. 2011). Aside from these, collagen membranes may also be used as resorbable membrane material (Letic-Gavrilovic et al. 2000; Irinakis 2006; Kim et al. 2011; Schulten et al. 2013) for both guided bone regeneration techniques (Irinakis 2006; Fei et al. 2008) and guided tissue regeneration techniques (Letic-Gavrilovic et al. 2000; Parrish et al. 2009). The placement of an enamel matrix derivative (EMD, enamel matrix protein exerting periodontal regenerative properties) may also be combined with the use of resorbable membranes (Sculean et al. 2001; Parrish et al. 2009), although EMD may also be used efficiently without membranes (Windisch et al. 2002; Parrish et al. 2009). Resorbable membranes may also be used for the delivery of several growth/morphogenetic substances.

3.6. Sutures

3.6.1. Non-Resorbable Sutures

There are a variety of non-resorbable materials used in manufacturing sutures, from which silk, nylon, and polytetrafluoroethylene (PTFE) are the most frequently occurring (Aderriotis and Sandor 1999). A silk suture is easy to tie and can be used efficiently to oppose wound edges; however, the braided nature of silk allows the accumulation of surface debris and/or bacteria, which may result in inflammation (Aderriotis and Sandor 1999). In contrast, nylon sutures are monofilament strands with no interstices; therefore they are less prone to cause inflammation due to the accumulation of debris/bacteria. However, their cut edges are very sharp and therefore may bother patients if used intraorally (Aderriotis and Sandor 1999). That is not the case for PTFE sutures, which are well tolerated and accompanied by almost no inflammation (Aderriotis and Sandor 1999).

3.6.2. Resorbable Sutures

Similar to non-resorbable sutures, there are also a variety of resorbable suture materials, from which animal-derivative gut, resorbable polymer PGLA, and combined PGLA-polyglactin sutures may be mentioned (Aderriotis and Sandor 1999). The disadvantage of gut sutures is that as this material breaks down, its by-products may result in wound inflammation (Aderriotis and Sandor 1999). In contrast, PGLA sutures are absorbed via enzymatic hydrolysis, resulting in less inflammation (Aderriotis and Sandor 1999). PGLA sutures are also well suited for deeper layer non-surface closures (Aderriotis and Sandor 1999). However, when used on the surface, the absorption of PGLA sutures may take a long time, which often necessitates manual removal (Aderriotis and Sandor 1999). The combined form of PGLA-polyglactin sutures are usually gamma irradiated; the irradiation alters the suture material's molecular structure and enhances its absorption rate (Aderriotis and Sandor 1999), which may overcome the premised problem of delayed suture resorption (Aderriotis and Sandor 1999).

3.7. Other Materials

3.7.1. Silicon Nitride Ceramics

Silicon nitride (Si_3N_4) is used in its ceramic form. This biomaterial is of good biocompatibility, with a mechanical strength roughly twice as large as the strength of aluminum-oxide (Al_2O_3) ceramics (Neumann and Kevenhoerster 2009). The major disadvantages of this material (similar to other ceramics) are its lack of ductility and the technical complexity of manufacturing ceramic screws. Despite the premised disadvantages, silicon nitride may be qualified for use as a bone substitute or implant fixture in the future (Neumann and Kevenhoerster 2009).

3.7.2. Aluminum Oxide Ceramics

The ceramic form of aluminum oxide (also referred to as "alumina") was once used as implant fixture material, but because of its insufficient physical properties it was withdrawn from the market (Yamashita et al. 2009). This biomaterial is practically poreless and has neither osteoconductive nor osteoinductive or osteostimulative properties (Neumann and Kevenhoerster 2009).

3.7.3. Calcium Sulfate (Gypsum)

Calcium sulfate (also called "plaster of Paris") is one of the oldest biomaterials used for bone substitution (Dreesmann 1892; Neumann and Kevenhoerster 2009). It is resorbed rather quickly, roughly within 2–6 months (Neumann and Kevenhoerster 2009). Calcium sulfate also exerts certain bacteriostatic properties; therefore it may be used for composites even today (Smeets et al. 2009). In certain cases, calcium sulfate may also be inserted into bone lesions in order to stop bleeding and accomplish hemostasis (Norholt and Christiansen 2013).

3.7.4. Plastics

Plastics like poly-methyl methacrylate (PMMA) and poly-hydroxyethyl methacrylate (PHEMA), as well as porous polyethylene (PPE) or high density polyethylene (HDPE), are used in maxillofacial surgery for permanent bone replacement in the form of blocks, granula, or via CAD-CAM technology performed implants (Nuss and von Rechenberg 2008; Neumann and Kevenhoerster 2009). Because of their porosity (roughly 250–500 μm pore size), they allow the ingrowth of bone or other tissues (i.e. blood vessels, connective tissue) and therefore facilitate a firm fixation to the surrounding tissue (Neumann and Kevenhoerster 2009). Plastic-type materials may be used as implant fixtures in the future, but by today's standards, they are not favored because they induce a fibrous layer at the bone-implant interface and cannot achieve osseointegration (Letic-Gavrilovic et al. 2000; Nuss and von Rechenberg 2008).

Conclusion

Many different biomaterials may be used for implant surgery, and the number of such biomaterials available is continuously increasing. Therefore, it is rather difficult for both researchers and clinicians to be caught up on such information in this field. Consequently, there is a need for general reviews on available current scientific data to keep related knowledge up-to-date and functional. In this chapter the most important current knowledge related to biomaterials used for implant surgery has been summarized.

References

Aderriotis, D; Sandor, GKB. Outcomes of irradiated polyglactin 910 Vicryl Rapide Fast-absorbing suture in oral and scalp wound. *J Can Dent Assoc*, 1999, 65, 345–347.

Akintoye, SO; Giavis, P; Stefanik, D; Levin, L; Mante, FK. Comparative osteogenesis of maxilla and iliac crest human bone marrow stromal cells attached to oxidized titanium – a pilot study. *Clin Oral Implant Res*, 2008, 19, 1197–1201.

Albrektsson, T; Branemark, PI; Hansson, HA; Lindstrom, J. Osseointegrated titanium implants. Requirements for ensuring a long-lasting direct bone anchorage in man. *Acta Orthop Scand*, 1981, 52, 155–170.

Albrektsson, T; Johansson, C. Osteoinduction, osteoconduction and osseointegration. *Eur Spine J*, 2001, 10, S96–S101.

Andersen, K; Norholt, SE; Knudsen, J; Kuseler, A; Jensen, J. Donor site morbidity after reconstruction of alveolar bone defects with mandibular symphyseal bone grafts in cleft patients – 111 consecutive patients. *Int J Oral Maxillofac Surg*, in press, DOI: 10.1016/j.ijom.2013.09.007.

Barboni, B; Mangano, C; Valbonetti, L; Marruchella, G; Berardinelli, P; Martelli, A; Muttini, A; Mauro, A; Bedini, R; Turriani, M; Pecci, R; Nardinocchi, D; Zizzari, VL; Tete, S; Piattelli, A; Mattioli, M. *PLoS ONE*, 2013, 8, e63256.

Barros, RRM; Novaes Jr., AB; Papalexiou, V; Souza, SLS; Taba Jr., M; Palioto, DB; Grisi, MFM. Effect of biofunctionalized implant surface on osseointegration – A histomorphometric study in dogs. *Braz Dent J*, 2009, 20, 91–98.

Berglund, F; Carlmark, B. Titanium, sinusitis and the yellow nail syndrome. *Biol Trace Elem Res*, 2011, 143, 1–7.

Borgonovo, AE; Fabbri, A; Vavassori, V; Censi, R; Maiorana, C. Multiple teeth replacement with endosseous one-piece yttrium-stabilized zirconia dental implants. *Med Oral Patol Oral Cir Bucal*, 2012, 17, e981–e987.

Bose, S; Tarafder, S. Calcium phosphate ceramic systems in growth factor and drug delivery for bone tissue engineering: A review. *Acta Biomater*, 2012, 8, 1401–1421.

Branemark, PI. Rehabilitation with a denture anchored to the jawbone. *Lakartidningen*, 1972, 69, 4813–4814.

Branemark, PI. Osseointegration and its experimental background. *J Prosthet Dent*, 1983, 50, 399–410.

Branemark, PI; Adell, R; Breine, U; Hansson, BO; Lindstrom, J; Ohlsson, A. Intra-osseous anchorage of dental prostheses. I. Experimental studies. *Scand J Plast Reconstr Surg*, 1969, 3, 81–100.

Branemark, PI; Hansson, BO; Adell, R; Breine, U; Lindstrom, J; Hallen O; Ohman, A. Osseointegrated titanium implants in the treatment of the edentulous jaw. *Scand J Plast Reconstr Surg*, 1977, 11, (Suppl. 16) 1–175.

Bressan, E; Sbricoli, L; Guazzo, R; Tocco, I; Roman, M; Vindigni, V; Stellini, E; Gardin, C; Ferroni, L; Sivolella, S; Zavan, B. Nanostructured surfaces of dental implants. *Int J Mol Sci*, 2013, 14, 1918–1931.

Brkovic, BMB; Prasad, HS; Konandreas, G; Milan, R; Antunovic, D; Sandor, GKB; Rohrer, MD. Simple preservation of a maxillary extraction socket using beta-tricalcium phosphate with type I collagen: Preliminary clinical and histomorphometric observations. *J Can Dent Assoc*, 2008, 74, 523–528.

Bueno, RBL; Adachi, P; Castro-Raucci, LMS; Rosa, AL; Nanci, A; Oliveira, PT. Oxidative nanopatterning of titanium surfaces promotes production and extracellular accumulation of osteopontin. *Braz Dent J*, 2011, 22, 179–184.

Carlsen, A; Gorst-Rasmussen, A; Jensen, T. Donor site morbidity associated with autogenous bone harvesting from the ascending mandibular ramus. *Implant Dent*, 2013, 22, 503–506.

Cabal, B; Cafini, F; Esteban-Tejeda, L; Alou, L; Bartolome, JF; Sevillano, D; Lopez-Piriz, R; Torrecillas, R; Moya, JS. Inhibitory effect on *in vitro Streptococcus oralis* biofilm of a soda-lime glass containing silver nanoparticles coating on titanium alloy. *PLoS ONE*, 2012, 7, e42393.

Cheng, Y; Wu, J; Gao, B; Zhao, X; Yao, J; Mei, S; Zhang, L; Ren, H. Fabrication and in vitro release behavior of a novel antibacterial coating containing halogenated furanone-loaded poly(L-lactic acid) nanoparticles on microarc-oxidized titanium. *Int J Nanomedicine*, 2012, 7, 5641–5652.

Davies, JE; Understanding peri-implant endosseous healing. *J Dent Education*, 2003, 67, 932–949.

Davies, JE; Matta, R; Mendes, VC; de Carvalho, PSP. Development, characterization and clinical use of a biodegradable composite scaffold for bone engineering in oro-maxillo-facial surgery. *Organogenesis*, 2010, 6, 161–166.

Depprich, R; Ommerborn, M; Zipprich, H; Naujoks, C; Handschel, J; Wiesmann, HP; Kubler, NR; Meyer, U. Behavior of osteoblastic cells cultured on titanium and structured zirconia surfaces. *Head & Face Medicine*, 2008/a, 4, 29.

Depprich, R; Zipprich, H; Ommerborn, M; Mahn, E; Lammers, L; Handschel, J; Naujoks, C; Wiesmann, HP; Kubler, N; Meyer, U. Osseointegration of zirconia implants: an SEM observation of the bone-implant interface. *Head & Face Medicine*, 2008/b, 4, 25.

Depprich, R; Zipprich, H; Ommerborn, M; Naujoks, C; Wiesmann, HP; Kiattavorncharoen, S; Laurer, HC; Meyer, U; Kubler, NR; Handschel, J. Osseointeration of zirconia implants compared with titanium: an in vivo study. *Head & Face Medicine*, 2008/c, 4, 30.

Dori, F; Huszar, T; Nikolidakis, D; Arweiler, NB; Gera, I; Sculean, A. Effect of platelet-rich plasma on the healing of intrabony defects treated with a natural mineral and collagen membrane. *J Clin Periodontol*, 2007, 34, 254–261.

Dori, F; Huszar, T; Niklidakis, D; Arweiler, NB; Gera, I; Sculean, A. Effect of platelet-rich plasma on the healing of intrabony defects treated with an anorganic bovine bone mineral and expanded polytetrafluoroethylene membranes. *J Periodontol*, 2007, 78, 983–990.

Dreesmann, H. Über Knochenplombierung. *Beitr Klin Chir*, 1892, 9, 804–810.

Dziedzich, DM; Savva, IH; Wilkinson, DS; Davies, JE. Osteoconduction on, and bonding to, calcium phosphate ceramic implants. *Mat Res Soc Symp Proc*, 1996, 414, 147–156.

Fei, W; Yang, XM; Li, Z; Yin, MP; Shen, ZH; Liao, CH. Experimental study of the bioresorbable collagen membrane used for guided bone regeneration around dental implants. *West China J Stomatol*, 2008, 26, 494–498.

Friedman, KE; Vernon, SE. Squamous cell carcinoma developing in conjunction with a mandibular staple bone plate. *J Oral Maxillofac Surg*, 1983, 41, 265–266.

Forni, F; Marzagalli, M; Tesei, P; Grassi, A. Platelet gel: applications in dental regenerative surgery. *Blood Transfus*, 2013, 11, 102–107.

Fu, DL; Jiang, QH; He, FM; Yang, GL; Liu, L. Fluorescence microscopic analysis of bone osseointegration of strontium-substituted hydroxyapatite implants. *J Zhejiang Univ-Sci B (Biomed & Biotechnol)*, 2012, 13, 364–371.

Fujikawa, K; Sugawara, A; Kusama, K; Nishiyama, M; Murai, S; Takagi, S; Chow LC. Fluorescent labeling analysis and electron probe microanalysis for alveolar ridge augmentation using calcium phosphate cement. *Dental Materials J*, 2002, 21, 296–305.

Hanawa, T. A comprehensive review of techniques for biofunctionalization of titanium. *J Periodontal Implant Sci.*, 2011, 41, 263–272.

Hashimoto, K; Yoshinari, M; Matsuzaka, K; Shiba, K; Inoue, T. Identification of peptide motif that binds to the surface of zirconia. *Dent Material J*, 2011 30, 935–940.

Hench, LL; Wilson, J, Surface-active biomaterials. *Science*, 1984, 226, 630–636.

Ho, SKC; Peel, SAF; Hu, ZM; Sandor, GKB; Clokie, CML. Augmentation of the maxillary sinus: Comparison of bioimplants containing bone morphogenetic protein and autogenous bone in a rabbit model. *J Can Dent Assoc*, 2010, 76, a108.

Iijama, T; Homma, S; Sekine, H; Sasaki, H; Yajima, Y; Yoshinari, M. Influence of surface treatment of yttria-stabilized tetragonal zirconia polycrystal with hot isostatic pressing on cyclic fatigue strength. *Dental Materials J*, 2013, 32, 274–280.

Irinakis, T. Rational for socket preservation after extraction of a single-rooted tooth when planning for future implant placement. *J Can Dent Assoc*, 2006, 72, 917–922.

Ishizaki, K; Sugita, Y; Iwasa, F; Minamikawa, H; Ueno, T; Yamada, M; Suzuki, T; Ogawa, T. Nanometer-thin TiO_2 enhances skeletal muscle cell phenotype and behavior. *Int J Nanomedicine*, 2011, 6, 2191–2203.

Ito, H; Sasaki, H; Saito, K; Honma, S; Yamija, Y; Yoshinari, M. Response of osteoblast-like cells to zirconia with different surface topography. *Dental Materials J*, 2013, 32, 122–129.

Iwasa, F; Tsukimura, N; Sugita, Y; Kanuru, RK; Kubo, K; Hasnain, H; Att, W; Ogawa, T. TiO_2 micro-nano-hybrid surface to alleviate biological aging of UV-photofunctionalized titanium. *Int J Nanomedicine*, 2011, 6, 1327–1341.

Jensen, T; Schou, S; Stavropoulos, A; Terheyden, H; Holmstrup, P. Maxillary sinus floor augmentation with Bio-Oss or Bio-Oss mixed with autogenous bone as graft in animals: a systematic review. *Int J Oral Maxillofac Surg*, 2012/a, 41, 114–120.

Jensen, T; Schou, S; Svendsen, PA; Forman, JL; Gundersen, HJG; Terheyden, H; Holmstrup, P. Volumetric changes of the graft after maxillary sinus floor augmentation with Bio-Oss and autogenous bone in different ratios: a radiographic study in minipigs. *Clin Oral Implants Res*, 2012/b, 23, 902–910.

Jensen, T; Schou, S; Stavropoulos, A; Terheyden, H; Holmstrup, P. Maxillary sinus floor augmentation with Bio-Oss or Bio-Oss mixed with autogenous bone as a graft: a systematic review. *Clin Oral Implant Res*, 2012/c, 23, 263–273.

Jung, UW; Hwang, JW; Choi, DY; Hu, KS; Kwon, MK; Choi, SH; Kim, HJ. Surface characteristics of a novel hydroxyapatite-coated dental implant. *J Periodontal Implant Sci*, 2012, 42, 59–63.

Kaigler, D; Avila, G; Wisler-Lynch, L; Nevins, ML; Nevins, M; Rasperini, G; Lynch, SE; Giannobile, WV. Platelet-derived growth factor applications in periodontal and peri-implant bone regeneration. *Expert Opin Biol Ther*, 2011, 11, 375–385.

Kammerer, PW; Heller, M; Brieger, J; Klein, MO; Al-Nawas, B; Gabriel, M. Immobilisation of linear and cyclic RGD-peptides on titanium surfaces and their impact on endothelial cell adhesion and proliferation. *Eur Cells Materials*, 2011, 21, 364–372.

Kang, MK; Lee, SB; Moon, SK; Kim, KM; Kim, KN. The biomimetic apatite-cefalotin coating on modified titanium. *Dental Materials J*, 2012, 31, 98–105.

Kim, D; Kang, T; Gober, D; Orlich, C. A liquid membrane as a barrier membrane for guided bone regeneration. *ISRN Dentistry*, 2011, Article ID: 468282. DOI: 10.5402/2011/468282.

Kim, KH; Ramaswamy, N. Electrochemical surface modification of titanium in dentistry. *Dental Material J*, 2009, 28, 20–36.

Kimura, I; Kanatani, M; Watanabe, K. Adhesion of hollow calcium-deficient hydroxyapatite microspheres onto titanium. *Dental Materials J*, 2009, 28, 700–707.

Koh, JW; Yang, JH; Han, JS; Lee, JB; Kim, SH. Biomechanical evaluation of dental implants with different surfaces: Removal torque and resonance frequency analysis in rabbits. *J Adv Prosthodont*, 2009, 1, 107–112.

Koyama, T; Sato, T; Yoshinari, M. Cyclic fatigue resistance of yttria-stabilized tetragonal zirconia polycrystals with hot isostatic press processing. *Dental Materials J*, 2012, 31, 1103–1110.

Kuwabara, A; Hori, N; Sawada, T; Hoshi, N; Watazu, A; Kimoto, K. Enhanced biological responses of a hydroxyapatite/TiO_2 hybrid structure when surface electric charge is controlled using radiofrequency sputtering. *Dental Materials J*, 2012, 31, 368–376.

Lavenus, S; Louarn, G; Layrolle, P. Nanotechnology and dental implants. *Int J Biomaterials*, 2010, Article ID: 915327. DOI: 10.1155/2010/915327.

Lavenus, S; Berreur, M; Trichet, V; Pilet, P; Louarn, G; Layrolle, P. Adhesion and osteogenic differentiation of human mesenchymal stem cells on titanium nanopores. *Eur Cells Materials*, 2011, 22, 84–96.

Lelli, M; Marchisio, O; Foltran, I; Genosevi, A; Montebugnoli, G; Marcaccio, M; Covani, U; Roveri, N. Different corrosive effects on hydroxyapatite nanocrystals and amine fluoride-based mouthwashes on dental titanium brackets: a comparative in vitro study. *Int J Nanomedicine*, 2013, 8, 307–314.

Letic-Gavrilovic, A; Scandurra, R; Abe, K. Genetic potential of interfacial guided osteogenesis in implant devices. *Dental Materials J*, 2000, 19, 99–132.

Liu, H; Webster, TJ. Mechanical properties of dispersed ceramic nanoparticles in polymer composites for orthopedic applications. *Int J Nanomedicine*, 2010, 5, 299–313.

Liu, Y; Li, JP; Hunziker, EB; de Groot, K. Incorporation of growth factors into medical devices via biomimetic coatings. *Phil Trans R Soc A*, 2006, 364, 233–248.

Liu, Y; Wu, G; de Groot, K. Biomimetic coatings for bone tissue engineering of critical-sized defects. *J R Soc Interface*, 2010, 7, S631–S647.

Ma, Q; Wang, W; Chu, PK; Mei, S; Ji, K; Jin, L; Zhang, Y. Concentration- and time-dependent response of human gingival fibroblasts to fibroblast growth factor 2 immobilized on titanium dental implants. *Int J Nanomedicine*, 2012, 7, 1965–1976.

Macewen, W. Illustrative cases of cerebral surgery. *Lancet*, 1885 1, 881–883.

Maiorana, C; Beretta, M; Grossi, GB; Santoro, F; Herford, AS; Nagursky, H; Cicciu, M. Histomorphometric evaluation of anorganic bovine bone coverage to reduce autogenous grafts resorption: Preliminary results. *The Open Dentistry J*, 2011 5, 71–78.

Mano, T; Ishikawa, K; Harada, K; Umeda, H; Ueyama, Y. Comparison of apatite-coated titanium prepared by blast coating and flame spray methods – Evaluation using simulated body fluid and initial histological study. *Dental Materials J*, 2011, 30, 431–437.

Marx, RE; Carlson, ER; Eichstaedt, RM; Schimmele, SR; Strauss, JE; Georgeff KR. Platelet-rich plasma: Growth factor enhancement for bone grafts. *Oral Surg Oral Med Oral Pathol Oral Radiol Endod*, 1998, 85, 638–646.

Masago, H; Shibuya, Y; Munemoto, S; Takeuchi, J; Umeda, M; Komori, T; Kuboki, Y. Alveolar ridge augmentation using various bone substitutes – A web form of titanium fibers promotes rapid bone development. *Kobe J Med Sci*, 2007, 53, 257–263.

Matsuno, T; Hashimoto, Y; Adachi, S; Omata, K; Yoshitaka, Y; Ozeki, Y; Umezu, Y; Tabata, Y; Nakamura, M; Satoh, T. Preparation of injectable 3D-formed β-tricalcium phosphate bead/alginate composite for bone tissue engineering. *Dental Materials J*, 2008, 27, 827–834.

Min, SK; Kang, HK; Jang, DH; Jung, SY; Kim, OB; Min, BM; Yeo, IS. Titanium surface coating with a laminin-derived functional peptide promotes bone cell adhesion. *BioMed Res International*, 2013, Article ID: 638348. DOI: 10.1155/2013/638348.

Moreau, JL; Weir, MD; Xu, HHK. Self-setting collagen-calcium phosphate bone cement: Mechanical and cellular properties. *J Biomed Mater Res A*, 2009, 91, 605–613.

Myshin, HL; Wiens, JP. Factors affecting soft tissue around dental implants: a review of the literature. *J Prosthet Dent*, 2005, 94, 440–444.

Neumann, A; Kevenhoerster, K. Biomaterials for craniofacial reconstruction. *GMS Curr Top Otorhinolaryngol Head Neck Surg*, 2009 8, Doc08. DOI: 10.3205/cto000060.

Norholt, SE; Christiansen, MLS. Application and use of hemostatic agents in dental practice. *Danish Dent J*, 2013, 117, 828–834.

Nuss, KMR; von Rechenberg, B. Biocompatibility issues with modern implants in bone – A review for clinical orthopedics. *The Open Orthop J*, 2008, 2, 66–78.

Osathanon, T; Bespinyowong, K; Arksornnukit, M; Takahashi, H; Pavasant, P. Human osteoblast-like cell spreading and proliferation on Ti-6Al-7Nb surfaces of varying roughness. *J Oral Sci*, 2011, 53, 23–30.

Palmquist, A; Grandfield, K; Norlindh, B; Mattsson, T; Branemark, R; Thomsen, P. Bone-titanium oxide interface in humans revealed by transmission electron microscopy and electron tomography. *J R Soc. Interface*, 2012, 9, 396–400.

Pamula, E; Kokoszka, J; Cholewa-Kowalska, K; Laczka, M; Kantor, L; Niedzwiedzki, L; Reilly, GC; Filipowska, J; Madej, W; Kolodziejczyk, M; Tylko, G; Osyczka, AM. Degradation bioactivity and osteogenic potential of composites made of PLGA and two different sol-gel bioactive glasses. *Annals Biomed Engineering*, 2011, 39, 2114–2129.

Parrish, LC; Miyamoto, T; Fong, N; Mattson, JS; Cerutis, DR. Non-bioabsorbable vs. bioabsorbable membrane: assessment of their clinical efficacy in guided tissue regeneration technique. A systematic review. *J Oral Sci*, 2009, 51, 383–400.

Petrie, TA; Raynor, JE; Reyes, CD; Burns, KL; Collard, DM; Garcia, AJ. The effect of integrin-specific bioactive coatings on tissue healing and implant osseointegration. *Biomaterials*, 2008, 29, 2849–2857.

Piemontese, M; Aspriello, SD; Rubini, C; Ferrantee, L; Procaccini, M; Treatment of periodontal infrabony defects with demineralized freeze-dried bone allograft in combination with platelet-rich plasma: a comparative clinical trial. *J Periodontol*, 2008, 79, 802–810.

Phemister, DB. The fate of transplanted bone and regenerative power of its various constituents. *Surg Gynecol Obstet*, 1914, 19, 303–333.

Rajesh, JB; Nandakumar, K; Varma, HK; Komath, M. Calciumphosphate cement as a "barrier-graft" for the treatment of human periodontal intraosseous defects. *Indian J Dental Res*, 2009, 20, 471–479.

Ramaglia, L; Postiglione, L; Di Spigna, G; Capece, G; Salzano, S; Rossi, G. Sandblasted-acid-etched titanium surface influences *in vitro* the biological behavior of SaOS-2 human osteoblast-like cells. *Dental Materials J*, 2011, 30, 183–192.

Renoud, P; Toury, B; Benayoun, S; Attik, G; Grosgogeat, B. Functionalization of titanium with chitosan via silanation: Evaluation of biological and mechanical performances. *PLoS ONE*, 2012, 7, e39367.

Roselino Ribeiro, AL; Noriega, JR; Dametto, FR; Vaz, LG. Compressive fatigue in titanium dental implants submitted to fluoride ions action. *J Appl Oral Sci*, 2007, 15, 299–304.

Roy, M; Bandyopadhyay, A; Bose, S. Induction plasma sprayed nano hydroxyapatite coatings on titanium for orthopaedic and dental implants. *Surf Coat Technol*, 2011, 205, 2785–2792.

Saini, N; Sikri, P; Gupta, H. Evaluation of the relative efficacy of autologous platelet-rich plasma in combination with β-tricalcium phosphate alloplast versus an alloplast alone in the treatment of human periodontal infrabony defects: A clinical and radiological study. *Indian J Dental Res*, 2011, 22, 107–115.

Saulacic, N; Bosshardt, DD; Bornstein, MM; Berner, S; Buser, D. Bone apposition to a titanium-zirconium alloy implant, as compared to two other titanium-containing implants. *Eur Cells Materials*, 2012, 23, 273–288.

Sasikumar, KP; Elavarasu, S; Gadagi, J. The application of bone morphogenetic proteins to periodontal and periimplant tissue regeneration: A literature review. *J Pharm Bioallied Sci*, 2012, 4, S427–S430.

Sculean, A; Windisch, P; Chiantella, G; Donos, N; Brecx, M; Reich, E. Treatment of intrabony defects with enamel matrix proteins and guided tissue regeneration. A prospective controlled clinical study. *J Clin Periodontol*, 2001, 28, 397–403.

Schulten, EAJM; Prins, HJ; Overman, JR; Helder, MN; ten Bruggenkate, CM; Klein-Nulend, J. A novel approach revealing the effect of a collagenous membrane on osteoconduction in maxillary sinus floor elevation with β-tricalcium phosphate. *Eur Cells Materials*, 2013, 25, 215–228.

Shigeishi, H; Takechi, M; Nishimura, M; Takamoto, M; Minami, M; Ohta, K; Kamata, N. Clinical evaluation of novel interconnected porous hydroxyapatite ceramics (IP-CHA) in a maxillary sinus floor augmentation procedure. *Dental Materials J*, 2012, 31, 54–60.

Simon, Z; Watson, PA. Biomimetic dental implants – New ways to enhance osseointegration. *J Can Dent Assoc*, 2002, 68, 286–288.

Smeets, R; Kolk, A; Gerressen, M; Driemel, O; Maciejewski, O; Hermanns-Sachweh, B; Riediger, D; Stein, JM. A new bisphasic osteoinductive calcium composite material with a negative Zeta potential for bone augmentation. *Head & Face Medicine*, 2009, 5, 13.

Song, K; Du, JM; Luo, RH; Cao, YG. Effect of Bio-Oss loading with rAAV-BMP7 on regeneration of bone defects around dental implant. *West China J Stomatol*, 2008, 26, 421–429.

Spin-Neto, R; Stavropoulos, A; Pereira, LAVD; Marcantonio Jr., E; Wenzel, A. Fate of autologous and fresh-frozen allogenic block bone grafts used for ridge augmentation. A CBCT-based analysis. *Clin Oral Implant Res*, 2013, 24, 167–173.

Sugawara, A; Fujikawa, K; Hirayama, S; Takagi, S; Chow, LC. In vivo characteristics of premixed calcium phosphate cements when implanted in subcutaneous tissues and periodontal bone defects. *J Res Natl Inst Stand Technol*, 2010, 115, 277–290.

Takagi, S; Frukhtbeyn, S; Chow, LC; Sugawara, A; Fujikawa, K; Ogata, H; Hayashi, M; Ogiso, B. In vitro and in vivo characteristics of fluorapatite-forming calcium phosphate cements. *J Res Natl Inst Stand Technol*, 2010, 115, 267–276.

Takahashi, K. Effect of new bone substitute materials consisting of collagen and tricalcium phosphate. *Bull Tokyo Dent Coll*, 2009, 50, 1–11.

Takechi, M; Ohta, K; Ninomiya, Y; Tada, M; Minami, M; Takamoto, M; Ohta, A; Nakagawa, T; Fukui, A; Miyamoto, Y; Kamata, N. 3-dimensional composite scaffolds consisting of apatite-PLGA-atelocollagen for bone tissue engineering. *Dental Materials J*, 2012, 31, 465–471.

Tamazawa, G; Ito, A; Miyai, T; Matsuno, T; Kitahara, K; Sogo, Y; Kimishima, K; Satoh, T. Gatifloxacine-loaded PLGA and β-tricalcium phosphate composite for treating osteomyelitis. *Dental Materials J.* 2011, 30, 264–273.

Teng, FY; Ko, CL; Kuo, HN; Hu, JJ; Lin, JH; Lou, CW; Hung, CC; Wang, YL; Cheng, CY; Chen, WC. A comparison of epithelial cells, fibroblasts and osteoblasts in dental implant titanium topographies. *Bioinorg Chemistry and Applications*, 2012, Article ID: 687291. DOI: 10.1155/2012/687291.

Thomas, NG; Sanil, GP; Rajmonah, G; Prabhakaran, JV; Panda, AK. Fabrication and anti-microbial evaluation of drug loaded polylactide space filler intended for ridge preservation following extraction. *J Indian Soc Periodontol*, 2011, 15, 260–264.

Thor, A. Porous titanium granules and blood for bone regeneration around dental implants: Report of four cases and review of the literature. *Case Reports in Dentistry*, 2013, Article ID: 410515. DOI: 10.1155/2013/410515.

Tiainen, H; Verket, A; Haugen, HJ; Lyngstadaas, SP; Wohlfahrt, JC. Dimensional ridge preservation with a novel highly porous TiO_2 scaffold: An experimental study in minipigs. *Int J Biomaterials*, 2012, Article ID: 851264. DOI: 10.1155/2012/851264.

Tomsia, AP; Launey, ME; Lee, JS; Mankani, MH; Wegst, UGK; Saiz, E. Nanotechnology approaches to improve dental implants. *Int J Maxillofac Implants*, 2011, 26(Suppl), 25–49.

Tsuruga, E; Takita, H; Itoh, H; Wakisaka, Y; Kuboki, Y. Pore size of porous hydroxyapatite as the cell-substratum controls BMP-induced osteogenesis. *J Biochem*, 1997, 121, 317–324.

Variola, F; Brunski, J; Orsini, G; Oliveira, PT; Wazen, R; Nanci, A. Nanoscale surface modifications of medically-relevant metals: state-of-the art and perspectives. *Nanoscale*, 2011, 3, 335–353.

Watanabe, H; Saito, K; Kokubun, K; Sasaki, H; Yoshinari, M. Change in surface properties of zirconia and initial attachment of osteoblast-like cells with hydrophilic treatment. *Dental Materials J*, 2012, 31, 806–814.

Windisch, P; Sculean, A; Klein, F; Toth, V; Gera, I; Reich, E; Eickholz, P; Comparison of clinical, radiographic, and histometric measurements following treatment with guided tissue regeneration or enamel matrix proteins in human periodontal defects. *J Periodontol*, 2002, 73, 409–417.

Wu, X; Liu, X; Wei, J; Ma, J; Deng, F; Wei, S. Nano-TiO_2/PEEK bioactive composite as a bone substitute material: in vitro and in vivo studies. *Int J Nanomedicine*, 2012, 7, 1215–1225.

Yamada, M; Ueno, T; Tsukimura, N; Ikeda, T; Nakagawa, K; Hori, N; Suzuki, T; Ogawa, T. Bone integration capability of nanopolymorphic crystalline hydroxyapatite coated on titanium implants. *Int J Nanomedicine*, 2012, 7, 859–873.

Yamamichi, N; Pugdee, K; Chang, WJ; Lee, SY; Yoshinari, M; Hayakawa, T; Abiko, Y. Gene expression monitoring in osteoblasts on titanium coated with fibronectin-derived peptide. *Dental Materials J*, 2008, 27, 744–750.

Yamashita, D; Machigashira, M; Miyamoto, M; Takeuchi, H; Noguchi, K; Izumi, Y; Ban, S. Effect of surface roughness on initial responses of osteoblast-like cells on two types of zirconia. *Dental Materials J*, 2009, 28, 461–470.

Yamazoe, J; Nakagawa, M; Matono, Y; Takeuchi, A; Ishikawa, K. The development of Ti alloys for dental implant with high corrosion resistance and mechanical strength. *Dental Materials J*, 2007, 26, 260–267.

Yoneyama, Y; Matsuno, T; Hashimoto, Y; Satoh, T. In vitro evaluation of H_2O_2 hydrothermal treatment of aged titanium surface to enhance biofunctional activity. *Dental Materials J*, 2013, 32, 115–121.

Yu, M; Hui, XM; Wang, F; Zhang, N; Zhang, HP; Song, YL. Effect of sustained release of recombinant rat insulin-like growth factor-1 from poly (lactide-CO-glycolide) microspheres on bone formation in the peri-implant areas in Goto-Kakizaki rats with type 2 diabetes. *Acta Acad Med Sin*, 2010, 32, 260–264.

Zhao, L; Burguera, EF; Xu, HHK; Amin, N; Ryou, H; Arola, DD. Fatigue and human umbilical cord stem cell seeding characteristics of calcium phosphate-chitosan-biodegradable fiber scaffolds. *Biomaterials*, 2010, 31, 840–847.

CHAPTER 4

OSSEOINTEGRATION

Abstract

Osseointegration is the stable and clinically asymptomatic rigid anchorage of an implant fixture achieved by direct bone-to-implant contact. In this chapter the most important mechanisms of osseointegration are summarized. The osseointegration process may be deconvoluted both phenomenologically and experimentally into distinct phases such as osteoinduction, osteoconduction, and *de novo* bone formation, which, in time, will be followed by the remodeling of the peri-implant bone tissue. The premised peri-implant healing phases, which include a cascade of recruitment, maturation, and migration of osteogenic cells followed by the bone formation of these cells on the implant surface, result in a specific type of osteogenesis, termed "contact osteogenesis." Although contact osteogenesis is currently considered as optimum, osseointegration may also occur via "distance osteogenesis." In this case, *osteoinduction* is followed by the laying down of bone on the old bone surface in the peri-implant site instead of on the implant surface itself. The produced new matrix encroaches on the implant, and in this way, the fixture becomes surrounded by bone, although there is no bone formation on the implant itself. Although the success rate of implant treatment is high, achieving osseointegration is still a challenging task for clinicians. Understanding the basic phenomena behind osseointegration may help a clinician solve more complex cases that appear in praxis. It may also help to be well informed in the rather complex market of various implant products, treatment trends, and related protocols. Although contact osteogenesis is considered the optimum solution, it is very likely that proper osseointegration may also occur via distance osteogenesis. The latter may gain more theoretical and clinical importance in the future if developments in relation to resorbable or partially resorbable coatings lead to a breakthrough.

4.1. Introduction

Osseointegration is the stable and clinically asymptomatic rigid anchorage of an implant fixture achieved by direct bone-to-implant contact (Branemark et al. 1969; Branemark 1972; Branemark et al. 1977; Branemark 1983; Albrektsson et al. 1981; Albrektsson and Johansson 2001; Davies 2003; Palmquist et al. 2012). In this chapter the most important mechanisms of osseointegration are summarized. The osseointegration process may be deconvoluted both phenomenologically and experimentally into distinct phases such as osteoinduction, osteoconduction, and *de novo* bone formation (Albrektsson and Johansson 2001; Davies 2003), which, in time, will be followed by the remodeling of the peri-implant bone tissue (Davies 2003). The latter, remodeling, is not discussed in this chapter, because it relies on slow processes influenced by different biomechanical stimuli from the developed healing site (Davies 2003); thus it is not closely related to the most critical early osseointegration phases.

Osteoinduction is the process by which osteogenesis is induced regularly in any type of bone healing (Albrektsson and Johansson 2001). Osteoinduction implies the recruitment, of immature mesenchymal cells and their stimulation to develop into preosteoblasts (Albrektsson and Johansson 2001). Osteoconduction is the second and considerably the most critical healing phase, which includes those important early events that will position the osteogenic cells on the surface of the implant (Davies 2003). It relies on the recruitment and maturation of osteogenic cells (i.e. osteoinduction), especially their migration to the implant surface through the residue of a peri-implant blood clot (Albrektsson and Johansson 2001; Davies 2003). The third healing phase, *de novo* bone formation, can be considered a separate and distinct phenomenon, which results in the appearance of a mineralized (Davies 2003; Palmquist et al. 2012) and collagen-free (Davies 2003) interfacial bone matrix on the surface of fixtures that continues on as a normal bone matrix farther away from the fixture (Davies 2003; Palmquist et al. 2012).

The three premised peri-implant healing phases, which include a succession of the recruitment, maturation, and migration of osteogenic cells followed by bone formation from these cells on the implant surface, result in a specific type of osteogenesis, termed "contact osteogenesis" (Osborn and Newesely 1980; Davies 2003). Although contact osteogenesis is considered currently as optimum, osseointegration may also occur via "distance osteogenesis" (Osborn and Newesely 1980; Davies 2003; Palmquist et al. 2012). In this case, *osteoinduction* is followed by the laying down of bone on the old bone surface at the peri-implant site (Albrektsson and Johansson 2001; Davies 2003) instead of on the implant surface itself. The newly produced matrix encroaches on the implant (Osborn and Newesely 1980; Albrektsson and Johansson 2001; Davies 2003; Palmquist et al. 2012), and in this way, the fixture becomes surrounded by bone, although there is no bone formation on the implant itself (Osborn and Newesely 1980; Albrektsson and Johansson 2001; Davies 2003; Palmquist et al. 2012). Even though most important aspects of osseointegration have been recognized in relation to the osseointegration of titanium implants (Branemark et al. 1969; Branemark 1972; Branemark et al. 1977; Branemark 1983; Albrektsson et al. 1981; Albrektsson and Johansson 2001; Davies 2003; Palmquist et al. 2012), it should be emphasized that the mechanism of osteogenesis seems to be rather similar in the case of many candidate implant materials, including newly developed metal alloys and ceramics (Pillar et al. 1991; de Bruijn et al. 1995; Davies and Baldan 1997; Davies 2003; Depprich et al. 2008/a, b, c), as well as in the case of implant-coating materials (Davies 2003; Lavenus et al. 2010) or bone substitutes.

4.2. Concept of Osseointegration

Osseointegration is the stable and clinically asymptomatic rigid anchorage of an implant achieved by direct bone-to-implant contact (Branemark et al. 1969; Branemark 1972;

Branemark et al. 1977; Branemark 1983; Albrektsson et al. 1981; Albrektsson and Johansson 2001; Davies 2003; Palmquist et al. 2012). The importance of osseointegration in other parts of the body (i.e. in relation to major arthroplasties) is under debate (Albrektsson and Johansson 2001), because the ingrowth of bone in a porous-coated prosthesis may or may not represent osseointegration (Albrektsson and Johansson 2001). However, in the case of implant dentistry, this mode of anchorage is the only one for which high success rates have been reported (Branemark et al. 1969; Branemark 1972; Branemark et al. 1977; Branemark 1983; Albrektsson et al. 1981; Albrektsson and Johansson 2001; Davies 2003; Lavenus et al. 2010; Palmquist et al. 2012).

The *classic concept* of osseointegration was based on the criterion that there be a direct contact between the living bone and implant without the appearance of fibrous tissue at the bone-implant interface at the *light microscope* level (Branemark et al. 1977; Albrektsson et al. 1981). Based on this definition, distance osteogenesis based fixation of implants may also be considered a form of osseointegration (Palmquist et al. 2012), but not necessarily in that sense of the word as is true in the case of contact osteogenesis (Davies 2003; Lavenus et al. 2010; Palmquist et al. 2012) and the current definition of osseointegration.

The *current concept* of osseointegration is based on the phenomenon of contact osteogenesis (Davies 2003; Lavenus et al. 2010) and the criterion that there be a real, direct intimate contact and bonding (Lavenus et al. 2010; Palmquist et al. 2012) between the living bone and implant without any cellular/tissue (or other not bone related) layer between the bone and implant surface either at the light microscope (microscale) or at the electron microscope (nanoscale) level (Davies 2003; Lavenus et al. 2010; Palmquist et al. 2012). The new concept of osseointegration implies that the biological response of the bone is not one kind of "inertness" toward a foreign material, but rather one kind of active integration of the implant (Letic-Gavrilovic et al. 2000; Davies 2003; Lavenus et al. 2010; Palmquist et al. 2012).

4.3. Bone Healing and Osteoinduction

Bone is a dynamic, vascular, living connective tissue, and as such comprises cells that become embedded in their own extracellular matrix (Davies 2003). Bone tissue is arranged into two major forms, like trabecular bone (also termed "cancellous" or "spongy bone") and cortical bone (also termed "compact bone"), which exist in various proportions and geometries in the individual bones (Davies 2003). There is a constant remodeling of bone tissue by means of bone destruction by osteoclasts followed by bone replacement by osteoblasts (Albrektsson and Johansson 2001; Davies 2003; Fabian et al. 2009), which results in the lamellar microarchitecture of both cortical and trabecular mature bone (Davies 2003) and provides a mechanism for scar-free healing and the regeneration of damaged bone tissue (Davies 2003). The relatively slow generation of peri-implant cortical bone relies exclusively on the premised lamellar remodeling, while the generation of peri-implant trabecular bone may involve both the remodeling of existing lamellar trabeculae and the rapid formation of new trabeculae through the recruitment of new populations of osteogenic cells (Davies 2003). In this latter case (during the rapid formation of new trabeculae), a woven bone of irregular architecture appears instead of a lamellar bone (Davies and Hosseini 2000; Davies 2003).

This woven structure is the result of rapid growth, but importantly, its structural immaturity should not be equated with a lack of functional utility (Davies and Hosseini 2000; Davies 2003). Even if the microstructure is different, the underlying histodynamics of the formation of woven and lamellar bone are remarkably similar (Davies and Hosseini 2000; Davies 2003).

Osteogenic cells are derived from both the endosteal trabecular surfaces and the bone marrow that fills the large interconnected pores of trabecular bone and contains mesenchymal progenitor cells that can give rise to osteoblasts (Albrektsson and Johansson 2001; Davies 2003; Fabian et al. 2009; Lavenus et al. 2010). Bone marrow also contains rich vasculature that can supply both the circulating mononuclear precursors to osteoclasts (being of hematopoietic origin) and the endothelial cells needed for angiogenesis (Albrektsson and Johansson 2001; Davies 2003; Fabian et al. 2009). It is no wonder that trabecular bone can remodel far more quickly than cortical bone and that bone healing may also vary in different bone sites (Davies 2003) depending on the macroarchitecture of the bone tissue within the healing compartment (Davies 2003). From this respect, trabecular bone represents a biologically superior tissue evolved for rapid peri-implant (or other) bone healing compared to the cortical bone, which typically has a slow remodeling healing pattern (Davies 2003; Lavenus et al. 2010).

In the case of bone trauma/injury, a large amount of immune mediators and growth factors including insulin-like growth factors (IGFs), a fibroblast growth factor (FGF), a platelet-derived growth factor, members of the transforming growth factor beta family, and others, are released (Albrektsson and Johansson 2001; Lavenus et al. 2010). The principle action of many growth factors is both mitogenic and angiogenic (Trippel et al. 1996; Albrektsson and Johansson 2001), which is crucial among other considerations for the (re)vascularization of the injured bone area and the newly forming bone tissue (Albrektsson 1980; Albrektsson and Johansson 2001). In relation to the new bone formation, bone morphogenetic proteins (also members of the TGF-β family) are of particular importance in the initial phase, because in the presence of BMPs, undifferentiated mesenchymal cells can be recruited and transformed into preosteoblasts (Urist et al. 1979; Albrektsson and Johansson 2001; Lavenus et al. 2010). This initial recruiting and transforming response within bone healing (termed "osteoinduction") starts immediately after an injury has occurred and is very active during the first week thereafter (Albrektsson and Johansson 2001) even though the action of the newly recruited and transformed preosteoblasts (their migration, transformation into osteoblasts, and bone formation) is not obvious for several weeks (Albrektsson and Johansson 2001). Consequently, a transient decrease in the stability of the newly inserted implant fixtures may appear (Lavenus et al. 2010), because the primary interlock (primary stability) of the newly inserted implant fixtures (related to the mechanical anchorage, design of the implant, and bone structure) decreases with time, whereas the secondary anchorage characterized by a stable biological bonding at the interface between bone tissues and the implant surface suffers an unavoidable delay (Lavenus et al. 2010).

4.4. Contact Osteogenesis

In the process of contact osteogenesis, new bone forms directly on the implant surface (Davies 2003; Lavenus et al. 2010). *Osteoinduction*, the process by which osteogenesis is induced regularly in any type of bone healing (Albrektsson and Johansson 2001), is also the first phase of healing in this case. Osteoinduction means that undifferentiated pluripotent cells are stimulated to develop into a bone-forming cell lineage (Albrektsson and Johansson 2001; Lavenus et al. 2010). Osteoinduction implies the recruitment of immature mesenchymal cells and their stimulation to develop into preosteoblasts (and later bone-forming osteoblasts), as would occur in any type of bone healing (Albrektsson and Johansson 2001; Lavenus et al. 2010).

However, in contrast to other types of bone healing, in the case of contact osteogenesis, osteoinduction is followed by *osteoconduction*, the second and probably most critical healing phase of contact osteogenesis, which relies on the recruitment and maturation of osteogenic cells (i.e. osteoinduction) and the migration of these osteogenic cells to the implant surface through the residue of a peri-implant blood clot (Davies 2003; Lavenus et al. 2010). Since there is no bone present on the surface of the fixture upon implantation, the implant surface has to become colonized by osteogenic cells before any bone matrix formation can begin (Davies 2003; Lavenus et al. 2010). Thus, the bone is formed for the first time at the appropriate site by differentiating osteogenic cells (Davies and Hosseini 2000; Davies 2003; Lavenus et al. 2010) in a process referred to as "*de novo* bone formation" (Davies and Hosseini 2000; Davies 2003). This is clearly an essential prerequisite of contact osteogenesis; bone cells must first get to the implant surface before extracellular matrix synthesis can be initiated. In this case, the implant bone interface is occupied by a thin mineralized (Davies 2003; Palmquist et al. 2012) and collagen-free (Davies 2003) bone matrix, which continues as a normal bone matrix farther away from the fixture (Davies 2003; Palmquist et al. 2012). This thin interfacial, collagen-free bone matrix is attached to the implant surface (Davies 2003; Lavenus et al. 2010) and is equivalent to a matrix seen as a cement line between the new and old bone tissue around the vascularized remodeling units (so-called osteons) of normal bone tissue (Davies 2003). Thus, in contrast to distance osteogenesis (which results in bone approximating the implant surface), contact osteogenesis results in bone apposition directly onto the implant surface (Davies 2003; Lavenus et al. 2010). Although it is inevitable that both distance and contact osteogenesis occurs in relation to the implant placement (Davies 2003; Lavenus et al. 2010; Palmquist et al. 2012), it seems reasonable to shift the peri-implant healing processes from a distance osteogenesis type toward a contact osteogenesis type by means of optimizing the implant surface design (Davies 2003; Lavenus et al. 2010; Palmquist et al. 2012).

In the case of contact osteogenesis, platelets are of considerable importance, because their activation leads to the release (degranulation) of their granular content, including a number of active factors (cytokines, vasoactive and growth factors) such as platelet-derived growth factor, transforming growth factor beta, serotonin, histamine, and others into the environment (Davies 2003; Lavenus et al. 2010). Besides several advantageous accelerating effects of the premised mediators on bone healing, including the stimulation of the proliferation of human osteoblasts in the surrounding bone (Davies 2003; Lavenus et al. 2010), importantly, they are also able to stimulate the recruitment, differentiation, and migration of bone marrow derived potentially-osteogenic cells (Davies 2003; Oprea et al. 2003; Lavenus et al. 2010). They can also stimulate the proliferation of matured osteoblasts appearing on the implant surface after surface attachment and the transformation of the arriving, recruited, potentially-osteogenic cells of mesenchymal origin (Lavenus et al. 2010).

Thus, one of the most important aspects of osseoconduction is the "knock-on" effect generated at the implant surface through the initiation of the activation of the surface-attached platelets, which results in directed osteogenic cell migration (Davies 2003; Lavenus et al. 2010,). The migration of osteogenic cells will occur through the peri-implant blood clot (or its residue) by means of the transient three-dimensional biological fibrin matrix formed (from fibrinogen) by the blood-clotting coagulation process (Davies 2003; Lavenus et al. 2010). Since fibrin can be expected to adhere to almost all surfaces, osteogenic cell migration may be expected in any implanted fixtures (Davies 2003; Lavenus et al. 2010). However, migrating cells can contract the fibrin matrix through which they migrate and this could cause the retraction of the transitory fibrin scaffold away from the implant surface (Davies 2003). In the case of such a retraction, the migrating osteogenic cells are not able to contact the surface of the implant, and consequently distance osteogenesis will occur instead of contact osteogenesis (Davies 2003; Lavenus et al. 2010). Therefore, in the case of contact osteogenesis, the ability of an implant surface to retain fibrin during the cell migration induced contraction phase of the peri-implant bone healing process is critical (Davies 2003; Lavenus et al. 2010).

Importantly, the roughened surfaces of greater micro-/nanotopography will exhibit an increased surface area and a resultant increase of fibrin attachment will lead to a stabler fixation of the fibrin matrix to the implant surface (Davies 2003; Lavenus et al. 2010). The increased available surface of roughened implant fixtures results in increased platelet absorption onto the fibrin-absorbed surface of the fixture as well (Davies 2003). Further, roughened surfaces also promote and accelerate the activation of attached platelets to a higher degree than smoother turned surfaces do (Park et al. 2001; Davies 2003; Lavenus et al. 2010), which accelerates the platelet-factor-induced osteogenic cell migration to the fixtures of a roughened surface. In this latter case, it is obvious that not only the increased available surface area, but also other micro- and nanotopographical parameters of roughened surfaces are of significant importance (Davies 2003; Lavenus et al. 2010). Similarly, the strength of the fibrin attachment as well as the efficiency of platelet absorption are also influenced by such (not only related to the available surface size) micro- and nanotopographical properties of the surface (Davies 2003; Lavenus et al. 2010).

Besides surface topography, surface chemistry seems to be also be very important (Albrektsson and Johansson 2001; Lavenus et al. 2010). For example, there is a significant difference in the amount of bone that grows on commercially pure titanium in comparison to several titanium alloys (Albrektsson and Johansson 2001). The difference may be even more obvious if several coatings are applied on the surface of titanium fixtures (Lavenus et al. 2010) regardless of the fact that in these cases it is rather difficult to find out whether the effect of a certain coating is a result of its chemical composition or a result of the specific surface topographical properties of the coating (Davies 2003). Calcium phosphate coatings, for example, readily absorb proteins to their surfaces (Davies 2003; Lavenus et al. 2010). Potentiating protein adsorption could be expected to increase the binding of fibrinogen and later fibrin (following blood clotting) to fixtures with a calcium phosphate coating (Davies 2003). This may lead to increased platelet adhesion, as well as to stronger fibrin matrix retention during the cell migration induced retraction phase of healing (Davies 2003). Calcium phosphate coatings may also have an effect on platelet activation (Davies 2003). A bone-bonding effect (Hench and Wilson 1984) of certain coating materials, including calcium phosphates, is also expected (Davies 2003). This bonding was hypothesized in relation to the bonding of collagen (Hench and Wilson 1984; Tomsia et al. 2011). However, in the case of contact osteogenesis, the primary chemical bonding could appear in the interface between the collagen-free *de novo* synthesized bone layer and the implant surface only (Davies 2003), which cannot be related to the collagen (Davies 2003) (because of the premised collagen-free character of the bone at the bone-implant interface). However, another (not collagen related) type of bonding between the implant fixture and the *de novo* synthesized bone may occur if an appropriate implant surface is provided (Davies 2003; Palmquist et al. 2012). But it seems rather difficult to evaluate the clinical importance of such chemical bonding compared to the micromechanical interdigitation of the collagen-free bone layer with a roughened implant surface (Dziedzich et al. 1996; Davies 2003). On the other hand, chemical bonding may be more important in improving distance osteogenesis related healing.

4.5. Distance Osteogenesis

Although contact osteogenesis is currently considered the optimum strategy, osseointegration may also occur via distance osteogenesis (Osborn and Newesely 1980; Davies 2003; Palmquist et al. 2012). Distance osteogenesis can be expected in relation to the peri-implant cortical bone healing since it occurs through a rather slow lamellar remodeling instead of through the rapid formation of new bone (Davies 2003). Distance osteogenesis is also expected in the case of machined (turned) titanium implants (Osborn and Newesely 1980; Davies 2003; Palmquist et al. 2012). It is also inevitable that a certain amount of distance osteogenesis occurs in relation to every implant placement, even if the peri-implant healing is shifted toward a contact osteogenesis type (Davies 2003; Lavenus et al. 2010; Palmquist et al. 2012).

The first phase of distance osteogenesis is also *osteoinduction* in this case, as induced regularly in any type of bone healing (Albrektsson and Johansson 2001). Osteoinduction includes the recruitment and maturation of immature mesenchymal cells and their stimulation to develop into preosteoblasts (Albrektsson and Johansson 2001). The bone surface provides a population of osteogenic cells that can give rise to osteoblasts, which lay down bone on the old bone surface in the peri-implant site instead of on the implant surface itself (Davies 2003). The newly produced matrix encroaches on the implant, and in this way, the fixture become surrounded by bone, although there is no bone formation on the implant itself. However, the implant surface is obscured from the bone by intervening cells (Osborn and Newesely 1980; Davies 2003; Lavenus et al. 2010), and in certain cases a *transitory* fibrous interface (Carmagnola et al. 2009; Neumann and Kevenhoester 2009; Tomsia et al. 2011) may also appear between the newly forming bone and the implant. Optimally the bone grows toward the implant subsequent to the death of the intervening cells/tissue, and in this way the bone can also become juxtaposed to the implant surface (Osborn and Newesely 1980; Davies 2003; Palmquist et al. 2012). This can be considered osseointegration (based on the *classic* concept), even though it is not necessarily in the same sense of the word as in the cases of contact osteogenesis (Davies 2003; Lavenus et al. 2010,) and the *current* concept of osseointegration (Letic-Gavrilovic et al. 2000; Davies 2003; Lavenus et al. 2010; Palmquist et al. 2012). This is especially true if the intervening cells (or fibrous interface) between the growing bone and the implant fixture do not disappear but persist (Letic-Gavrilovic et al.

2000; Lavenus et al. 2010). In the latter cases the bone healing should not be considered as osseointegration in the sense of the *classic* concept but should certainly be considered as an instance of fibrous encapsulation (Letic-Gavrilovic et al. 2000; Neumann and Kevenhoester 2009; Lavenus et al. 2010).

Even if contact osteogenesis is considered the optimum option, it is inevitable that distance osteogenesis also occurs to a certain extent after every implant placement (Davies 2003; Lavenus et al. 2010; Palmquist et al. 2012). Therefore it seems reasonable to optimize this kind of healing by means of proper implant surface design. This is especially true because the resorbable (Lavenus et al. 2010; Tomsia et al. 2011) or partially resorbable (Tomsia et al. 2011) calcium phosphate coatings should dissolve or degrade under osteoclastic activity followed by bone apposition due to osteoblasts (Lavenus et al. 2010; Tomsia et al. 2011), which can be considered as a kind of distance osteogenesis.

The expected bone-bonding effect (Hench and Wilson 1984; Tomsia et al. 2011) of certain coating materials, including calcium phosphates, may also be of importance in distance osteogenesis. This bonding was hypothesized in relation to the bonding of collagen present in the bone (Hench and Wilson 1984; Davies 2003; Tomsia et al. 2011). In contrast to contact osteogenesis in which chemical bonding to collagen seems to be of no significance because of the collagen-free character of the bone at the bone-implant interface (Davies 2003), the binding of collagen may be of importance in the case of distance osteogenesis by means of optimizing the production of a new bone matrix that encroaches on the implant (Tomsia et al. 2011).

Conclusion

Although the success rate of implant treatment is high, achieving osseointegration is still a challenging task for clinicians. The understanding of basic phenomena behind osseointegration may help clinicians solve more complex cases appearing in praxis. It may also help to be well informed about the rather complex market of various implant products, treatment trends, and related protocols. Although contact osteogenesis is currently considered the optimum strategy, it is very likely that proper osseointegration may also occur via distance osteogenesis. The latter may gain more theoretical and clinical importance in the future if developments in relation with resorbable or partially resorbable coatings lead to a breakthrough.

References

Albrektsson, T. The healing of autologous bone grafts after varying degrees of surgical trauma. *J Bone Joint Surg (Br)*, 1980, 32, 403–410.

Albrektsson, T; Branemark, PI; Hansson, HA; Lindstrom, J. Osseointegrated titanium implants. Requirements for ensuring a long-lasting direct bone anchorage in man. *Acta Orthop Scand*, 1981, 52, 155–170.

Albrektsson, T; Johansson, C. Osteoinduction, osteoconduction and osseointegration. *Eur Spine J*, 2001, 10, S96–S101.

Branemark, PI. Rehabilitation with a denture anchored to the jawbone. *Lakartidningen*, 1972, 69, 4813–4814.

Branemark, PI. Osseointegration and its experimental background. *J Prosthet Dent*, 1983, 50, 399–410.

Branemark, PI; Adell, R; Breine, U; Hansson, BO; Lindstrom, J; Ohlsson, A. Intra-osseous anchorage of dental prostheses. I. Experimental studies. *Scand J Plast Reconstr Surg*, 1969, 3, 81–100.

Branemark, PI; Hansson, BO; Adell, R; Breine, U; Lindstrom, J; Hallen O; Ohman, A. Osseointegrated titanium implants in the treatment of the edentulous jaw. *Scand J Plast Reconstr Surg*, 1977, 11, (Suppl. 16) 1–175.

Carmagnola, D; Abati, S; Addis, A; Ferreri, G; Chiapasco, M; Romeo, E; Vogel, G. Time sequence of bone healing around two implant systems in minipigs: preliminary histologic results. *Int J Periodontics Restorative Dent*, 2009, 29, 549–555.

de Bruijn, JD; van Blitterswijk, CA; Davies, JE. Initial bone matrix formation at the hydroxyapatite interface in vivo. *Biomed Mater Res*, 1995, 29, 89–99.

Davies, JE; Understanding peri-implant endosseous healing. *J Dent Education*, 2003, 67, 932–949.

Davies, JE; Baldan, N. Scanning electron microscopy of the bone-bioactive implant interface. *J Biomed Mater Res*, 1997, 36, 429–440.

Davies, JE; Hosseini, MM. Histodynamics of endosseous wound healing. In Davies JE, editor. *Bone engineering*. Toronto: em squared Inc.; 2000, 1–14.

Depprich, R; Ommerborn, M; Zipprich, H; Naujoks, C; Handschel, J; Wiesmann, HP; Kubler, NR; Meyer, U. Behavior of osteoblastic cells cultured on titanium and structured zirconia surfaces. *Head & Face Medicine*, 2008/a, 4, 29.

Depprich, R; Zipprich, H; Ommerborn, M; Mahn, E; Lammers, L; Handschel, J; Naujoks, C; Wiesmann, HP; Kubler, N; Meyer, U. Osseointegration of zirconia implants: an SEM observation of the bone-implant interface. *Head & Face Medicine*, 2008/b, 4, 25.

Depprich, R; Zipprich, H; Ommerborn, M; Naujoks, C; Wiesmann, HP; Kiattavorncharoen, S; Laurer, HC; Meyer, U; Kubler, NR; Handschel, J. Osseointeration of zirconia implants compared with titanium: an in vivo study. *Head & Face Medicine*, 2008/c, 4, 30.

Dziedzich, DM; Savva, IH; Wilkinson, DS; Davies, JE. Osteoconduction on, and bonding to, calcium phosphate ceramic implants. *Mat Res Soc Symp Proc*, 1996, 414, 147–156.

Fabian, TK; Csermely, P; Fabian, G; Fejerdy, P. Spondiloarthropaties and bone resorption: A possible role of heat shock protein (Hsp70) (Review). *Acta Physiol Hungarica*, 2009, 96, 149–155.

Hench, LL; Wilson, J. Surface-active biomaterials. *Science*, 1984, 226, 630–636.

Lavenus, S; Louarn, G; Layrolle, P. Nanotechnology and dental implants. *Int J Biomaterials*, 2010, Article ID: 915327. DOI: 10.1155/2010/915327.

Letic-Gavrilovic, A; Scandurra, R; Abe, K. Genetic potential of interfacial guided osteogenesis in implant devices. *Dental Materials J*, 2000, 19, 99–132.

Neumann, A; Kevenhoerster, K. Biomaterials for craniofacial reconstruction. *GMS Curr Top Otorhinolaryngol Head Neck Surg*, 2009, 8, Doc08. DOI: 10.3205/cto000060.

Oprea, WE; Karp, JM; Hosseini, MM; Davies, JE. Effect of platelet relelasate on bone cell migration and recruitment in vitro. *J Craniofac Surg*, 2003, 14, 292–300.

Osborn, F; Newesely, H. Dynamic aspects of the implant-bone interface. In: Heimke G, editor. *Dental Implants: materials and systems.* Munchen: Carl Hanser Verlag, 1980, 111–123.

Palmquist, A; Grandfield, K; Norlindh, B; Mattsson, T; Branemark, R; Thomsen, P. Bone-titanium oxide interface in humans revealed by transmission electron microscopy and electron tomography. *J R Soc. Interface*, 2012, 9, 396–400.

Park, JY; Gemmell, CH; Davies, JE. Platelet interactions with titanium: modulation of platelet activity by surface topography. *Biomaterials*, 2001, 22, 2671–2682.

Pillar, RM; Davies, JE; Smith, DC. The bone-biomaterial interface for load-bearing implants. *MRS Bulletin*, 1991, 9, 55–61.

Tomsia, AP; Launey, ME; Lee, JS; Mankani, MH; Wegst, UGK; Saiz, E. Nanotechnology approaches to improve dental implants. *Int J Maxillofac Implants*, 2011, 26(Suppl), 25–49.

Trippel, SE; Coutts, RD; Einhorn, TA; Mundy, GR; Rosenfeld, RG. Growth factors as therapeutic agents. *J bone Joint Surg (Am)*, 1996, 78, 1272–1286.

Urist, MR; Mikulski, A; Lietze, A. Solubilized bone morphogenetic protein. *Proc Natl Acad Sci USA*, 1979, 76, 1828–1832.

CHAPTER 5

PERI-IMPLANT GINGIVAL HEALING

Abstract

Successful dental implant treatment depends on the attachment of three basic components of healing peri-implant tissues, including the peri-implant bone, the peri-implant connective tissue, and the peri-implant gingival epithelium, which is composed of the apically located junctional epithelium (JE) and the peri-implant epithelium (PIE) located farther away toward the peri-implant gingival sulcus. In the microenvironment of the peri-implant healing area, mesenchymal stem cells are stimulated by specific factors to differentiate into the adequate cell lineage. Under the influence of these factors, mesenchymal stem cells switch to osteoblastic cells in contact to bone tissue while they differentiate into the fibroblastic lineage in the gingival tissue region. The migration, early attachment, and proliferation of gingival epithelial cells also occur at the same time. Although bone and soft tissue processes are interconnected and thus cannot be isolated in reality, this chapter will focus on the healing and attachment of peri-implant gingival tissues only, because processes of peri-implant bone healing and attachment (i.e. osseointegration) are discussed in detail elsewhere.

5.1. Introduction

Successful dental implant treatment depends on the attachment of three basic components of healing peri-implant tissues, including the peri-implant bone, the peri-implant connective tissue, and the peri-implant gingival epithelium (Teng et al. 2012), which is composed of the apically located junctional epithelium and the peri-implant epithelium located farther away toward the peri-implant gingival sulcus (Ikeda et al. 2000; Larjava et al. 2011). In the microenvironment of the peri-implant healing area, mesenchymal stem cells are stimulated by specific factors to differentiate into the adequate cell lineage (Lavenus et al. 2010). Under the influence of these factors, mesenchymal stem cells switch to osteoblastic cells that are in contact with bone tissue while they differentiate into the fibroblastic lineage in the gingival tissue region (Lavenus et al. 2010). The migration, early attachment, and proliferation of gingival epithelial cells also occur at the same time (Teng et al. 2012). Although bone and soft tissue processes are interconnected and thus cannot be isolated in reality, this chapter will focus on the healing and attachment of peri-implant gingival tissues only, because processes of peri-implant bone healing and attachment (i.e. osseointegration) are discussed in detail elsewhere.

5.2. Implanto-Gingival Complex

The concept of the implanto-gingival complex is rather similar to the concept of the dento-gingival complex, with the difference being that in this case the concept is related to *implants* and their surrounding (peri-implant) gingival tissues. The implanto-gingival complex can be considered an optimal connection between the implant and gingival tissues. This connection appears by the time the gingival healing processes are finished. The implanto-gingival complex includes the trans-gingival surface of the implant fixture and/or the abutment as well as the peri-implant connective tissue, the junctional epithelium, the peri-implant epithelium, the peri-implant gingival sulcus (gingival crevice), and the crevicular fluid (Mobelli et al. 1995; Khoury et al. 2008). The latter seems to be rather similar to the periodontal crevicular fluid with respect to flow and microflora (Mobelli et al. 1995; Khoury et al. 2008; de Oliveira et al. 2012).

In the case of smooth trans-gingival surfaces, the presence of hemidesmosomal attachment of the junctional epithelium to the implant surface is well documented, and the peri-implant epithelium also appears to be attached at the light microscopic level (Rompen et al. 2006; Larjava et al. 2011). However, recent data indicate that there may be an attached epithelium in the lower (apical) third of the surrounding epithelium only, which corresponds to the junctional epithelium (Ikeda et al. 2000; Larjava et al. 2003); whereas the peri-implant epithelium appears to just "lean on" but not really attach to the implant (Fujiseki et al. 2003; Larjava et al. 2011; Ma et al. 2012). Accordingly, the internal basal lamina is also likely to be present in the junctional epithelium only (Ikeda et al. 2000; Larjava et al. 2011); and there are also certain differences between the cell differentiation markers of cells present in the peri-implant epithelium compared to those present in the junctional epithelium (Fujiseki et al. 2003; Larjava et al. 2011).

In the case of smooth titanium trans-gingival implant surfaces, the "height" of the implanto-gingival complex (i.e. the vertical distance from the gingival margin to the bone) seems to be slightly greater (*usually* between 2.85–3.80 mm) than the corresponding dimension of the dento-gingival complex around the teeth (ca. 2.73–3.25 mm) regardless of whether the implants have been submerged or not (Hermann et al. 2001; Larjava et al. 2011). The difference likely originates from the size difference between the biological width (Ikeda et al. 2000; Larjava et al. 2011), which in the case of implants is composed of the vertical dimensions of the gingival connective tissue, the junctional epithelium, and the peri-implant epithelium located farther away toward the peri-implant gingival sulcus (Ikeda et al. 2000; Larjava et al. 2011); whereas in the case of natural teeth it is composed of the vertical dimensions of the gingival connective tissue attachment and the junctional epithelial attachment (Hermann et al. 2001; Larjava et al. 2011). In the case of natural teeth, the biological width is roughly 2 mm and is composed of ca. 1 mm of gingival connective tissue attachment and ca. 1 mm of a junctional epithelial attachment (Gargiulo et al. 1961; Vacek et al. 1994; Larjava et al. 2011). With implants (of smooth trans-gingival titanium surface), the width of the gingival connective tissue attachment remains roughly the same (Rompen et al.

2006; Larjava et al. 2011) but the epithelial attachment (i.e. the JE and the PIE together) is somewhat longer.

5.3. Healing Process

In the microenvironment of the gingival peri-implant healing area, mesenchymal stem cells in contact with gingival tissue are stimulated by specific factors to differentiate into the adequate fibroblastic cell lineage (Lavenus et al. 2010). In response to cytokines and other factors like fibroblast growth factor (Ma et al. 2012), fibroblastic cells migrate and generate a capsule of collagen attached around the trans-gingival implant surface located next to the osseointegrating bone, which may be considered the most determinative step in the peri-implant gingival connective tissue attachment (Lavenus et al. 2010). The migration, early attachment, and proliferation of gingival epithelial cells also occur at the same time, leading to the formation of the junctional epithelium and peri-implant epithelium next to the attached connective tissue and farther away toward the peri-implant gingival sulcus, respectively (Teng et al. 2012).

Importantly, the surface roughness properties of implants also strongly influence the premised processes (Eisenbarth et al. 1996; Cohen et al. 2007; Lavenus et al. 2010; Teng et al. 2012); and it is also obvious that the properties of surface morphology are equally important at both the microscale and nanoscale levels (Eisenbarth et al. 1996; Cohen et al. 2007; Lavenus et al. 2010). The early attachment of epithelial cells seems to be higher in the case of smooth surfaces; however, their proliferation is slower on smooth surfaces in comparison to roughened surfaces (Teng et al. 2012). In contrast, the early attachment of fibroblasts is higher in the case of roughened surfaces, but they proliferate quicker on smooth surfaces when compared to rough surfaces (Teng et al. 2012). Conventionally smooth surfaces are used in the trans-gingival region (Teng et al. 2012); however, taking into account the above data, it seems to be rather difficult to find out which surface structure could be considered the optimal one for gingival closure. This is especially true, because it is rather difficult to find out whether it would be desirable to enhance epithelial attachment while suppressing connective tissue attachment (Teng et al. 2012) or to achieve a relatively strong connective tissue attachment (Ma et al. 2012) at the expense of the peri-implant epithelium. (There is no doubt that enhancing the junctional epithelium at the expense of the peri-implant epithelium would be desirable.)

Besides surface roughness, chemical composition and physical properties like hydrophilicity and others also affect the behavior of peri-implant tissues (Ma et al. 2012; Teng et al. 2012). However there are currently only a few relevant data sets available in the literature; therefore, it is difficult to draw conclusions on this topic.

5.4. The Importance of Gingival Healing

Although the stability of implant fixtures relies primarily on the attachment of peri-implant bone (i.e. osseointegration), the proper healing and attachment of peri-implant gingival tissues are also crucial for the success of implant placement. The optimal attachment of the connective tissue, the junctional epithelium, and the peri-implant epithelium to the implant surface is very important for the prevention of the apical migration of bacteria and the subgingival formation of their bacterial biofilm (plaque) (Larjava et al. 2011), thus contributing to the prevention of peri-implant inflammatory lesions and consequent bone loss (Larjava et al. 2011). Further, the esthetic outcome also relies heavily on the healing characteristics of peri-implant gingival tissues, such as the connective tissue and gingival epithelium, including the JE and PIE (Teng et al. 2012). Therefore, future research should focus on improving connective tissue and epithelial attachment on implant fixtures and also on abutments in the case of two-piece implant systems (Larjava et al. 2011; Teng et al. 2012; Ma et al. 2012).

Conclusion

The surface roughness properties of implants strongly influence peri-implant gingival healing processes (Eisenbarth et al. 1996; Cohen et al. 2007; Lavenus et al. 2010; Teng et al. 2012); and it is also obvious that the properties of surface morphology are equally important at both microscale and nanoscale levels (Eisenbarth et al. 1996; Cohen et al. 2007; Lavenus et al. 2010). Although smooth titanium surfaces are used conventionally in the trans-gingival region (Teng et al. 2012), it seems rather difficult to find out which surface properties could be considered as optimal for gingival closure, especially because not only surface roughness, but also chemical composition and physical properties like hydrophilicity and others, affect the behavior of peri-implant gingival tissues (Ma et al. 2012; Teng et al. 2012). Since proper healing and the attachment of peri-implant gingival tissues are crucial for the success of implant placement, future research should focus on improving the connective tissue and epithelial attachment on implant fixtures and also on abutments in the case of two-piece implant systems (Larjava et al. 2011; Teng et al. 2012; Ma et al. 2012).

References

Cohen, A; Liu-Synder, P; Storey, D; Webster, TJ. Decreased fibroblasts and increased osteoblast functions on ionic plasma deposited nanostructured Ti coatings. *Nanoscale Research Letters*, 2007, 2, 385–390.

de Oliveira, GR; Pozzer, L; Cavalieri-Pereira, L; de Moraes, PH; Olate, S; de Albergaria Barbosa, JR. Bacterial adhesion and colonization differences between zirconia and titanium implant abutments: an in vivo human study. *J Periodontal Implant Sci*, 2012, 42, 217–223.

Eisenbarth, E; Meyle, J; Nachtigall, W; Breme, J. Influence of the surface structure of titanium materials on the adhesion of fibroblasts. *Biomaterials*, 1996, 17, 1399–1403.

Fujiseki, M; Matsuzaka, K; Yoshinary, M; Shimono, M; Inoue, T. An experimental study on the features of peri-implant epithelium: immunohistochemical and electron-microscopic observations. *Bull Tokyo Dent Coll*, 2003, 44, 185–199.

Gargiulo, AW; Wentz, FM; Orban, B. Dimensions and relations of the dentogingival junction in humans. *J Periodontol*, 1961, 32, 261–267.

Hermann, JS; Buser, D; Schenk, RK; Schoolfield, JD; Cochran, DL. Biological width around one- and two-piece titanium implants. *Clin Oral Implant Res* 2001, 12, 559–571.

Ikeda, H; Shiraiwa, M; Yamaza, T; Yoshinari, M; Kido, MA; Ayukawa, Y; Inoue, T; Koyano, K; Tanaka, T. Difference in penetration of horseradish peroxidase tracer as a foreign substance into the peri-implant or juntional epithelium of rat gingivae. *Clin Oral Implant Res*, 2002, 13, 243–251.

Khoury, SB; Thomas, L; Walters, JD; Sheridan, JF; Leblebicioglu, B. Early wound healing following one-stage dental implant placement with and without antibiotic prophylaxis: A pilot study. *J Periodontol*, 2008, 79, 1904–1912.

Larjava, H; Koivisto, L; Hakkinen, L; Heino, J. Epithelial integrins with special reference to oral epithelia. *J Dent Res*, 2011, 90, 1367–1376.

Lavenus, S; Louarn, G; Layrolle, P. Nanotechnology and dental implants. *Int J Biomaterials*, 2010, Article ID: 915327. DOI: 10.1155/2010/915327.

Ma, Q; Wang, W; Chu, PK; Mei, S; Ji, K; Jin, L; Zhang, Y. Concentration- and time-dependent response of human gingival fibroblasts to fibroblast growth factor 2 immobilized on titanium dental implants. *Int J Nanomedicine*, 2012, 7, 1965–1976.

Mobelli, A; Marxer, M; Gaberthuel, T; Grunder, U; Lang, NP. The microbiota of osseointegrated implants in patients with a history of periodontal disease. *J Clin Periodontol*, 1995, 22, 124–130.

Rompen, E; Domken, O; Degidi, M; Pontes, AE; Piatelli, A. The effect of material characteristics, of surface topography and of implant components and connections on soft tissue integration: a literature review. *Clin Oral Implant Res*, 2006, 17 (Suppl. 2), 55–67.

Teng, FY; Ko, CL; Kuo, HN; Hu, JJ; Lin, JH; Lou, CW; Hung, CC; Wang, YL; Cheng, CY; Chen, WC. A comparison of epithelial cells, fibroblasts and osteoblasts in dental implant titanium topographies. *Bioinorg Chemistry and Applications*, 2012, Article ID: 687291. DOI: 10.1155/2012/687291.

Vacek, JS; Gher, ME; Assad, DA; Richardson, AC; Giambarresi, LI. The dimensions of human dentogingival junction. *Int Periodontics Restorative Dent*, 1994, 14, 154–165.

Chapter 6

Alveolar Ridge Preservation

Abstract

Bone formation in the alveolar socket is a naturally occurring event as long as the surrounding alveolar walls remain intact. However, the volumetric contraction of the alveolar ridge may impair implant placement; therefore, several surgical techniques have been proposed to reduce loss of the alveolar bone to an acceptable level. The primary aim of all these techniques is to reduce the postextraction loss of the alveolar bone and hereby enable the installation, primary stability, and osseointegration of dental implants as well as to improve the esthetic outcome of the final prosthesis, to reduce the need for additional bone grafting procedures, and to enable faster bone regeneration, allowing earlier prosthetic restoration. The preservation of the alveolar ridge may be crucial for successful implant placement in many cases. For the preservation of the alveolar bone following tooth extraction, the use of common preservation techniques like "socket grafting," guided bone regeneration, immediate implant placement, and (in certain cases) forced eruption of compromised teeth may be used. In general, less invasive techniques like "socket grafting" and forced eruption are preferred; whereas guided bone regeneration and immediate implant placement should be used only if indicated. Invasive techniques should be used very carefully, as the advancement of flaps may result in an increased inflammatory response, in a decrease in vestibular dimension, and in the creation of unesthetic scars. Reducing the extraction trauma and limiting flap elevation (if any) are essentials for each of these procedures.

6.1. Introduction

Bone formation in the alveolar socket is a naturally occurring event as long as the surrounding alveolar walls remain intact. However, the volumetric contraction of the alveolar ridge may impair implant placement (Irinakis 2006; Brkovic et al. 2008; Almasri et al. 2012; Pagni et al. 2012); therefore, several surgical techniques have been proposed to reduce the loss of the alveolar bone to an acceptable level (Irinakis 2006; Brkovic et al. 2008; Almasri et al. 2012; Pagni et al. 2012). The primary aim of all these techniques is to reduce the postextraction loss of the alveolar bone and thereby enable the installation, primary stability, and osseointegration of dental implants as well as to improve the esthetic outcome of the final prosthesis, to reduce the need for additional bone grafting procedures, and to enable faster bone regeneration, allowing earlier prosthetic restoration (Irinakis 2006; Brkovic et al. 2008; Almasri et al. 2012; Pagni et al. 2012).

In general, a labial bone thickness of more than 1.91 mm following implant placement could prevent a failure of the implant resulting from severe labial bone resorption (Cho et al. 2011; Kim et al. 2012). However, the buccal wall of the frontal/premolar region can be thinner, averaging ca. 0.8 mm in the anterior and ca. 1.1 mm in the premolar sites (Pagni et al. 2012). Further, after tooth extraction, the alveolar bone undergoes sequential reparative resorption and in particular, the labial cortical bone and alveolar crest resorb (Kim et al. 2012), which may compromise both implant stability and esthetics (especially in the case of anterior maxilla). Therefore, the preservation of the alveolar ridge may be crucial for successful implant placement in these regions in many cases. Similarly, postextraction alveolar ridge resorption is also an inevitable process in the molar region (Brkovic et al. 2008; Almasri et al. 2012; Pagni et al. 2012), and molar ridges present higher degrees of resorption than premolar areas (Pagni et al. 2012).

For the preservation of the alveolar bone following tooth extraction, the use of common preservation techniques like "socket grafting," guided bone regeneration, immediate implant placement, and (in certain cases) forced eruption of compromised teeth may be used (Covani et al. 2003, 2007; McNutt and Chou 2003; Irinakis 2006; Nevins et al. 2006; Yoo et al. 2006; Brkovic et al. 2008; Fabian et al. 2012; Almasri et al. 2012; Pagni et al. 2012). In general, less invasive techniques like "socket grafting" and forced eruption are preferred (Brkovic et al. 2008; Fabian et al. 2012; Pagni et al. 2012); whereas guided bone regeneration and immediate implant placement should be used only if indicated (McNutt and Chou 2003; Irinakis 2006; Pagni et al. 2012). Reducing the extraction trauma and limiting flap elevation (if any) are essentials for each of these procedures (Irinakis 2006; Brkovic et al. 2008; Fickl et al. 2008; Almasri et al. 2012; Pagni et al. 2012).

6.2. Healing of Extraction Socket

Following tooth extraction, the alveolar ridge undergoes an inevitable remodeling process that influences the implant therapy of the edentulous area at issue (Brkovic et al. 2008; Pagni et al. 2012). Socket grafting, guided bone regeneration and/or immediate implant placement, and (in certain cases) forced eruption of compromised teeth are available therapies for the preservation of the alveolar bone (Irinakis 2006; Brkovic et al. 2008; Almasri et al. 2012; Fabian et al. 2012; Pagni et al. 2012). In the case of the mandible the thinner of the two alveolar walls is a labial wall in the anterior and a lingual wall in the molar regions (Williams and Warwick 1980); whereas in the case of the maxilla, the labial alveolar wall is thinner everywhere (Williams and Warwick 1980). A thin layer of the alveolar bone is the bundle bone that lines the alveolar socket and extends coronally, forming the alveolar crest (Pagni et al. 2012) and also making up part of the periodontal structure as it encloses the external terminations of Sharpey's (periodontal) fibers (Pagni et al. 2012).

After tooth extraction, the initial reparative bone resorption/remodeling occurs in two phases. *During the first phase* (immediately after tooth extraction), the alveolar socket is filled by a blood clot that is replaced with granulation tissue within a week (Pagni et al.

2012), and the epithelium migrates over the granulation tissue to cover the healing socket afterward (Pagni et al. 2012). Simultaneously, the granulation tissue is rapidly remodeled into a provisional matrix followed by mineralization processes that lead to the formation of woven bone, which eventually is replaced by mature lamellar bone (Trombelli et al. 2008; Pagni et al. 2012). Thus, during the first phase, initially the blood clot, subsequently the granulation tissue, and later the provisional matrix and the woven bone fill up the alveolus (Pagni et al. 2012). These processes lead to the rapid resorption of the bundle bone and the consequently rather quick resorption of the thin alveolar crest, leading to a great reduction in bone height, especially in the thinner regions of the alveolar wall (Williams and Warwick 1980; Pagni et al. 2012) since their crestal portion is comprised nearly "solely" of the bundle bone in many cases (Pagni et al. 2012). *During the second phase*, the outer surface of the alveolar bone is remodeled, which causes further overall horizontal and vertical bone tissue contraction (Pagni et al. 2012); therefore, the height of the socket never reaches the coronal level of bone attached to the extracted tooth. Interestingly, the horizontal bone tissue contraction is greater in the molar region compared to the premolar area (Pagni et al. 2012).

Following the initial bone resorption/remodeling, the remaining parts of the alveolar bone are gradually absorbed throughout life (Williams and Warwick 1980; Pagni et al. 2012). The resorption rate of the alveolar ridges is faster during the first six months following the extraction and proceeds at an average of 0.5%–1.0% per year over an entire lifespan (Williams and Warwick 1980; Nagaraj et al. 2010; Pagni et al. 2012). The process of resorption primarily affects the thinner of the two alveolar walls (Williams and Warwick 1980), which is the labial wall of both the mandible and maxilla in the anterior region (Williams and Warwick 1980; Pagni et al. 2012) as opposed to the lingual wall of the mandible and the buccal wall of the maxilla in the molar region (Williams and Warwick 1980).

6.3. Reducing Surgical Trauma

Bone formation in the alveolar socket is a naturally occurring event as long as the surrounding alveolar walls remain intact. However, the volumetric contraction of the alveolar ridge may impair implant placement (Irinakis 2006; Brkovic et al. 2008; Almasri et al. 2012; Pagni et al. 2012); therefore, several surgical techniques have been proposed to reduce the loss of the alveolar bone to an acceptable level (Irinakis 2006; Brkovic et al. 2008; Almasri et al. 2012; Pagni et al. 2012). Reducing the extraction trauma and limiting flap elevation (if any) are essentials for each of these procedures (Irinakis 2006; Brkovic et al. 2008; Fickl et al. 2008; Pagni et al. 2012). It may be hypothesized that disrupting the thin layer of cells that comprise the osteogenic layer of an adult periosteum through flap elevation might diminish the ability of periosteal cells to regenerate bone (Pagni et al. 2012); in such a situation, the undisturbed periosteum (i.e. flapless extraction/preservation techniques) might maintain its full osteogenic potential (Pagni et al. 2012). However, animal studies show confusing results when evaluating differences in ridge remodeling between flapped and nonflapped extraction sockets (Pagni et al. 2012). It may be held that flap elevation affects alveolar dimensional alterations only in the short term (Tan et al. 2012; Pagni et al. 2012), while there is no significant difference in the long term (Caneva et al. 2010/a; Pagni et al. 2012). However, the use of invasive techniques is hardly recommended as the advancement of flaps may result in an increased inflammatory response, in a decrease in vestibular depth, and in the creation of unesthetic scars (Pagni et al. 2012).

6.4. "Socket Grafting"

In the case of socket grafting, the extraction socket is filled up either with bone grafts or with bone substitutes (or other biomaterials). The inserted bone graft or bone substitute may be covered by a flap, but may also be covered with nothing but a collagen plug (Brkovic et al. 2008; Pagni et al. 2012). In certain cases it may also be enough if the inserted bone substitute/graft material is secured with a simple suture placed over the extraction site but without a barrier membrane or flap (Brkovic et al. 2008). Since not only grafts but also bone substitutes or other biomaterials may be used (and because the socket itself is not "grafted" at all), the terms "socket grafting" as well as "grafted socket" or "grafted site" are rather confusing and questionable. On the other hand, the premised terms seem to be commonly accepted and are frequently used in the related literature; therefore, they may also be used in this chapter.

As indicated above, the first phase of initial healing at the extraction site leads to rapid resorption of the bundle bone, leading to a great reduction in bone height, especially in the thinner regions of the alveolar wall (Williams and Warwick 1980; Pagni et al. 2012). If "socket grafting" is used, this first phase of initial bone resorption still occurs (Pagni et al. 2012); therefore, the height of the healed ridge never reaches the original level of bone attached to the extracted tooth (Pagni et al. 2012). However, further overall horizontal and vertical bone tissue contractions caused by the alveolar bone remodeling during the second phase of healing can be reduced significantly by means of "socket grafting" techniques (Brkovic et al. 2008; Pagni et al. 2012).

Many articles reported only a partial resorption of bone substitutes at short and long intervals, raising doubts concerning the achievement of osseointegration when using implants inserted in augmented sites; however experimental (Fiorellini et al. 2007; de Santis et al. 2011; Pagni et al. 2012) and clinical (Carmagnola et al. 2003; Molly et al. 2008; Almasri et al. 2012; Pagni et al. 2012) data indicate that the grafting procedure does not impair primary stability or osseointegration (Carmagnola et al. 2003; Fiorellini et al. 2007; Brkovic et al. 2008; Molly et al. 2008; de Santis et al. 2011; Almasri et al. 2012; Pagni et al. 2012). Accordingly, implants placed in grafted sites are able to sustain loading and provide similar long-term results as those placed in pristine bone (Fiorellini and Nevins 2003; Brkovic et al. 2008; Almasri et al. 2012; Pagni et al. 2012).

6.5. Guided Bone Regeneration

Guided bone regeneration techniques utilize barrier membranes to keep gingival cells from penetrating into the defect to be regenerated (Irinakis 2006; Almasri et al. 2012; Pagni et al. 2012). Importantly, the use of guided bone regeneration for ridge preservation is based on slightly different principles than the original principles (Melcher et al. 1976) underlying guided tissue regeneration techniques (Melcher 1976) because the extraction socket per se will not be filled up with gingival soft tissue (i.e. epithelial cells and/or connective tissue); instead, it tends to heal through the regeneration of bone as summarized above (Irinakis 2006; Pagni et al. 2012). However, barrier membranes seem to minimize alveolar resorption (Lekovic et al. 1997) if the membranes are covered with full-thickness soft tissue flaps (elevated buccally and lingually/palatinally and mobilized by means of periosteal releasing incision), especially if the membranes are not exposed during the healing period (Lekovic et al. 1997; Irinakis 2006,). The use of additional grafting/bone-substituting material does not seem to be a crucial factor of success (Pinho et al. 2006) but the maintenance of space is of consequence (Pinho et al. 2006; Pagni et al. 2012), at least if a nonresorbable membrane is used (Lekovic et al. 1997; Pinho et al. 2006; Pagni et al. 2012). If resorbable membranes are used (Lekovic et al. 1998; Luczyszyn et al. 2005; Neiva et al. 2011; Almasri et al. 2012) there may be an additional benefit gained from the administration of bone substitutes like resorbable hydroxyapatite (Luczyszyn et al. 2005; Irinakis 2006) or a demineralized freeze-dried bone matrix (Irinakis 2006; Almasri et al. 2012).

Importantly, if the guided bone generation technique is used properly, there will only be insignificant changes made to the alveolar ridge's dimensions in comparison to the original dimensions of any bone attached to the extracted tooth (Irinakis 2006; Neiva et al. 2011; Pagni et al. 2012). In other words, GBR techniques effectively prevent bone resorption and bone tissue contraction during both the first and second phases of initial bone healing (Irinakis 2006; Neiva et al. 2011; Pagni et al. 2012). An adequate bone formation for implant placement occurs roughly as early as 12 weeks following a tooth extraction if guided bone regeneration techniques are used (Neiva et al. 2011; Pagni et al., 2012). However, it should also be considered that the improper use of a GBR technique may result in an increased inflammatory response, in a decrease in vestibular dimension, and in the creation of unesthetic scars (Irinakis 2006; Pagni et al. 2012).

6.6. Immediate Implant Placement

To prevent the resorption of the maxillary labial cortical bone from the crestal region following tooth extraction, immediate implant placement (Schulte et al. 1978/a, b, c) should also be considered (Barzilay et al. 1991, 1996/a, b; Covani et al. 2003, 2007; McNutt and Chou 2003; Yoo et al. 2006; Pagni et al. 2012), because substantially less ridge remodeling may occur if an implant is placed immediately (and properly) into the extraction site (Barzilay et al. 1991, 1996/a, b; Pagni et al., 2012). Importantly, the closer the implant is to the buccal bony plate, the more the buccal bone resorbs (Sanz et al. 2010; Tomasi et al. 2010; Pagni et al. 2012). Accordingly, an implant position 0.8 mm deeper and more lingual/palatinal in relation to the center of the socket results in a lesser degree of buccal bone dehiscence (Caneva et al. 2010/b; Pagni et al. 2012); and smaller (3.3 mm) diameter cylindrical implants may be more advantageous than larger (5 mm) diameter root-formed implants (McNutt and Chou 2003; Caneva et al. 2010/c; Pagni et al. 2012). Smaller size implants seem to be more advantageous in this case as well in relation to soft tissue healing, because soft tissue follows bone level; therefore, it is more apically located in the case of larger-sized implants with a higher degree of buccal dehiscence (McNutt and Chou 2003; Caneva et al. 2012/a; Pagni et al. 2012).

The placement of a collagen membrane over the buccal gap (advantageously with a graft/substitute filling the buccal dehiscence) of immediately placed implants advantageously modifies hard tissue healing (Caneva et al. 2010/d, 2012/b; Pagni et al. 2012). This treatment is likely to provide additional amounts of hard tissue at the entrance of the previous socket, impede the buccal bone wall remodeling process (and the following horizontal contraction), and improve the level of marginal bone-to-implant contact and consequently the soft tissue contour (Araujo et al. 2011; Pagni et al. 2012).

Although immediate implant placement may be used with a high success rate if properly indicated (McNutt and Chou 2003; Khanifam et al. 2013), for more predictable results, it is recommended that proper time be allowed for bone healing prior to proceeding with implant treatment (Nagaraj et al. 2010; Pagni et al. 2012; Khanifam et al. 2013). This may be especially important from an esthetic point of view in the case of a thin gingival biotype (Nagaraj et al. 2010); whereas in the case of a thick gingival biotype, the esthetic results may be more predictable (Nagaraj et al. 2010). If there was no implant placed into the socket *immediately* (Type-1 implant) it may be advantageous in certain cases to place an implant *early* into the extraction site during early stage healing (within 4–8 weeks; Type-2 implant) or during the "partial bone" stage (within 12–16 weeks; Type-3 implant). This may be advantageous because bone augmentation around the premised early inserted implants (i.e. Type-2 and Type-3 implants) may provide better hard tissue dimensions and less postoperative complications compared to those that appear around *delayed* (Type-4) implants (Hammerle et al. 2004; Pagni et al. 2012; Sanz et al. 2012).

6.7. Forced Eruption of Compromised Teeth

The use of forced eruption followed by the extraction of buried or periodontally compromised teeth provides the opportunity to permanently increase the vertical and/or horizontal dimensions of hard and soft tissues at the site of the tooth undergoing this procedure (Atherton 1970; Heithersay 1973; Ingber 1974, 1989; Mantzikos and Shamus 1997; Capri et al. 2003; Fabian et al. 2012).

In the case of buried teeth, forced eruption generates an alteration of the periodontal tissues, resulting in a coronal shift of periodontal fibers, marginal gingiva, and bone, coupled with a somewhat more pronounced coronal shift of the erupted tooth (Fabian et al. 2012). The coronal movement of the bone may produce both the necessary height and width for the alveolar crest (Fabian et al. 2012). Forced eruption of buried roots can be carried out with a simplified eruption procedure using a horizontal bar fixed between the neighboring teeth, a hook cemented into the root canal of the buried root, and an elastic band responsible for the tooth movement (Stein and Sidley 1997; Ziskind et al. 2000). Brackets bounded to two–three adjacent neighboring teeth on both sides together with a 0.016 inch nickel titanium wire (Ziskind et al. 2000; Chambrone and Chambrone 2005) fixed to the hook cemented into the root canal may also be used (Fabian et al. 2012). Since in the case of buried teeth an extrusion of a few millimeters is usually enough, the orthodontic procedure may only take roughly a month (Fabian et al. 2012).

In the case of periodontally compromised teeth, the bone that moves coronally is attached to the apical third of the root (because of the advanced periodontal disease of the tooth at issue) where the root diameter is relatively narrow (Capri et al. 2003). Therefore, the coronal movement of the bone may produce the necessary height in the edentulous ridge for the insertion of an implant (Capri et al. 2003; Chambrone and Chambrone 2005; Holst et al. 2007; Kim et al. 2011); but the width may remain deficient in many cases because of the narrow root diameter (Capri et al. 2003; Fabian et al. 2012). To increase the buccolingual bulk of the alveolar bone, a buccal root torque component may be applied concomitantly (Korayem et al. 2008; Fabian et al. 2012), but a mucogingival surgery to widen the ridge may also be needed in certain cases to develop the desired ridge width (Capri et al. 2003). For tooth eruption, light, constant extrusive forces are recommended (i.e. 15 g for anterior and 50 g for posterior teeth) (Korayem et al. 2008; Fabian et al. 2012). The extrusion rate is roughly 2.0 mm per month. A retention/stabilization phase of the same length as the active extrusion phase is recommended prior to extraction (Korayem et al. 2008; Fabian et al. 2012). The desired movement can usually be achieved in roughly three months with another three month retention phase before extraction (Capri et al. 2003; Chambrone and Chambrone 2005; Fabian et al. 2012).

Conclusion

The preservation of the alveolar ridge may be crucial for successful implant placement in many cases. For the preservation of the alveolar bone following tooth extraction, the use of common preservation techniques like "socket grafting," guided bone regeneration, immediate implant placement, and (in certain cases) forced eruption of compromised teeth may be used (Covani et al. 2003, 2007; McNutt and Chou 2003; Irinakis 2006; Nevins et al. 2006; Yoo et al. 2006; Brkovic et al. 2008; Fabian et al. 2012; Almasri et al. 2012; Pagni et al. 2012). Invasive techniques should be used very carefully, as the advancement of flaps may result in an increased inflammatory response, in a decrease in vestibular dimension, and in the creation of unesthetic scars (Irinakis 2006; Pagni et al. 2012). Therefore guided bone regeneration and immediate implant placement should be used only if indicated (McNutt and Chou 2003; Pagni et al. 2012). Reducing the extraction trauma and limiting flap elevation (if any) are essentials for each of these procedures (Irinakis 2006; Brkovic et al. 2008; Fickl et al. 2008; Pagni et al. 2012).

References

Araujo, MG; Linder, E; Lindhe, J. Bio-Oss collagen in the buccal gap at immediate implants: a 6-month study in the dog. *Clin Oral Implants Res*, 2011, 22, 1–8.

Almasri, M; Camarda, AJ; Ciaburro, H; Chouikh, F; Dorismond, SJ. Preservation of posterior mandibular extraction site with allogenic demineralized freeze-dried bone matrix and calcium sulphate graft binder before eventual implant placement: A case series. *J Can Dent Assoc*, 2012, 78, c15.

Atherton, JD. The gingival response to orthodontic tooth movement. *Am J Orthod*, 1970, 58, 179–186.

Barzilay, I; Graser, GN; Iranpour, B; Natiella, JR. Immediate implantation of a pure titanium implant into an extraction socket: report of a pilot procedure. *Int J Oral Maxillofac Implants*, 1991, 6, 277–284.

Barzilay, I; Graser, GN; Iranpour, B; Proskin, HM. Immediate implantation of pure titanium implants into extraction sockets of Macaca fascicularis. Part I: clinical and radiographic assessment. *Int J Oral Maxillofac Implants*, 1996/a, 11, 299–310.

Barzilay, I; Graser, GN; Iranpour, B; Natiella, JR; Proskin, HM. Immediate implantation of pure titanium implants into extraction sockets of Macaca fascicularis. Part II: histologic observations. *Int J Oral Maxillofac Implants*, 1996/b, 11, 489–497.

Brkovic, BMB; Prasad, HS; Konandreas, G; Milan, R; Antunovic, D; Sandor, GKB; Rohrer, MD. Simple preservation of a maxillary extraction socket using beta-tricalcium phosphate with type I collagen: Preliminary clinical and histomorphometric observations. *J Can Dent Assoc*, 2008, 74, 523–528.

Caneva, M; Botticelli, D; Salata, LA; Souza, SLS; Bressan, E; Lang, NP. Flap vs. "flapless" surgical approach at immediate implants: a histomorphometric study in dogs. *Clin Oral Implant Res*, 2010/a, 21, 1314–1319.

Caneva, M; Salata, LA; de Souza, SS; Baffone, G; Lang, NP; Botticelli, D. Influence of implant positioning in extraction sockets on osseointegration: histomorphometric analyses in dogs. *Clin Oral Implant Res*, 2010/b, 21, 43–49.

Caneva, M; Salata, LA; de Souza, SS; Bressan, E; Botticelli, D; Lang, NP. Hard tissue formation adjacent to implants of various size and configuration immediately placed into extraction sockets: an experimental study in dogs. *Clin Oral Implants Res*, 2010/c, 21, 885–890.

Caneva, M; Botticelli, L; Salata, LA; Scombatti Souza, SL; Carvalho Cardoso, L; Lang, NP. Collagen membranes at immediate implants: a histomorphometric study in dogs. *Clin Oral Implants Res*, 2010/d, 21, 891–897.

Caneva, M; Botticelli, D; Rossi, F; Cardoso, LC; Pantani, F; Lang, NP. Influence of implants with different sizes and configurations installed immediately into extraction sockets on peri-implant hard and soft tissues: an experimental study in dogs. *Clin Oral Implants Res*, 2012/a, 23, 396–401.

Caneva, M; Botticelli, D; Pantani, F; Baffone, GM; Rangel, IG; Lang, NP. Deproteinized bovine bone mineral in marginal defects at implants installed immediately into extraction sockets: an experimental study in dogs. *Clin Oral Implants Res*, 2012/b, 23, 106–112.

Capri, D; Albehbehani, Y; Smukler, H. Augmentation of an anterior edentulous ridge for fixed prosthodontics with combined use of orthodontics and surgery: A clinical report. *J Prosthet Dent*, 2003, 90, 111–115.

Carmagnola, D; Adriaens, P; Berglundh, T. Healing of human extraction sockets filled with Bio-Oss®. *Clin Oral Implant Res*, 2003, 14, 137–143.

Chambrone, L; Chambrone, LA. Forced orthodontic eruption of fractured teeth before implant placement: Case report. *J Can Dent Assoc*, 2005, 71, 257–261.

Cho, YB; Moon, SJ; Chung, CH; Kim, HJ. Resorption of labial bone in maxillary anterior implant. *J Adv Prosthodont*, 2011, 3, 85–89.

Covani, U; Cornelini, R; Barone, A. Bucco-lingual bone remodeling around implants placed into immediate extraction sockets: a case series. *J Periodontol*, 2003, 74, 268–273.

Covani, U; Cornelini, R; Barone, A. Vertical crestal bone changes around implants placed into fresh extraction sockets. *J Periodontol*, 2007, 78, 810–815.

de Santis, E; Botticelli, D; Pantani, F; Pereira, FP; Beolchini, M; Lang, NP. Bone regeneration at implants placed into extraction sockets of maxillary incisors in dogs. *Clin Oral Implant Res*, 2011, 22, 430–437.

Fabian, TK; Beck, A; Rencz, B; Fejerdy, P; Hermann, P; Fabian, G. Orthodontics for patients of prosthetic dentistry. Possibilities and complications of psychosomatic origin. In: Fabian TK, Fejerdy P, Hermann P, editors. *Dentures. Types, benefits and potential complications.* New York: Nova Science Publishers, 2012, 15–26.

Fickl, S; Zuhr, O; Wachtel, H; Bolz, W; Huerzeler, M. Tissue alterations after tooth extraction with and without surgical trauma: a volumetric study in the beagle dog. *J Clin Periodontol*, 2008, 35, 356–363.

Fiorellini, JP; Kim, DM; Nakajima, Y; Weber, HP. Osseointegration of titanium implants following guided bone regeneration using expanded polytetrafluoroethylene membrane and various bone fillers. *Int J Periodontics & Restorative Dent*, 2007, 27, 287–294.

Fiorellini, JP; Nevins, ML. Localized ridge augmentation/preservation. A systematic review. *Annals Periodontol*, 2003, 8, 321–327.

Hammerle, CHF; Chen, ST; Wilson Jr., TG. Consensus statements and recommended clinical procedures regarding the placement of implants in extraction sockets. *Int J Oral Maxillofac Implants*, 2004, 19, 26–28.

Heithersay, GS. Combined endodontic-orthodontic treatment of transverse root fractures in the region of the alveolar crest. *Oral Surg Oral Med Oral Pathol*, 1973, 36, 404–415.

Holst, S; Hegenbarth, EA; Schlegel, KA; Holst, AI. Restoration of a nonrestorable central incisor using forced orthodontic eruption, immediate implant placement, and an all-ceramic restoration: A clinical report. *J Prosthet Dent*, 2007, 98, 251–255.

Ingber, JS; Forced eruption. Part I. A method of treating isolated one and two wall infrabony osseus defects – Rational and case report. *J Periodontol*, 1974, 45, 199–206.

Ingber, JS. Forced eruption: alteration of soft tissue cosmetic deformities. *Int J Periodontics Restorative Dent*, 1989, 9, 416–425.

Irinakis, T. Rationale for socket preservation after extraction of a single-rooted tooth when planning for future implant placement. *J Can Dent Assoc*, 2006, 72, 917–922.

Khanifam, P; Pullisaar, H; Leknes, K. Dental implant placement in fresh extraction sockets. *Danish Dent J*, 2013, 117, 1002–1007.

Kim, SH; Tramontina, VA; Papalexiou, V; Luczyszyn, SM. Orthodontic extrusion and implant site development using an interocclusal appliance for a severe mucogingival deformity: A clinical report. *J Prosthet Dent*, 2011, 105, 72–77.

Kim, HJ; Yu, SK; Lee, MH; Lee, HJ; Kim, HJ; Chung, CH. Cortical and cancellous bone thickness on the anterior region of alveolar bone in Korean: a study of dentate human cadavers. *J Adv Prosthodont*, 2012, 4, 146–152.

Korayem, M; Flores-Mir, C; Nassar, U; Olfert, K. Implant site development by orthodontic extrusion. A systematic review. *Angle Orthodontist*, 2008, 78, 752–760.

Lekovic, V; Kenney, EB; Weinlander, M, Han, T. Klokkevold, P; Nedic, M; Orsini, M. A bone regenerative approach to alveolar ridge maintenance following tooth extraction. Report of 10 cases. *J Periodontol*, 1997, 68, 563–570.

Lekovic, V; Camargo, PM; Klokkevold, PR. Weinlander, M; Kenney, EB; Dimitrijevic, B; Nedic, M. Preservation of alveolar bone in extraction sockets using bioabsorbable membranes. *J Periodontol*, 1998, 69, 1044–1049.

Luczyszyn, SM; Papalexiou, V; Novaes, AB; Grisi, MFM; Souza, SLS; Taba, M. Acellular dermal matrix and hydroxyapatite in prevention of ridge deformities after tooth extraction. *Implant Dent*, 2005, 14, 176–184.

Mantzikos, T; Shamus, I. Forced eruption and implant site development: soft tissue response. *Am J Orthod Dentofacial Orthop*, 1997, 112, 596–606.

McNutt, MD; Chou, CH. Current trends in immediate osseous dental implant case selection criteria. *J Dent Education*, 2003, 67, 850–859.

Melcher, AH. On the repair potential of periodontal tissues. *J Periodontol*, 1976, 47, 256–260.

Molly, L; Vandromme, H; Quirynen, M; Schepers, E; Adams, JL; van Steenberghe, D. Bone formation following implantation of bone biomaterials into extraction sites. *J Periodontol*, 2008, 79, 1108–1115.

Nagaraj, KR; Savadi, RC; Savadi, AR; Parashanth Reddy, GT; Srilakshmi, J; Dayalan, M; John, J. Gingival biotype – Prosthodontic perspective. *Ind J Prosthodontic Soc.* 2010, 10, 27–30.

Neiva, R; Pagni, G; Duarte, F; Park, CH; Yi, E; Holman, LA; Giannobile, WV. Analysis of tissue neogenesis in extraction sockets treated with guided bone regeneration: clinical, histologic, and micro-CT results. *Int J Periodontics & Restorative Dent*, 2011, 31, 457–469.

Nevins, M; Camelo, M; De Paoli, S; Friedland, B; Schenk, RK; Parma-Benfenati, S; Simion, M; Tinti, C; Wagenberg, B. A study of the fate of the buccal wall of extraction sockets of teeth with prominent roots. *Int J Periodontics Restorative Dent*, 2006, 26, 19–29.

Pagni, G; Pellegrini, G; Giannobile, WV; Rasperini, G. Postextraction alveolar ridge preservation: Biological basis and treatments. *Int J Dentistry*, 2012, Article ID: 151030. DOI: 10.1155/2012/151030.

Pinho, MN; Roriz, VM; Novaes Jr., AB; Taba Jr., M; Grisi, MF; de Souza, SL; Palioto, DB. Titanium membranes in prevention of alveolar collapse after tooth extraction. *Implant Dentistry*, 2006, 15, 53–61.

Sanz, M; Cecchinato, D; Ferrus, J; Pjeturson, EB; Lang NP; Lindhe, J. A prospective, randomized-controlled clinical trial to evaluate bone preservation using implants with different geometry placed into extraction sockets in the maxilla. *Clin Oral Implants Res*, 2010, 21, 13–21.

Sanz, I; Garzia-Gargallo, M; Herrera, D; Martin, C; Figuero, E; Sanz, M. Surgical protocols for early implant placement in post-extraction sockets: a systematic review. *Clin Oral Implants Res*, 2012, 23, 67–79.

Schulte, W; Kleineikenscheidt, H; Schareyka, R; Heimke, G. Concept and testing of the Tubingen immediate implant. *Deutsche zahnarztl Zeitschrift*, 1978/a, 33, 319–325.

Schulte, W; Kleineikenscheidt, H; Lindner, K; Schareyka, R; Heimke, G; Gerlach, C; Hrdegg, W. Animal experiments on the question of healing around the Tubingen immediate implant. *Deustche zahnarztl. Zeitschrift*, 1978/b, 33, 326–331.

Schulte, W; Kleineikenscheidt, H; Linder, K; Schareyka, R. The Tubingen immediate implant in clinical studies. *Deutsche zahnarztl Zeitschrift*, 1978/c, 33, 348–859.

Stein, E; Sidley, C. Orthodontic extrusion – a new and simplified aesthetic technique. *J Dent Assoc*, 1997, 52, 287–293.

Tan, WL; Wong, TLT; Wong, MCM; Lang, NP. A systemic review of post-extractional alveolar hard and soft tissue dimensional changes in humans. *Clin Oral Implants Res*, 2012, 23, 1–21.

Tomasi, C; Sanz, M; Cecchinato, D; Pjetursson, B; Ferrus, J; Lang, NP; Lindhe, J. Bone dimensional variations at implants placed in fresh extraction sockets: a multilevel multivariate analysis. *Clin Oral Implants Res*, 2010, 21, 30–36.

Trombelli, L; Farina, A; Marzola, A; Bozzi, L; Liljenberg, B; Lindhe, J. Modelling and remodeling of human extraction sockets. *J Clin Periodontol*, 2008, 35, 630–639.

Williams, PL; Warwick, R. (Ed-in-chiefs). *Gray's Anatomy*. Thirty-sixth edition. Edinburgh-London-Melbourne-New York: Churchill Livingstone, 1980, 319.

Yoo, RH; Chuang, SK; Erakat, MS; Weed, M; Dodson, TB. Changes in crestal bone levels for immediately loaded implants. *Int J Oral Maxillofac Implants*, 2006, 21, 253–261.

Ziskind, D; Sharon, E; Hirschfeld, Z; Becker, A. Analysis of lateral tooth movement during forced orthodontic eruption. *J Prosthet Dent*, 2000, 84, 462–466.

CHAPTER 7

PHYSIOTHERAPY FOR PERI-IMPLANT HEALING

Abstract

Physiotherapies were found to be beneficial in a wide variety of therapeutic processes over the last few decades. Data in the literature revealed that bone formation and soft tissue healing around dental implants can also be significantly promoted through physiotherapeutic treatment. There are various physiotherapeutic modalities that may be used in certain stages of implant-related treatments, including ultrasound, low-intensity pulsed ultrasound (LIPU), electric fields, light-emitting diode (LED) photomodulation therapy (LPT), and others. Some of them may be used before implant placement only (i.e. to promote bone augmentation before implant placement) and should not be used thereafter. Others may have compromised efficiency in deeper-located healing bone areas. Two major tools, namely pulsed electromagnetic field (PEMF) therapy and low level laser therapy (LLLT), seem to be highly applicable in relation to implant dentistry; therefore, this chapter will focus on these two modalities only. Although the exact mechanisms by which they affect alveolar bone and other peri-implant tissues is far from fully understood, certain mechanisms have already been recognized and the increased amount of knowledge may be utilized in clinical practice. In this chapter, scientific data pertaining to clinical relevance are collected and discussed.

7.1. Introduction

There are various physiotherapeutic modalities that may be used in certain stages of implant-related treatments, including ultrasound (Fabian and Fejerdy 2010), low-intensity pulsed ultrasound (Ustun et al. 2008; Ding et al. 2010; Kim and Hong 2010), electric fields (Fabian and Fejerdy 2010; Gittens et al. 2011; Mohn et al. 2011), light-emitting diode photomodulation therapy (Cankaya et al. 2011; Uysal et al. 2012), and others (Fabian and Fejerdy 2010). Some of them may be used before implant placement only (i.e. to promote bone augmentation before implant placement) and should not be used thereafter (Fabian and Fejerdy 2010). Others may have compromised efficiency in deeper-located healing bone areas (Fabian and Fejerdy 2010). Two major tools, namely pulsed electromagnetic field therapy and low level laser therapy, seems to be highly applicable in any relation to implant dentistry

(Fabian and Fejerdy 2010; Fabian et al. 2012); therefore, this chapter will focus on these two modalities only.

7.2. Pulsed Electromagnetic Field (PEMF) Therapy

7.2.1. General Effects of PEMF on Cells

How a cell detects a pulsed electromagnetic field signal is currently unknown, but some mechanisms have been proposed to account for the interaction of PEMF with cells (Fabian and Fejerdy 2010; Fabian et al. 2012). It is very likely that PEMF interacts with moving charges and changes their velocities, as in the classic interaction of magnetic fields with any moving charge (Blank 1995; Goodman and Blank 1998). Besides this, the resonance-interaction of PEMF fields with Earth's magnetic field (Goodman and Blank 1998) as well as the phenomenon of ion-cyclotron resonance (Liboff et al. 1987; Lednev 1991; Blanchard and Blackman 1994) may also be responsible for several biological responses (Fabian and Fejerdy 2010; Fabian et al. 2012).

Importantly, a PEMF penetrates the cell (unlike electric fields); therefore, its interaction with cells can occur anywhere inside (or outside) the cell (Goodman and Blank 1998). It is also very likely that a PEMF signal exhibits sufficient energy to elicit a transient activation/alteration of membrane-bound receptors or their inner associated proteins (Luben 1982; Varani et al. 2003; Schnoke and Midura 2007) and may also alter the density of certain receptors of the cells (Varani et al. 2003); therefore, PEMF is believed to influence the function of the receptor-coupled signal transduction pathways of cells (Luben 1982; Goodman and Blank 1998; Varani et al. 2003; Schnoke and Midura 2007; Fabian and Fejerdy 2010; Fabian et al. 2012). The alteration of cell communication via the PEMF-induced alteration of local factor production and gap junction signaling is also very likely (Lohmann et al. 2003). Further, a wide variety of cell-membrane structural and functional properties (Lednev 1991; Balcavage et al. 1996), signal transduction processes (Satake et al. 1990; Schnoke and Midura 2007), and the activity of several ATPases and enzymes (Blank 1995; Goodman and Blank 1998) as well as gene activation (McClellan et al. 1990; Blank and Goodman 1997), transcription (Blank and Goodman 1997; Tuinstra et al. 1997; Solazzo et al. 2010), translation, and protein synthesis (Goodman et al. 1993; Goodman and Blank 1998) are also altered by PEMF. The above data clearly indicate the rather complex effect of PEMF stimulation on cells, which serves as a good basis for the understanding of how PEMF stimulation may influence the functions of those cells that are present and participate in peri-implant healing (Fabian and Fejerdy 2010; Fabian et al. 2012).

7.2.2. Effect of PEMF on Osteoclasts

Osteoclasts are large bone-resorptive multinucleated cells derived from bone marrow hematopoietic stem cells of the monocyte-macrophage lineage (Chang et al. 2005; Fabian et al. 2009/a; Barnaba et al. 2012) and are responsible for both bone demineralization and collagen degradation in the bone (Chang et al. 2005; Fabian et al. 2009/a; Barnaba et al.

2012). PEMF treatment is likely to cause a delay in osteoclast differentiation (Chang et al. 2004/a, 2005; Barnaba et al. 2012) and increases the production of osteoprotegerin (OPG) in osteoblasts without any change in the secretion of RANKL (receptor activator of nuclear factor-κβ ligand), leading to the increase of the OPG/RANKL ratio, which leads decreased osteoclast maturation and decreased bone resorption (Schwartz et al. 2009). However, the effect may be transitory in nature and may disappear thereafter (Barnaba et al. 2012); it also seems to be coupled with the PEMF stimulation of lower energy only (Chang et al. 2003, 2005). In certain cases, the PEMF may also increase the apoptotic rate of osteoclasts, which may also lead to the decrease of bone degradation (Chang et al. 2006). The PEMF is also likely to inhibit the parathyroid hormone (PTH) induced release of the osteoclast activating factor (Luben et al. 1982; Spadaro and Bergstrom 2002), which prevents PTH-induced Ca^{2+} mobilization by inhibiting the resorption of the bone by osteoclasts (Spadaro and Bergstrom 2002). In contrast, stimulation with a PEMF of higher energy may lead to increased osteoclast differentiation (Chang et al. 2003, 2005) and the decreased secretion of the OPG and OPG/RANKL ratio (Chang et al. 2005), resulting in increased osteoclast maturation and increased bone resorption (Fabian et al. 2012).

7.2.3. Effect of PEMF on Osteoblasts

Osteoblasts arise from multipotential mesenchymal (stromal) cells in bone marrow (Chang et al. 2005; Fabian et al. 2009/a) and their primary function is to produce a bone matrix during development, after bone injury, and during normal bone remodeling (Chang et al. 2005; Fabian et al. 2009/a). PEMF exposure likely decreases the rate of proliferation of bone marrow-derived mesenchymal stem cells and speeds up their osteogenic differentiation (Tsai et al. 2009; Jansen et al. 2010) together with a simultaneous increase of OPG/RANKL ratio (Chang et al. 2004/b; Schwartz et al. 2009; Jansen et al. 2010). However these effects may be transitory in nature and may disappear thereafter (Tsai et al. 2009; Jansen et al. 2010) in accordance with the effect of a PEMF on osteoclast maturation (as mentioned above). There is also a transitory stimulatory effect from a PEMF on the proliferation (Diniz et al. 2002; Chang et al. 2004/b; Lin and Lin 2011) and extracellular matrix formation (Diniz et al. 2002; Solazzo et al. 2010) of matured osteoblasts, but notably, this effect also disappears thereafter (Diniz et al. 2002; Chang et al. 2004/b; Lin and Lin 2011). PEMF stimulation also induces the release of a soluble factor from osteoblasts, which significantly increases vascular endothelial proliferation (a major factor of angiogenesis) in a paracrine manner (Hopper et al. 2009).

7.2.4. PEMF Therapy and Peri-Implant Healing

Data in the literature has revealed that bone formation around dental implants, including both bone coverage and osseointegration (Matsumoto et al. 2000; Chan and Bergman 2008; Grana et al. 2008; Fabian et al. 2012), as well as peri-implant soft tissue healing, can be significantly promoted through PEMF treatment. Besides its effect on the osteoclasts and osteoblasts (summarized above), PEMF also promotes angiogenesis (Tepper et al. 2004; Hopper et al. 2009), which is an important factor in peri-implant bone and soft tissue healing

(Fabian et al. 2012). PEMF also improves the wound healing of the gastrointestinal mucosa (Mentes et al. 1996) and the skin (Patino et al. 1996; Scardino et al. 1998); therefore it may be hypothesized that PEMF improves the formation of the implanto-gingival complex (Fabian et al. 2012). This is especially likely because PEMF stimulation seems to have a significant effect on fibroblasts (Satake et al. 1990) and increases the release of their local factors, including those influencing cell attachment and the spreading of both periodontal ligament fibroblasts and osteoblasts (Kim 1990). Further, PEMF reverses the proliferative defects of lymphocytes in aged subjects (Cossarizza et al. 1989/a, b) and induces the expression (and consequent release) of immune activator/modulator HSP70/HSPA-type stress proteins (Goodman and Blank 1998; Heredia-Rojas et al. 2010) that are likely to improve proper bone (Fabian et al. 2009/a, b) and mucosal healing (Fabian et al. 2003, 2007, 2009/b, 2011) around the implants (Fabian et al. 2012).

Since a PEMF decreases the rate of residual ridge resorption following tooth extraction (Ortman et al. 1992), it is likely that a PEMF improves the peri-implant healing of implants inserted immediately into extraction sites (Fabian et al. 2012). Besides this, a PEMF may also be used advantageously for the acceleration of bone healing following advanced implant surgery (Fabian et al. 2012). PEMF treatment enhances the healing of osteotomy gaps (Pienkowski et al. 1992; Darendelier et al. 1997; Fredericks et al. 2000; Inoue et al. 2002; Grana et al. 2008) and accelerates bone formation and the total recovery of bone tissue in bone defects filled with hydroxyapatite (Ottani et al. 2002) or with a demineralized bone matrix (Takano-Yamamoto et al. 1992). Similarly, a PEMF can also accelerate bone graft incorporation (Kold et al. 1987). Further, a PEMF accelerates the consolidation of regenerate bone during distraction osteogenesis (Fredericks et al. 2003) and accelerates the healing of both fresh (Grace et al. 1998) and ununited bone fractures (Gossling et al. 1992). PEMFs also alleviate postoperative pain (Heden and Pilla 2008; Strauch et al. 2009) and decrease postoperative edema (Strauch et al. 2009), which could also be rather advantageous following implant surgery (Fabian et al. 2012). Further, a PEMF also improves the regeneration of injured nerves (Raji and Bowden 1983; Raji 1984; Zienowicz et al. 1991; Kanje et al. 1993).

It is likely that the energy value of PEMF stimulation as well as the pattern of waveform characteristics, including the shape and amplitude of the bursts, the pulse frequency of the bursts, the duration of the bursts, and the length of burst on-off periods (burst on-off frequency) are rather important factors with regard to the PEMF-induced promotion of bone healing (Leisner et al. 2002; Midura et al. 2005; Fabian et al. 2012). It is also likely that the high-amplitude narrow-pulse portions of PEMF stimulation are especially advantageous in producing a beneficial bone response (Pienkowski et al. 1992); whereas the symmetry/asymmetry relations of the stimulus pulse waveform may be of less importance (Pienkowski et al. 1992). Further, low values (15 Hz) of burst on-off frequencies seem to be more efficient than high values (50–150 Hz) of burst on-off frequencies (Rubin et al. 1993); although higher burst on-off frequencies also promote bone healing significantly (Rubin et al. 1993; Matsumoto et al. 2000). Moreover, low energy fields 0.2–0.3 mT (Matsumoto et al. 2000) seem to be more efficient than high energy fields 0.8 mT (Matsumoto et al. 2000) in promoting bone healing procedures (Rubin et al. 1993; Matsumoto et al. 2000; Fabian et al. 2012). The authors' own experiences indicate that PEMF stimulation with very low energy fields (0.05–0.1 mT) also appears to be promising for clinical use (Fabian et al. 2012).

In general, daily PEMF exposure of 1 to 2 hours may be recommended (Fabian et al. 2012) based on the scientific literature: 2 x 30 min. (Grana et al. 2008), 1 hour (Fredericks et al. 2000; Inoue et al. 2002), or 2 hours (Chan and Bergman 2008). However, the authors' own experiences have indicated that PEMF stimulation of 10–15 minutes three times a week also appears to be promising for clinical use (Fabian et al. 2012). Although stimulations during the first two weeks after surgery seem to be the most efficient (Matsumoto et al. 2000), the later phases of bone healing (even 4–8 weeks after surgery) may also be accelerated with PEMF administration (Inoue et al. 2002; Chan and Bergman 2008), leading to somewhat greater new bone formation, an increased mineral apposition rate, and the decreased porosity of the cortex adjacent to the healing area (Inoue et al. 2002).

7.2.5. PEMF Therapy and Peri-Implant Bone Remodeling

Bone is remodeled continuously throughout life through the resorption of old bone by osteoclasts and the subsequent formation of new bone by osteoblasts (Chang et al. 2004/a; Fabian et al. 2009/a; Fabian et al. 2012); these two events are tightly coupled to each other and are responsible for the renewal of bone while maintaining its anatomical and structural integrity (Chang et al. 2004/a; Fabian et al. 2009/a; Fabian et al. 2012). As indicated above, PEMF stimulation with low energy fields usually leads to the suppression of osteoclast function (Chang et al. 2003, 2005), which may be advantageous in the acceleration of early phase peri-implant bone healing (Rubin et al. 1993; Matsumoto et al. 2000; Fabian et al. 2012). However, stimulation with a PEMF of higher energy (Chang et al. 2003, 2005) and/or with certain specific patterns of PEMF waveform characteristics (Leisner et al. 2002; Midura et al. 2005) may speed up osteoclast function and bone remodeling (Fabian et al. 2012). It may also lead to increased osteoclast differentiation (Stark and Sinclair 1987; Chang et al. 2003, 2005), coupled with an increased proinflammatory cytokine (TNF-α, IL-1β) production (Chang et al. 2003) and a decreased secretion of OPG and of the OPG/RANKL ratio (Chang et al. 2005), which are likely to stimulate osteoclast function and bone remodeling (Fabian et al. 2009/a; Fabian et al. 2012). This is especially true if the premised PEMF stimulation that induces a moderate increase of osteoclast function is coupled with a somewhat more increased osteoblast function (Fabian and Fejerdy 2010; Fabian et al. 2012), as can be seen clearly in the case of PEMF-accelerated orthodontic tooth movement and coupled periodontal processes (Stark and Sinclair 1987; Kim 1990; Satake et al. 1990; Chen 1991; Darendeliler et al. 1995, 2007; Showkatbakhsh et al. 2010). This kind of accelerated bone remodeling may be of clinical importance in relation to the later phases of peri-implant healing and to the improvement of bone remodeling around the implants after their loading with masticatory forces.

7.3. Low Level Laser (Soft Laser) Therapy

7.3.1. General Considerations

Laser light is unique in that it is monochromatic (i.e. light of one specific wavelength), directional (i.e. has low divergence), and coherent (i.e. wave-synchronized). Clinical applications of lasers are largely divided into high level laser (HLL) therapy (HLLT) and low level laser (LLL) therapy. In general, HLLT is useful for cutting biologic materials and producing coagulation necrosis in target tissues with a subsequent reaction in the surrounding tissues; whereas LLLT provides photobiological and photochemical effects (Naka and Yokose 2012). Thus low level laser therapy (also referred to as "soft laser therapy") is a treatment with athermic low power lasers (Fabian and Fejerdy 2010; Beck et al. 2012).

There are many different types of low level lasers may be used for LLLT, including either pulsed or continuous LLLs with wavelengths in both the visible and invisible range (Khullar et al. 1995; Kimura et al. 2000; Fabian and Fejerdy 2010; Beck et al. 2012; Elavarasu et al. 2012). The most commonly used laser types are the HeNe laser (wavelength: 632 nm), Ar laser (wavelength: 514 nm), GaAlAs laser (wavelengths: 780, 830, or 900 nm), ruby laser (wavelength: 694 nm), Nd:YAG laser (wavelength: 1060 nm) ErCr:YSGG laser (wavelength: 2780 nm), and the CO_2 laser (wavelength: 10600 nm) (Khullar et al. 1995; Kimura et al. 2000; Fabian and Fejerdy 2010; Gomez-Santos et al. 2010). Although the usual output power of CO_2 lasers (Kimura et al. 2000), Nd:YAG lasers (Kimura et al. 2000), ErCr:YSGG lasers (Gomez-Santos et al. 2010), and Ar lasers is mostly at the middle level or higher (therefore these lasers are typically not referred to as "low level lasers"), they may be used at a lower level output power suitable for LLLT as well (Fabian and Fejerdy 2010; Naka and Yokose 2012).

Although the biological mechanisms behind the effect of the low level laser stimulation is far from fully understood, in general, an increase of cell metabolism, collagen synthesis, and activity from immune cells are the most important pathways behind the efficiency of low level laser therapy (Qadri et al. 2005). Besides, these LLLTs also stimulate osteoblastic differentiation (Petri et al. 2010). Further, LLLT also induces the long-lasting expression of HSP70-/HSPA-type stress proteins (Souil et al. 2001). There is also a prominent placebo effect coupled with low laser therapy (Kimura et al. 2000; Payer et al. 2005). Notably, it is very likely that both the wavelength (of a laser) and the cell type (of the irradiated tissue) significantly influence its biological effect (Moore et al. 2005). Therefore, it is no wonder that there is still controversy regarding which wavelength would be the most appropriate for various orofacial applications (Khullar et al. 1995; Fabian et al. 2010).

7.3.2. LLLT and Peri-Implant Healing

LLLT may be used to improve both implant-tissue interaction in the bone (Khadra 2005; Kim et al. 2007; Lopes et al. 2007) and the interaction at the implant-soft tissue interface (Khadra et al. 2005/a, b; Schwarz et al. 2005). LLLT may facilitate bone metabolism during bone healing at the sites of deproteinized bone grafts (Kim et al. 2009) and bone defects filled with hydroxyapatite (Pinheiro et al. 2009) or enamel matrix protein derivatives (Ozcelik et al. 2008/a). LLLT may also be used to facilitate bone remodeling, as is obvious in relation to the facilitation of orthodontic tooth movement and related alveolar bone remodeling (Kawasaki and Shimizu 2000; Fujita et al. 2008; Kim et al. 2010). LLLT may also be used advantageously to control periodontal inflammation (Qadri et al. 2005; de Almeida et al. 2008; Schwarz et al. 2008) and more severe inflammatory and/or necrotizing bone pathologies (Vescovi et al. 2008).

Besides its advantageous effect in the bone, LLLT improves postsurgical trismus and facial swelling (Aras and Gungormus 2010) and may also be used to improve the functional recovery of injured peripheral nerves (Khullar et al. 1995; Ozen et al. 2006). LLLT also accelerates oral wound healing (Neiburger 1999; Amorim et al. 2006; Ozcelik et al. 2008/b) as well as the healing of oral ulcerations (Sharon-Buller and Sela 2004; Navarro et al. 2007).

LLLT may also be used to treat several orofacial pain manifestations, like myofascial pain (de Medeiros et al. 2005; Shirani et al. 2009), temporomandibular joint pain (Dahlstrom 1992; Mazzetto et al. 2007), and other TMD (temporomandibular disorder) symptoms (Carrasco et al. 2008) as well as the dentinal hypersensitivity of exposed dentin (Gerschman et al. 1994; Kimura et al. 2000; Pesevska et al. 2010). Although these applications are not closely related to peri-implant healing, they may be significant in the case of the implant treatment of problem patients and/or patients with strongly compromised oral health.

7.3.3. LLLT and Peri-Implantitis

Peri-implantitis can be understood as an inflammatory process affecting the tissues around an osseointegrated implant that is associated with the suppuration of deepened pockets and the loss of supporting marginal bone (Lindhe and Meyle 2008; Marotti et al. 2013). The treatment of this condition includes the elimination of bacterial biofilm (plaque) and calculus, the decontamination of the implant surface, and guided tissue/bone regeneration (Marotti et al. 2013). The effective decontamination of titanium surfaces is a crucial and rather difficult step, which may be carried out by mechanical cleaning (i.e. dental curettes, ultrasonic scalers, air flow glycine-powdering) and/or by means of chemical procedures (i.e. citric acid, H_2O_2, chlorhexidine digluconate, EDTA), and may be supplemented with local or systemic antibiotics (Marotti et al. 2013). Higher energy lasers may also be used advantageously based on their hemostatic, selective calculus ablative, and bactericidal properties (Marotti et al. 2013); however high level lasers can promote an undesirable increase in temperature (Gomez-Santos et al. 2010; Geminiani et al. 2012). To overcome this weakness, an alternative approach may be photodynamic therapy (PDT) carried out by means of LLLT combined with a suitable photosensitizer dye in the presence of oxygen (Takasaki et al. 2009; Marotti et al. 2013). With the use of roughly a 30 mW energy LLL (660 nm, continuous) for 3–5 min. in the frame of PDT, efficient decontamination can be obtained (Marotti et al. 2013) based on the principle that a photosensitizer binds to bacteria, and when irradiated (with a LLL) in the presence of oxygen, it undergoes a transition to an excited singlet state, leading to the production of singlet oxygen and other very reactive products that are toxic to bacteria (Takasaki et al. 2009; Marotti et al. 2013).

Although this chapter focuses on low level laser applications and how the premised LLL-based photodynamic therapy may overcome the problem of temperature rise, for the sake of comparison, it may be mentioned that somewhat higher (1.5–2 W) energy laser applications frequently used in the treatment of peri-implantitis may lead to the significant heating of the implants (Gomez-Santos et al. 2010; Geminiani et al. 2012). An *in vitro* study revealed that the irradiation of implants with a 2 W energy (810 nm or 980 nm, continuous) lasers can induce a 10°C increase in the temperature of implants within 10–20 sec. (Geminiani et al. 2012); and the rise of implant temperature could reach 30°C–40°C after 60 sec. of irradiation (Geminiani et al. 2012). A temperature rise of more than 10°C can compromise bone vitality (Erikson and Albrektsson 1983; Gomez-Santos et al. 2010; Geminiani et al. 2012); therefore, great care should be taken if such laser therapies are used even if the rise of temperature seems to be somewhat slower *in vivo* (Gomez-Santos et al. 2010). Similarly, great care should be taken regarding temperature rise if higher energy lasers, i.e. 4–10 W CO_2 lasers (Gomez-Santos et al. 2010; Lambrecht et al. 2012), are used to expose implants after the osseointegration/incorporation phase (Lambrecht et al. 2012). A water spray applied to the sealing cap or coronal zone of the implants may be used as an efficient refrigerator in such cases (Gomez-Santos et al. 2010).

7.4. Contraindications

There are some general safety considerations that should be considered before using any kind of physiotherapy (Fabian and Fejerdy 2010; Fabian et al. 2012). In general, physiotherapy should not be used in the case of patients with any severe systemic diseases or with strongly compromised health (Fabian and Fejerdy 2010; Fabian et al. 2012). In the case of such patients, the use of physiotherapy should be avoided in the absence of a clear agreement with the medical professional(s) responsible for the treatment of the systemic disease(s) at issue and/or responsible for the medical care of the individual with strongly compromised health (Fabian and Fejerdy 2010; Fabian et al. 2012). Similarly, physiotherapy is usually contraindicated in the cases of patients with any hemorrhagic diathesis, precancerosis, or malignancy as well as in the case of patients having any oncologic treatment in the anamnesis (at least in the absence of a clear agreement with the oncologist or other responsible medical professional) (Fabian and Fejerdy 2010; Fabian et al. 2012).

Importantly, the use of *any* physiotherapy should be *strictly* avoided near to a nevus (Fabian and Fejerdy 2010; Fabian et al. 2012). In the absence of clear evidence concerning their innocuousness, several forms of physiotherapy may be contraindicated for patients with a pacemaker or with another implanted electric instrument (Fabian and Fejerdy 2010; Fabian et al. 2012). Similarly, physiotherapeutic treatment should be avoided near the ear, eye, brain, or spinal cord (i.e. temporal or paravertebral use) in the absence of clear evidence about the innocuousness of the chosen treatment modality. Those modalities utilizing electric impulses or irradiative energy with a significant heat generating effect like laser or ultrasound (the latter is not discussed in this chapter) should be considered in this respect (Fabian and Fejerdy 2010; Fabian et al. 2012). Certain forms of physiotherapies are also contraindicated for patients with any implants, including dental implants (Fabian and Fejerdy 2010; Fabian et al. 2012), but these kinds of physicotherapies will not be discussed in this chapter.

Besides the premised general considerations, the use of a PEMF should also be avoided in the condylar area during the growth period (Wilmot et al. 1993). The use of a PEMF *may* also be contraindicated for patients with a pacemaker, especially in the case of unipolar electrode configuration (Gwechenberger et al. 2006), or with any other implanted electric instruments (Gwechenberger et al. 2006; Fabian and Fejerdy 2010; Fabian et al. 2012); therefore, its use should be avoided in the absence of clear evidence about its innocuousness (Fabian et al. 2012).

In the case of low level laser therapy, the eyes (of both the patient and the therapist) should be defended properly. In the case of higher energy lasers, applications near the ear, eye, brain, or spinal cord (i.e. temporal or paravertebral use) should also be avoided (Fabian and Fejerdy 2010; Fabian et al. 2012); however higher level laser applications are not discussed in this chapter in further detail.

Conclusion

Physiotherapies have been found to be beneficial for a wide variety of therapeutic processes over the last few decades. Data in the literature revealed that bone formation and soft tissue healing around dental implants can be significantly promoted through physiotherapeutic treatment (Fabian and Fejerdy 2010; Fabian et al. 2012). Although various modalities of physiotherapy have been found to be beneficial for a wide variety of therapeutic processes in implant dentistry (Fabian and Fejerdy 2010; Fabian et al. 2012), the exact mechanisms by which they affect alveolar bone and other peri-implant tissues are still not fully understood. However, certain mechanisms have already been recognized and the increased amount of knowledge may be utilized for clinical practice (Fabian and Fejerdy 2010; Fabian et al. 2012). Although physiotherapies in general can be seen as noninvasive tools, the few contraindications related to their use should be considered carefully for safe and successful implementation.

References

Amorim, JC; de Sousa, GR; de Barros Silveira, L; Prates, RA, Pinotti, M; Ribeiro, MS. Clinical study of the gingiva healing after gingivectomy and low-level laser therapy. *Photomed Laser Surg*, 2006, 24, 588–594.

Aras, MH; Gungormus, M. Placebo-controlled randomized clinical trial of the effect of two different low-level laser therapies (LLLT) - intraoral and extraoral - on trismus and facial swelling following surgical extraction of the lower third molar. *Lasers Med Sci*, 2010, 25, 641–645.

Balcavage, W; Alvager, T; Swez, J; Goff, C; Fox, M; Abdullyava, S; King, M. A mechanism for action of extremely low frequency electromagnetic fields on biological systems. *Biochem Biophys Res Communication*, 1996, 222 (suppl.), 374–378.

Barnaba, SA; Ruzzini, L; Di Martino, A; Lanotte, A; Sgambato, A; Denaro, V. Clinical significance of different effects of static and pulsed electromagnetic fields on human osteoclast cultures. *Rheumatol Int*, 2012, 32, 1025–1031.

Beck, A; Varga, G; Hermann, P; Fabian, G; Fejerdy, P; Fabian, TK. Methods for the treatment of denture induced psychogenic symptoms. In: Fabian TK, Fejerdy P, Hermann P, editors. *Dentures. Types, benefits and potential complications.* New York: Nova Science Publishers, 2012, 165–197.

Blanchard, J; Blackman, CF. Clarification and application of an ion parametric resonance model for magnetic field interactions with biological systems. *Bioelectromagnetics*, 1994, 15, 205–216.

Blank, M. Na/K-adenosine-triphosphatase. *Adv Chem*, 1995, 250, 339–348.

Blank, M; Goodman, R. Do electromagnetic fields interact directly with DNA? *Bioelectromagnetics*, 1997, 18, 111–115.

Cankaya, AB; Erdem, MA; Erdem, AP; Erguven, M; Aybar, B; Kasapoglu, C; Bilir, A. Evaluation of light-emitting diode (LED-660 nm) application over primary osteoblast-like cells on titanium surfaces: An in vitro study. *Int J Med Sci*, 2011, 8, 584–593.

Carrasco, TG; Mazzeto, MO; Mazzetto, RG; Mestriner Jr., W. Low intensity laser therapy in temporomandibular disorder: a phase II double-blind study. *Cranio*, 2008, 26, 274–281.

Chan, AY; Bergman, H. Performance verification of a prototype non-invasive intra-oral bone growth stimulator for titanium dental implants. *Conf Proc IEEE Eng Med Biol Soc*, 2008, 5624–5627.

Chang, K; Chang, WHS; Wu, ML; Shih, C. Effects of different intensities of extremely low frequency pulsed electromagnetic fields on formation of osteoclast-like cells. *Bioelectromagnetics*, 2003, 24, 431–439.

Chang, K; Chang, WHS; Yu, YH; Shih, C. Pulsed electromagnetic field stimulation of bone marrow cells derived from ovariectomized rats affects osteoclast formation and local factor production. *Bioelectromagnetics*, 2004/a, 25, 134–141.

Chang, WHS, Chen LT; Sun, JS; Lin, FH. Effect of pulse-burst electromagnetic field stimulation on osteoblast cell activities. *Bioelectromagnetics*, 2004/b, 25, 457–465.

Chang, K; Chang, WHS; Huang, S; Huang, S; Shih, C. Pulsed electromagnetic fields stimulation affects osteoclast formation by modulation of osteoprotegerin, RANK ligand and macrophage colony-stimulating factor. *J Orthop Res*, 2005, 23, 1308–1314.

Chang, K; Chang, WHS; Tsai, MT; Shih, C. Pulsed electromagnetic fields accelerate apoptotic rate in osteoclasts. *Connect Tissue Res*, 2006, 47, 222–228.

Chen, Q. Effect of pulsed electromagnetic field on orthodontic tooth movement through transmission electronmicroscopy. *Zhonghua Kou Quiang Yi Xue Za Zhi*, 1991, 26, 7–10, 61.

Cossarizza, A; Monti, D; Bersani, F; Cantini, M; Cadossi, R; Sacchi, A; Franceschi, C. Extremely low frequency pulsed electromagnetic fields increase cell proliferation in lymphocytes from young and aged subjects. *Biochem Biophys Res Commun*, 1989/a, 160, 692–698.

Cossarizza, A; Monti, D; Bersani, F; Paganelli, R; Montagnani, G; Cadossi, R; Cantini, M; Franceschi, C. Extremely low frequency pulsed electromagnetic fields increase interleukin-2 (IL-2) utilization and IL-2 receptor expression in mitogen-stimulated human lymphocytes from old subjects. *FEBS Lett*, 1989/b, 248, 141–144.

Dahlstrom, L. Conservative treatment methods in craniomandibular disorder. *Swed Dent J*, 1992, 16, 217–230.

Darendeliler, MA; Sinclair, PM; Kusy, RP. The effects of samarium-cobalt magnets and pulsed electromagnetic fields on tooth movement. *Am J Orthod Dentofacial Orthop*, 1995, 107, 578–588.

Darendelier, MA; Darendelier, A; Sinclair, PM. Effects of static magnetic and pulsed electromagnetic fields on bone healing. *Int J Adult Orthodont Orthognath Surg*, 1997, 12, 43–53.

Darendelier, MA; Zea, A; Shen, G; Zoellner, H. Effects of pulsed electromagnetic field vibration on tooth movement induced by magnetic and mechanical forces: a preliminary study. *Australian Dent J*, 2007, 52, 282–287.

Ding, Y; Li, G; Ao, J; Zhou, L; Ma, Q; Liu, Y. 99m Technetium-methylene disphosphonate bone imaging using low-intensity pulsed ultrasound: promotion of bone formation during mandibular distraction osteogenesis in dogs. *Br J Oral Maxillofac Surg*, 2010, 48, 94–99.

Diniz, P; Shomura, K; Soejima, K; Ito, G. Effects of pulsed electromagnetic field (PEMF) stimulation on bone tissue like formation are dependent on the maturation stages of the osteoblasts. *Bioelectromagnetics*, 2002, 23, 398–405.

de Almeida, JM; Theodoro, LH; Bosco, AF; Nagata, MJH; Oshiiwa, M; Garcia, VG. In vivo effect of photodynamic therapy on periodontal bone loss in dental furcations. *J Periodontol*, 2008, 79, 1081–1088.

de Medeiros, JS; Vieira, GF; Nishimura, PY. Laser application effects on the bite strength of the masseter muscle, as an orofacial pain treatment. *Photomed Laser Surg*, 2005, 23, 373–376.

Elavarasu, S; Naveen, D; Thangavelu, A. Lasers in periodontics. *J Pharm Bioallied Sci*, 2012, 4, S260–S263.

Eriksson, AR; Albrektsson, T. Temperature threshold levels for heat-induced bone tissue injury: a vital-microscopic study in the rabbit. *J Prosthet Dent*, 1983, 50, 101–107.

Fabian, TK; Gaspar, J; Fejerdy, L; Kaan, B; Balint, M; Csermely, P; Fejerdy, P. Hsp70 is present in human saliva. *Med Sci Monit*, 2003, 9, BR62–65.

Fabian, TK; Fejerdy, P; Nguyen, MT; Soti, C; Csermely, P. Potential immunological functions of salivary Hsp70 in mucosal and periodontal defense mechanisms. *Arch Immunol Ther Exp*, 2007, 55, 91–98.

Fabian, TK; Csermely, P; Fabian, G; Fejerdy, P. Spondyloarthropathies and bone resorption: A possible role of heat shock protein (Hsp70). (Review). *Acta Physiol Hungarica*, 2009/a, 96, 149–155.

Fabian, TK; Gotai, L; Beck, A; Fabian, G; Fejerdy, P. The role of molecular chaperones (HSPAs/HSP70s) in oral health and oral inflammatory diseases. A review. *Eur J Inflammation*, 2009/b, 7, 53–61.

Fabian, TK; Fejerdy P. *Psychogenic denture intolerance. Theoretical background, prevention and treatment possibilities*. New York: Nova Science Publishers, 2010, 162–170.

Fabian, TK; Soti, C; Nguyen, MT; Csermely, P; Fejerdy, P. Expected functions of salivary HSP70 in the oral cavity. In: Berhardt LV editor. *Advances in Medicine and Biology*. Vol. 19. New York: Nova Science Publishers, 2011, 289–308.

Fabian, TK; Beck, A; Fabian, G; Fejerdy, P; Hermann, P. Pulsed electromagnetic field (PEMF) therapy for peri-implant healing and bone remodeling. In: Fabian TK, Fejerdy P, Hermann P, editors. *Dentures. Types, benefits and potential complications*. New York: Nova Science Publishers, 2012, 243–254.

Fujita, S; Yamaguchi, M; Utsunomiya, T; Yamamoto, H; Kasai, K. Low-energy laser stimulates tooth movement velocity via expression of RANK and RANKL. *Orthod Craniofac Res*, 2008, 11, 143–155.

Fredericks, DC; Nepola, JV; Baker, JT; Abbott, J; Simon, B. Effects of pulsed electromagnetic fields on bone healing in a rabbit tibial osteotomy model. *J Orthop Trauma*, 2000, 14, 93–100.

Fredericks, DC; Piehl, DJ; Baker, JT; Abbott, J; Nepola, JV. Effects of pulsed electromagnetic field stimulation on distraction osteogenesis in the rabbit tibial leg lengthening model. *J Pediatr Orthop*, 2003 23, 478–483.

Geminiani, A; Caton, JG; Romanos, GE. Temperature change during non-contact diode laser irradiation of implant surfaces. *Laser Med Sci*, 2012, 27, 339–342.

Gerschman, JA; Ruben, J; Gebart-Eaglemont, J. Low level laser therapy for dentinal tooth hypersensitivity. *Australian Dent J*, 1994, 39, 353–357.

Gittens, RA; Olivares-Navarrete, R; Tannenbaum, R; Boyan, BD; Schwartz, Z. Electrical implications of corrosion for osseointegration of titanium implants. *J Dent Res*, 2011, 90, 1389–1397.

Gomez-Santos, L; Arnabat-Dominguez, J; Sierra-Rebolledo, A; Gay-Escoda, C. Thermal increment due to ErCr: YSGG and CO_2 laser irradiation of different implant surfaces. A pilot study. *Med Oral Patol Oral Cir Bucal*, 2010, 15, e782–787.

Gossling, HR; Bernstein, RA; Abbott, J. Treatment of ununited tibial fractures: a comparison of surgery and pulsed electromagnetic fields (PEMF). *Orthopedics*, 1992, 15, 711–719.

Goodman, R; Blank, M. Magnetic field stress induces expression of hsp70. *Cell Stress & Chaperones*, 1998, 3, 79–88.

Goodman, EM; Greenbaum, B; Marron, MT. Altered protein synthesis in a cell-free system exposed to a sinusoidal magnetic field. *Biochim Biophys Acta*, 1993, 1202, 107–112.

Grace, KL; Revell, WJ; Brookes, M. The effects of pulsed electromagnetism on fresh fracture healing: osteochondral repair in the rat femoral groove. *Orthopedics*, 1998, 21, 297–302.

Grana, DR; Marcos, HJ; Kokubu, GA. Pulsed electromagnetic fields as adjuvant therapy in bone healing and peri-implant bone formation: an experimental study in rats. *Acta Odontol Latinoam*, 2008, 21, 77–83.

Gwechenberger, M; Rauscha, F; Stix, G; Schmid, G; Strametz-Juranek, J. Interference of programmed electromagnetic stimulation with pacemakers and automatic implantable cardioverter defibrillators. *Bioelectromagnetics*, 2006, 27, 365–377.

Heden, P; Pilla, AA. Effects of pulsed electromagnetic fields on postoperative pain: A double-blind randomized pilot study in breast augmentation patients. *Aesth Plast Surg*, 2008, 32, 660–666.

Heredia-Rojas, JA; de la Fuente, AOR; Gonzalez, JMA; Rodriguez-Flores, LE; Rodriguez-Padilla, C; Santoyo-Stephano, MA; Castaneda-Graza, E; Tamez-Guerrra, RS. Effect of 60 Hz magnetic fields on the activation of hsp70 promoter in cultured INER-37 and RMA E7 cells. *In Vitro Cell Dev Biol – Animal*, 2010, 46, 758–763.

Hopper, RA; VerHalen, JP; Tepper, O; Mehrara, BJ; Detch, R; Chang, EI; Baharestani, S; Simon, BJ; Gurtner, GC. Osteoblasts stimulated with pulsed electromagnetic fields increase HUVEC proliferation via a VEGF-A independent mechanism. *Bioelectromagnetics*, 2009, 30, 189–197.

Inoue, N; Ohnishi, I; Chen, D; Deitz, LW; Schwardt, JD; Chao, EY. Effect of pulsed electromagnetic fields (PEMF) on late-phase osteotomy gap healing in a canine tibial model. *J Orthop Res*, 2002, 20, 1106–1114.

Jansen, JHW; van der Jagt, OP; Punt, BJ; Verhaar, JAN; van Leeuwen, JPTM; Weinans, H; Jahr, H. Stimulation of osteogenic differentiation in human osteoprogenitor cells by pulsed electromagnetic fields: an in vitro study. *BMC Musculoskeletal Disorders*, 2010, 11, 188.

Kanje, M; Rusovan, A; Sisken, B; Lundborg, G. Pretreatment of rats with pulsed electromagnetic fields enhances regeneration of the sciatic nerve. *Bioelectromagnetics*, 1993, 14, 353–359.

Kawasaki, K; Shimizu, N. Effects of low-energy laser irradiation on bone remodeling during experimental tooth movement in rats. *Lasers Surg Med*, 2000, 26, 282–291.

Khadra, M. The effect of low level laser irradiation on implant-tissue interaction. In vivo and in vitro studies. *Swed Dent J Suppl*, 2005, 172, 1–63.

Khadra, M; Kasem, N; Lyngstadaas, SP; Haanæs HR; Mustafa, K. Laser therapy accelerates initial attachment and subsequent behavior of human fibroblasts cultured on titanium implant material. *Clin Oral Impl Res*, 2005/a, 16, 168–175.

Khadra, M; Lyngstadaas, SP; Hans, R; Haanæs, Mustafa, K. Effect of laser therapy on attachment, proliferation and differentiation of human osteoblast-like cells cultures on titanium implant material. *Biomaterials*, 2005/b, 26, 3503–3509.

Khullar, SM; Brodin, P; Messelt, EB; Haanæs, HR. The effects of low level laser treatment on recovery of nerve conduction and motor function after compression injury in the rat sciatic nerve. *Eur J Oral Sci*, 1995, 103, 299–305.

Kim, KT. Biochemical study of human periodontal ligament: preparation of cell attachment materials induced by pulsed electromagnetic fields. *Bull Kanagawa Dent Coll*, 1990, 18, 89–98.

Kim, SH; Hong, KS. Histologic evaluation of low-intensity pulsed ultrasound effects on bone regeneration in sinus lift. *J Periodontal Implant Sci*, 2010, 40, 271–275.

Kim, YD; Kim, SS; Hwang, DS; Kim, SG; Kwon, YH; Shin, SH; Kim, UK; Kim, JR; Chung, IK. Effect of low-level laser treatment after installation of dental titanium implant - immunohystochemical study of RANKL, RANK, OPG: an experimental study in rats. *Lasers Surg Med*, 2007, 39, 441–450.

Kim, YD; Song, WW; Kim, SS; Kim, GC; Hwang, DS; Shin, SH; Kim, UK; Kim, JR; Chung, IK. Expression of receptor activator of nuclear factor -κB ligand, receptor activator of nuclear factor -κB, and osteoprotegerin, following low-level laser treatment on deproteinized bovine bone graft in rats. *Lasers Med Sci*, 2009, 24, 577–84.

Kim, YD; Kim, SS; Kim, SJ; Kwon, DW; Jeon, ES; Son, WS. Low-level laser irradiation facilitates fibronectin and collagen type I turnover during tooth movement in rats. *Lasers Med Sci*, 2010, 25, 25–31.

Kimura, Y; Wilder-Smith, P; Yonaga, K; Matsumoto, K. Treatment of dentine hypersensitivity by lasers: a review. *J Clin Periodontol*, 2000, 27, 715–721.

Kold, SE; Hickman, J; Meisen, F. Preliminary study of quantitative aspects and the effect of pulsed electromagnetic field treatment on the incorporation of equine cancellous bone grafts. *Equine Vet J*, 1987, 19, 120–124.

Lambrecht, JT; Nyffeler, T; Linder, M. Thermal conduction of titanium implants under CO_2 laser irradiation in vitro. *Ann Maxillofac Surg*, 2012, 2, 12–16.

Lednev, VV. Possible mechanism for influence of weak magnetic fields on biosystems. *Bioelectromagnetics*, 1991, 12, 71–76.

Leisner, S; Shahar, R; Aizenberg, I; Lichovsky, D; Levin-Harrus, T. The effect of short-duration, high-intensity electromagnetic pulses on fresh ulnar fractures in rats. *J Vet Med*, 2002, 49, 33–37.

Liboff, AR; Rozek, RJ; Sherman, ML; McLeod, BR; Smith, SD. Ca^{2+} cyclotron resonance in human lymphocytes. *J Bioelectricity*, 1987, 6, 12–22.

Lin, HY; Lin, YJ. In vitro effects of low frequency electromagnetic fields on osteoblast proliferation and maturation in an inflammatory environment. *Bioelectromagnetics*, 2011, 32, 552–560.

Lindhe, J; Meyle, J; Peri-implant diseases: consensus report of the Sixth European Workshop on Periodontology. *J Clin Periodontol*, 2008, 35, 282–285.

Lohmann, CH; Schwartz, Z; Liu, Y; Li, Z; Simon, BJ; Sylvia, VL; Dean, DD; Bonewald, LF; Donahue, HJ; Boyan, BD. Pulsed electromagnetic fields affect phenotype and connexin 43 protein expression in MLO-Y4 osteocyte-like cells and ROS 17/2.8 osteoblast like cells. *J Orthop Res*, 2003, 21, 326–334.

Lopes, CB; Pinheiro, AL; Sathaiah, S; Da Silva, NS; Salgado, MA. Infrared laser photobiomodulation (lambda 830 nm) on bone tissue around dental implants: a Raman spectroscopy and scanning electronic microscopy study in rabbits. *Photomed Laser Surg*, 2007, 25, 96–101.

Luben, RA; Cain, CD; Chen, MCY; Rosen, DM; Adey, WR. Effects of electromagnetic stimuli on bone and bone cells in vitro: Inhibition of responses to parathyroid hormone by low-energy low-frequency fields. *Proc Natl Acad Sci USA*, 1982 79, 4180–4184.

Marotti, J; Tortamano, P; Cai, S; Ribeiro, MS; Franco, JEM; de Campos, TT. Decontamination of dental implant surfaces by means of photodynamic therapy. *Lasers Med Sci*, 2013, 28, 303–309.

Matsumoto, H; Ochi, M; Abiko, Y; Hirose, Y; Kaku, T; Sakaguchi, K. Pulsed electromagnetic fields promote bone formation around dental implants inserted into the femur of rabbits. *Clin Oral Implant Res*, 2000, 11, 354–360.

Mazzetto, MO; Carrasco, TG; Bidinelo, EF; de Andrade Pizzo, RC; Mazzetto, RG. Low intensity laser application in temporomandibular disorders: a phase I double-blind study. *Cranio*, 2007, 25, 186–192.

McClellan, JA; Boublikova, P; Palcek, E; Lilley, DMJ. Superhelical torsion in cellular DNA responds directly to environmental and genetic factors. *Proc Natl Acad Sci USA*, 1990, 87, 8373–8377.

Mentes, BB; Tascilar, O; Tatlicioglu, E; Bor, MV; Isman, F; Turkozkan, N; Celebi, M. Influence of pulsed electromagnetic fields on healing of experimental colonic anastomosis. *Dis Colon Rectum*, 1996, 39, 1031–1038.

Midura, RJ; Ibiwoye, MO; Powell, KA; Sakai, Y; Doehring, T; Grabiner, MD; Patterson, TE; Zborowski, M; Wolfman, A. Pulsed electromagnetic field treatments enhance the healing of fibular osteotomies. *J Orthop Res*, 2005, 23, 1035–1046.

Mohn, D; Zehnder, M; Stark, WJ; Imfeld, T. Electrochemical disinfection of dental implants – a proof of concept. *PLoS ONE*, 2011, 6, e16157.

Moore, P; Ridgway, TD; Higbee, RG; Howard, EW; Lucroy, MD. Effect of wavelength on low-intensity laser irradiation-stimulated cell proliferation in vitro. *Lasers Surg Med*, 2005, 36, 8–12.

Naka, T; Yokose, S. Application of laser-induced bone therapy by carbon dioxide laser irradiation in implant therapy. *Int J Dentistry*, 2012, Article ID: 409496. DOI: 10.1155/2012/409496.

Navarro, R; Marquezan, M; Cerqueira, DF; Silveira, BL; Correa, MS. Low-level-laser therapy as an alternative treatment for primary herpes simplex infection: a case report. *J Clin Pediatr Dent*, 2007, 31, 225–228.

Neiburger, EJ. Rapid healing of gingival incisions by helium-neon diode laser. *J Mass Dent Soc*, 1999, 48, 8–13, 40.

Ortman, LF; Casey, DM; Deers, M. Bioelectric stimulation and residual ridge resorption. *J Prosthet Dent*, 1992, 67, 67–71.

Ottani, V; Raspanti, M; Martini, D; Tretola, G; Ruggeri Jr., A; Franchi, M; Giuliani Piccari, G; Ruggeri, A. Electromagnetic stimulation on the bone growth using backscattered electron imaging. *Micron*, 2002, 33, 121–125.

Ozcelik, O; Cenk Haytac, M; Seydaoglu, G. Enamel matrix derivative and low-level laser therapy in the treatment of intra-bony defects: a randomized placebo-controlled clinical trial. *J Clin Periodontol*, 2008/a, 35, 147–156.

Ozcelik, O; Haytac, MC; Kunin, A; Seydaoglu, G. Improved wound healing by low-level laser irradiation after gingivectomy operations: a controlled clinical pilot study. *J Clin Periodontol*, 2008/b, 35, 250–254.

Ozen, T; Orhan, K; Gorur, I; Ozturk, A. Efficacy of low level laser therapy on neurosensory recovery after injury to the inferior alveolar nerve. *BMC Head Face Med*, 2006, 2, 3.

Patino, O; Grana, D; Bolgiani, A; Prezzavento, G; Mino, J; Merlo, A; Benaim, F. Pulsed electromagnetic fields in experimental cutaneous wound healing in rats. *J Burn Care Rehabil*, 1996, 17, 528–531.

Payer, M; Jakse, N; Pertl, C; Truschnegg, A; Lechner, E; Eskici, A. The clinical effect of LLLT in endodontic surgery: A prospective study on 72 cases. *Oral Surg Oral Med Oral Pathol Oral Radiol Endod*, 2005, 100, 375–379.

Pesevska, S; Nakova, M; Ivanovski, K. Angelov, N; Kesic, L; Obradovic, R; Mindova, S; Nares, S. Dentinal hypersensitivity following scaling and root planing: comparison of low level laser and topical fluoride treatment. *Lasers Med Sci*, 2010, 25, 647–650.

Petri, AD; Teixeira, LN; Crippa, GE; Beloti, MM; de Oliveira, PT; Rose, AL. Effects of low-level laser therapy on human osteoblastic cells grown on titanium. *Braz Dent J*, 2010, 21, 491–498.

Pienkowski, D; Pollack, SR; Brighton, CT; Griffith, NJ. Comparison of asymmetrical and symmetrical pulse waveforms in electromagnetic stimulation. *J Orthop Res*, 1992, 10, 247–255.

Pinheiro, ALB; Martinez Gerbi, ME; de Assis Limeira Jr., F; Carneiro Ponzi, EA; Marques, AMC; Carvalho, CM; de Carneiro Santos, R; Oliveira, PC; Noia, M; Ramalho, LMP. Bone repair following bone grafting hydroxyapatite guided bone regeneration and infra-red laser photobiomodulation: a histological study in a rodent model. *Lasers Med Sci*, 2009, 24, 234–240.

Qadri, T; Miranda, L; Tuner, J; Gustafsson, A. The sort-term effects of low-level lasers as adjunct therapy in the treatment of periodontal inflammation. *J Clin Periodontol*, 2005, 32, 714–719.

Raji, AM. An experimental study of the effects of pulsed electromagnetic field (Diapulse) on nerve repair. *J Hand Surg Br*, 1984, 9, 105–112.

Raji, AR; Bowden, RE. Effects of high-peak pulsed electromagnetic field on the degeneration and regeneration of the common peroneal nerve in rats. *J Bone Joint Surg Br*, 1983, 65, 478–492.

Rubin, CT; Donahue, HJ; Rubin, JE; McLeod, KJ. Optimization of electric field parameters for the control of bone remodeling: exploitation of an indigeous mechanism for the prevention of osteopenia. *J Bone Miner Res*, 1993, 8, S573–S581.

Satake, T; Yasu, N; Kakai, Y; Kawamura, T; Sato, T; Nakano, T; Amino, S; Ishiwata, Y; Saito, S. Effect of pulsed electromagnetic fields (PEMF) on human periodontal ligament in vitro. Alterations of intracellular Ca^{2+}. *Kanagawa Shikagu*, 1990, 24, 735–742.

Scardino, MS; Swaim, SF; Sartin, EA; Steiss, JE; Spano, JS; Hoffman, CE; Coolman, SL; Peppin, BL. Evaluation of treatment with a pulsed electromagnetic field on wound healing, clinicopathologic variables, and central nervous system activity of dogs. *Am J Vet Res*, 1998, 59, 1177–1181.

Schnoke, M; Midura, RJ. Pulsed electromagnetic fields rapidly modulate intracellular signaling events in osteoblastic cells: Comparison to parathyroid hormone and insulin. *J Orthop Res*, 2007, 25, 933–940.

Schwarz, F; Sculean, A; Rothamel, D; Schwenzer, K; Georg, T; Becker, J. Clinical evaluation of an Er:YAG laser for nonsurgical treatment of peri-implantitis: a pilot study. *Clin Oral Implant Res*, 2005, 16, 44–52.

Schwarz, F; Aoki, A; Becker, J; Sculean, A. Laser application in non-surgical periodontal therapy: a systematic review. *J Clin Periodontol*, 2008 35(8 Suppl), 29–44.

Schwartz, Z; Fisher, M; Lohmann, CH; Simon, BJ; Boyan, BD. Osteoprotegerin (OPG) production by cells in the osteoblast lineage is regulated by pulsed electromagnetic fields in cultures grown on calcium phosphate substrates. *Annals Biomed Engineering*, 2009, 37, 437–444.

Sharon-Buller, A; Sela, M. CO_2-laser treatment of ulcerative lesions. *Oral Surg Oral Med Oral Pathol Oral Radiol Endod*, 2004, 97, 332–334.

Shirani, AM; Gutknecht, N. Taghizadeh, M; Mir, M. Low-level laser therapy and myofacial pain dysfunction syndrome: a randomized controlled clinical trial. *Lasers Med Sci*, 2009, 24, 715–720.

Showkatbakhsh, R; Jamilian, A; Showkatbakhsh, M. The effect of pulsed electromagnetic fields on the acceleration of tooth movement. *World J Orthod*, 2010, 11, e52–e56.

Solazzo, V; Palmieri, A; Pezzetti, F; Massari, L. Carinci, F. Effects of pulsed electromagnetic fields on human osteoblastic cells (Mg-63). A pilot study. *Clin Orthop Relat Res*, 2010, 468, 2260–2277.

Souil, E; Capon, A; Mordon, S; Dinh-Xuan, AT; Polla, BS. Bachelet, M. Treatment with 815-nm diode laser induces long-lasting expression of 72-kDa heat shock protein in normal rat skin. *Brit J Dermatol*, 2001, 144, 260–266.

Spadaro, JA; Bergstrom, WH. In vivo and in vitro effects of a pulsed electromagnetic field on net calcium flux in rat calvarial bone. *Calcif Tissue Int*, 2002, 70, 496–502.

Stark, TM; Sinclair, PM. Effect of pulsed electromagnetic fields on orthodontic tooth movement. *Am J Orthod Dentofacial Orthop*, 1987, 91, 91–104.

Strauch, B; Herman, C; Dabb, R; Ignarro, LJ; Pilla, AA. Evidence-based use of pulsed electromagnetic field therapy in clinical plastic surgery. *Aesthet Surg J*, 2009, 29, 135–143.

Takano-Yamamoto, T; Kawakami, M; Sakuda, M. Effect of a pulsing electromagnetic field on demineralized bone-matrix-induced bone formation in a bony defect in the premaxilla of rats. *J Dent Res*, 1992, 71, 1920–1925.

Takasaki, AA; Aoki, A; Mizutani, K; Schwarz, F; Sculean, A; Wang, CY; Koshy, G; Romanos, G; Ishikawa, I; Izumi, Y. Application of antimicrobial photodynamic therapy in periodontal and peri-implant diseases. *Periodontol*, 2009, 51, 109–140.

Tepper, OM; Callaghan, MJ; Chang, EI; Galiano, RD; Bhatt, KA; Baharestani, S; Gan, J; Simon, B; Hopper, RA; Levine, JP; Gurtner, GC. Electromagnetic fields increase in vitro and in vivo angiogenesis through endothelial release of FGF-2. *FASEB J*, 2004, 18, 1231–1233.

Tsai, MT; Li, WJ; Tuan, RS; Chang, WH. Modulation of osteogenesis in human mesenchimal stem cells by specific pulsed electromagnetic field stimulation. *J Orthop Res*, 2009, 27, 1169–1174.

Tuinstra, R; Greenbaum, B; Goodman, EM. Effects of magnetic fields on cell-free transcription in *E. Coli* and HeLaextracts. *Bioelectrochem Bioenerg*, 1997, 43, 7–12.

Ustun, Y; Erdogan, O; Kurkcu, M; Akova, T; Damlar, I. Effects of low-intensity pulsed ultrasound on dental implant osseointegration: A preliminary report. *Eur J Dentistry*, 2008, 2, 254–262.

Uysal, T; Ekizer, A; Akcay, H; Etoz, O; Guray, E. Resonance frequency analysis of orthodontic miniscrews subjected to light-emitting diode photomodulation therapy. *Eur J Orthodontics*, 2012, 34, 44–51.

Varani, K; Gessi, S; Merighi, S; Iannota, V; Cattabriga, E; Pancaldi, C; Cadossi, R; Borea, PA. Alteration of A3 adenosine receptors in human neutrophils and low frequency electromagnetic fields. *Biochem Parmachol*, 2003, 66, 1897–1906.

Vescovi, P; Merigo, E; Manfredi, M; Meleti, M; Fornaini, C; Bonanini, M; Rocca, JP; Nammour, S. Nd:YAG laser biostimulation in the treatment of bisphosphonate-associated osteonecrosis of the jaw: clinical experience in 28 cases. *Photomed Laser Surg*, 2008, 26, 37–46.

Wilmot, JJ; Chiego Jr., DJ; Carlson, DS; Hanks, CT; Moskwa, JJ. Autoradiographic study of the effects of pulsed electromagnetic fields on bone and cartilage growth in juvenile rats. *Arch Oral Biol*, 1993, 38, 67–74.

Zienowicz, RJ; Thomas, BA; Kurtz, WH; Orgel, MG. A multivariate approach to the treatment of peripheral nerve transection injury: the role of electromagnetic field therapy. *Plast Reconstr Surg*, 1991, 87, 122–129.

CHAPTER 8

IMPLANT SURGERY

Abstract

The surgical aspects of implant dentistry are of primary importance. It is no wonder that there are huge amounts of data in the scientific literature in relation to this important topic. In this chapter the most important surgical aspects will be introduced. Principles of implant site preparation and implant placement, the timing of site preparation (i.e. immediate, early, and delayed placement), the timing of loading (i.e. immediate, early, and delayed loading), the surgical management of various implant failures, several forms of bone augmentation, sinus floor elevation (including management of sinus membrane perforation), and soft tissue surgery as well as certain important related topics like the assessment of bone quality and primary stability will be discussed in detail. Besides these, several other surgical techniques like alveolar distraction osteogenesis, alveolar nerve lateralization, alveolar nerve transposition, the use of tilted, zygomatic, and tuberal implantation, and the removal of fractured implant fixtures as well as the principles of virtual implant placement and navigational surgery will also be introduced. Although the aim of this chapter is to present a complete and comprehensive overview of implant surgery, specific aspects of alveolar ridge preservation in relation to immediate implant placement in the esthetic zone and bone augmentation of the extraction socket ("socket grafting") will not be discussed in this chapter.

8.1. Introduction

It is obvious that the surgical aspects of implant dentistry are of primary importance; therefore the primary aim of this chapter is to present a complete and comprehensive overview of several surgical techniques used in implant dentistry. Certain closely related topics, like the assessment of bone quality and primary stability as well as the complex problems of timing and the type of loading (i.e. functional, nonfunctional or progressive loading) used are also discussed in this chapter. This is because bone quality and primary stability can best be evaluated by the surgeon during surgery, and a surgeon's concrete observations in this regard should influence the surgical technique and surgical decision making as well as any decision making related to the timing and type of loading of the implants.

Although the aim of this chapter is to present a complete and comprehensive overview of implant surgery, specific surgical aspects of alveolar ridge preservation in relation to immediate implant placement in the esthetic zone and bone augmentation of the extraction sockets ("socket grafting") will not be discussed in this chapter, because these topics are discussed in detail elsewhere with regard to the complex field of alveolar ridge preservation.

8.2. Bone Quality and Primary Stability

8.2.1. Assessment of Bone Quality

A higher failure rate seems to be associated with the implants if the surgeon observes a poor degree of bone mineralization or limited bone resistance through tactile assessment while drilling (Turkyilmaz and McGlumphy 2008; Ihde et al. 2009). Since the premised mechanical behavior of bone seems to be a vital factor in the achievement of primary stability and osseointegration, several classification systems and procedures have been suggested for assessing bone quality (Turkyilmaz and McGlumphy 2008; Ihde et al. 2009).

The most popular system (Lekholm and Zarb 1985) is based on both the sensation of resistance experienced by the surgeon when preparing the implant site and on the radiographic assessment (Lekholm and Zarb 1985); it comprises four classes, including: Lekholm-Zarb type I, type II, type III, and type IV, from which the first (type I) refers to the highest, whereas the last (type IV) refers to the lowest, level of bone quality (Lekholm and Zarb 1985). Briefly: *type I bone* = entire jaw comprised of homogenous compact bone; *type II bone* = thick cortical layer surrounds a core of dense trabecular bone; *type III bone* = thin cortical layer surrounds a layer of low-density trabecular bone; and *type IV bone* = thin layer of cortical bone surrounds a core of low density trabecular bone (Lekholm and Zarb 1985). Although this classification is currently the most widely used, it has recently been questioned, because the grading refers to individual experience and provides only a rough mean value of the entire jaw, which may lead to poor objectivity and reproducibility (Turkyilmaz and McGlumphy 2008). It also has the disadvantage that the evaluation is (at least partially) retrospective, because the osteotomy has to be done before the evaluation.

Another popular system (Johansson and Strid 1994) evaluates bone quality as a function of density and hardness can be derived from the torque forces needed during implant site preparation and implant insertion (Johansson and Strid 1994). In this system, the evaluation of cutting resistance during implant insertion (insertion torque) especially seems to be an accurate measure of bone quality (Johansson and Strid 1994; Friberg et al. 1995). For such an evaluation, the measurement of the "maximum insertion torque" (the highest insertion torque value needed to continue implant insertion when the rotation has stopped because of friction) may be used if the available surgical equipment provides a well-controlled, adjustable insertion torque to avoid the mechanical overload of the equipment and/or bone (Turkyilmaz and McGlumphy 2008). The maximum insertion torque values usually range roughly between 20 and 45 Ncm (Turkyilmaz and McGlumphy 2008). Values lower than 30 Ncm indicate low quality bone, values between 30 and 40 Ncm indicate medium level bone quality, and values over 40 Ncm can be considered representative of high-level bone quality (Andres-Garcia et al. 2009). Although, this method may provide helpful information about bone density, it has the disadvantage of being retrospective to patient assessment; thus, the osteotomy has to be performed and the implant has to be screwed in before the evaluation (Turkyilmaz and McGlumphy 2008; Andres-Garcia et al. 2009).

Importantly, bone quality can also be evaluated *before* surgery by means of CBCT images. In this case the value is expressed in Hounsfield units, which are standard numbers originating from medical CT images and represent the relative density of tissues according to a calibrated gray-level scale (de Carvalho Crusoe Silva 2012) that ranges from minus (-)1000 (air) to plus (+)3000 (enamel) (Turkyilmaz and McGlumphy 2008). When compared with the Misch classification of bone density (Misch 1990), < 150 HU refers to D5, 150–350 HU refers to D4, 350–850 HU refers to D3, 850–1250 HU refers to D2, and > 1250 refers to a D1 Misch bone density class (Turkyilmaz and McGlumphy 2008; de Carvalho Crusoe Silva 2012). The values correlate well with real bone quality (Homolka et al. 2002; Turkyilmaz and McGlumphy 2008; Farre-Pages et al. 2011) and may predict implant insertion torque and implant stability (Homolka et al. 2002; Turkyilmaz and McGlumphy 2008; Farre-Pages et al. 2011).

8.2.2. Assessment of Primary Stability

Primary stability is a prerequisite in establishing mechanical rest, which is essential for undisturbed healing and osseointegration; therefore, it is one of the main factors influencing implant survival rates (Turkyilmaz and McGlumphy 2008). Primary stability is influenced by factors like implant geometry and micromorphology, surgical preparation technique, and the quality and quantity of the available bone (Turkyilmaz and McGlumphy 2008; Moon et al. 2010). There are several non-invasive clinical methods available to measure primary stability. The evaluation of the insertion torque (Johansson and Strid 1994), as described above in relation to the evaluation of bone quality, can also be used to evaluate primary stability (Johansson and Strid 1994; Friberg et al. 1995; Turkyilmaz and McGlumphy 2008); and the "maximum insertion torque" (the highest insertion torque value needed to continue implant insertion when the rotation has stopped because of friction) may also be a good measure in this case (Turkyilmaz and McGlumphy 2008). The maximum insertion torque ranges roughly between 20 and 45 Ncm (Turkyilmaz and McGlumphy 2008); and it is thought that the torque necessary to achieve an optimal primary stability should be roughly 30 Ncm or higher (Andres-Garcia et al. 2009).

Another method, termed "Periotest" may also be used to measure the stiffness of the bone-implant interface (Olive and Aparicio 1990). The instrument measures the contact time of an accelerated small pistil to the implant which moves according to the strike, and this is calculated into a value (called the "Periotest value") that reflects the deflection/deceleration of the implant that has been struck by the premised small pistil from inside the instrument's hand piece (Olive and Aparicio 1990). Although Periotesting has the advantage that it may be used for both the evaluation of the primary stability of an implant and also the evaluation of the periodontal integration of a natural tooth (Olive and Aparicio 1990), primary implant stability related values include only a narrow range over the scale of the instrument (Olive and Aparicio 1990). Thus, it provides relatively less sensitive information about primary implant stability (Olive and Aparicio 1990), and therefore its benefit in this regard is a matter of debate (Turkyilmaz and McGlumphy 2008).

Primary stability can also be measured through the mean of the implant stability quotient (ISQ) level measured *via* resonance frequency analysis (RFA) (Meredith et al. 1996). In this method, an L-shaped transducer tightened to the abutment or implant is used. Two piezoceramic components are attached to the vertical beam of the transducer: one is vibrated with a sinusoidal wave of 5–15 kHz and the first flexural resonance frequency is identified as a peak (Meredith et al. 1996). This resonance frequency value can be expressed as an implant stability quotient value on a scale from 3.500 Hz, corresponding to 1 ISQ unit, to 8.500 Hz, corresponding to 100 ISQ units. In the premised system, higher ISQ values correspond to greater implant stability. Currently, the measurement of resonance frequency analysis expressed in implant stability quotient values seems to be the most accepted method for the evaluation of primary implant stability (Turkyilmaz and McGlumphy 2008; Kim et al. 2009/a; Kang et al. 2011).

8.2.3. The Increase of Primary Stability in Poor Bone Quality

Most implants available currently provide good primary stability in cases of favorable bone density; however, inserting implants with good primary stability even in poor bone quality is still a challenge for both manufacturers and dentists (Moon et al. 2010). Tapered-screw type implants have been designed for immediate implantation after extraction but are also used to increase primary stability by providing pressure on the cortical bone of regions with poor bone qualities (O'Sullivan et al. 200, 2004; Moon et al. 2010). Tapered-screws are also known to distribute the occlusal force to surrounding bone more equally than straight-type screws (Glauser et al. 2004; Moon et al. 2010), which may be especially advantageous if the fixture is loaded immediately after insertion in poor quality bone. Besides implant design, there are also various surgical techniques to improve the primary stability of fixtures placed into poor quality bone, such as obtaining bicortical anchorage (Martinez et al. 2001; Wang et al. 2006) and using thinner drills than normal (Martinez et al. 2001) as well as self-tapping implantation, the cancellous compaction (osteotome) technique (Martinez et al. 2001; Moon et al. 2010; Yoon et al. 2011), and vertical under-preparation for tapered-screws (Moon et al. 2010).

8.3. Flap vs. Flapless Surgery

Reducing surgical trauma and limiting flap elevation (if any) are essentials in every procedure (Irinakis 2006; Brkovic et al. 2008; Fickl et al. 2008; Pagni et al. 2012). However, animal studies have shown confusing results when evaluating the differences in ridge remodeling between flapped and nonflapped surgery (Pagni et al. 2012). It may be that flap elevation affects alveolar dimensional alterations only in the short term (Tan et al. 2012; Pagni et al. 2012), while there is no significant difference in the long term (Caneva et al. 2010; Pagni et al. 2012). On the other hand, it may be hypothesized that by disrupting the thin layer of cells that comprise the osteogenic layer of periosteum by flap elevation, one might diminish the ability of the periosteal cells to regenerate bone (Pagni et al. 2012), while undisturbed periosteum (i.e. flapless techniques) might maintain its full osteogenic potential

(Pagni et al. 2012) as well as blood supply to the bone (Williams and Warwick 1980; Penarrocha et al. 2012).

The advancement of the flaps may result in increased inflammatory response, in a decrease in vestibular depth, and in the creation of unesthetic scars (Pagni et al. 2012). However, proper elevation of the flap is necessary to gain enough of a view of the surgical field (Park et al. 2012; Penarrocha et al. 2012) to avoid missing anatomical deformities (if any) and to facilitate the irrigation of the bone during drilling (Park et al. 2012).

Taking altogether the above data, it may be concluded that flapless techniques (i.e. punching, punch drilling for guided surgery, and minimally invasive mini-flap preparation) should be preferred if there is no concrete reason for flap elevation; and if there is a need for flap elevation, then any *unnecessary* advancement of the flaps should be avoided.

8.4. Implant Site Preparation

8.4.1. General Considerations

It should be considered first that *all preparations should be carried out under sterile saline irrigation* (Turkyilmaz and McGlumphy 2008; Park et al. 2012), excessive heating must be avoided at all times, and drilling must be performed with the highest precision in order to avoid unstable implant placement or over-tensioned fixation (Park et al. 2012). The implant positioning should be decided based on the individual anatomical and clinical situation but (with the exception of the frontal region of maxilla), it may be considered as a general rule that the implant should be preferably placed in the natural tooth position both in the mesio-distal and bucco-lingual/palatal dimensions (Park et al. 2012). However, the intraoral environment for working with the drills should also be considered and included in the planning (Arataki et al. 2007), because the position, depth, and direction of the implant placement determine the adequate working space needed for precise and careful drilling of the implant site (Arataki et al. 2007).

The distance between two implants should not be less than about 7 mm (measured from center to center), and the center of the drilling point should be 3.5–4.0 mm away from the prominence of the neighboring tooth (Park et al. 2012). Usually, the mesial implant site is determined first and the following implant positions are then marked in a distal direction until all planned implant sites have been determined (Park et al. 2012). For implant-supported overdenture in the edentulous mandible, a position 7 mm distal to the midline on each side may be considered optimal for implant placement (McCracken et al. 2006). In the case of a "knife-edge shaped" alveolar bone, the height of the bone should be reduced and shaped to reach an evenly made bone surface with a bucco-lingual diameter of a minimum 5–6 mm, which in general is considered necessary for successful implant placement into edentulous arches (Madrigal et al. 2008; Bassetti et al. 2010). This means that the mandibular bone height may need to be reduced by up to roughly 3–5 mm, which corresponds to a rather significant reduction of total bone height in certain cases (Madrigal et al. 2008). If two-stage surgery is used, the flaps should be closed with minimum tension and a distance of 3–5 mm may be considered proper for suture spacing (Park et al. 2012).

After having confirmed proper bucco-lingual (as well as mesio-distal) bone dimensions, in general, three basic techniques may be used: the conventional tapping technique, self-tapping technique, or cancellous compaction (osteotome) technique (Yoon et al. 2011). The basic principles of the premised techniques will be briefly introduced below; however it should be noted that manufacturers' instructions may differ from these, and in such a case, the manufacturer's instructions for site preparation and implant placement should certainly be followed (Kang et al. 2011).

8.4.2. Basic Techniques for Site Preparation

In the *conventional tapping technique*, the implant site is marked first by a round bur (i.e. 1.5 mm diameter) with a low (i.e. 1000 rpm) drill speed, followed by twist drills of increasing diameter (i.e. 2 mm, followed by 3 mm, etc.) with a somewhat lower (i.e. 500 rpm) speed until a hole size of a somewhat smaller (i.e. 0.5–0.75 mm smaller) diameter than the diameter of the fixture itself is reached (Yoon et al. 2011). Finally, tapping is performed in the drilled holes before implant fixture installation. The fixture is installed with a very low (i.e. 30 rpm) speed (Yoon et al. 2011). In the case of the *self-tapping technique*, the process is basically the same, with the only important difference being that the tapping step is omitted, because a self-tapping should occur during the installation (very low speed, i.e. 30 rpm) of the fixture (Yoon et al. 2011). In the case of the *cancellous compaction (osteotome) technique*, the implant site is marked first by a round bur (i.e. 1.5 mm diameter) with a low (i.e. 1000 rpm) drill speed, followed by twist drill(s) of increasing diameter (i.e. 2 mm, followed by 3 mm, etc.) with a somewhat lower (i.e. 500 rpm) speed, similar to the previous techniques (Yoon et al. 2011). However, in this case, the diameter of the last twist drill should be significantly smaller (i.e. 1.5–1.75 mm smaller) than the diameter of the fixture (Yoon et al. 2011). As a last step, taper-type osteotomes of increasing diameter (i.e. 2.5 mm, followed by 3.0 mm, followed by 3.5 mm, etc.) are used with light malleting until a final hole size that is somewhat smaller (i.e. 0.5–0.75 mm smaller) in diameter than the diameter of the fixture itself is reached (Yoon et al. 2011). Finally, the implant fixture is inserted with a very low (i.e. 30 rpm) speed into the prepared holes (Yoon et al. 2011). Notably, the fixtures should be inserted immediately after preparing the implant site to avoid the collapse of the prepared hole (Rambla-Ferrer et al. 2006).

As indicated above, manufacturers' instructions may differ from the above protocols, and in such a case, the manufacturer's instructions for site preparation and implant placement should certainly be followed (Kang et al. 2011). The manufacturers' instructions may also include the use of other types of instruments (i.e. pilot drills, tap drills, cortical drills, etc.), which should also be rigorously followed (Kang et al. 2011).

8.4.3. The Vertical Position of the Fixture-Abutment Interface

During the first year after implant loading, a typical pattern of bone loss referred to as "saucerization" occurs (Yi et al. 2010) that includes a marginal bone loss of 0.9–1.6 mm during the first year and 0.05–0.13 mm annually thereafter (Adell et al. 1981; Cox and Zarb 1987; Jemt et al. 1990; Yi et al. 2010). The success of an implant is defined as having less than 1.5 mm of marginal bone loss during the first year after functional loading (insertion of the prosthesis) and less than 0.2 mm annual bone loss thereafter (Albrektsson and Isidor 1993). The vertical position of the implant-abutment interface may significantly influence both the osseointegration of and initial marginal bone loss (i.e. bone loss in the first year after loading) around the implant fixtures (Yi et al. 2010). If the fixture-abutment interface is placed above the bone level, the implant stability quotient level measured by means of resonance frequency analysis (Meredith et al. 1996) may decrease significantly (Meredith et al. 1997; Kang et al. 2011). Increasing the effective length (i.e. the length over the bone level) with each 1 mm may lead to a decrease of 3–7 ISQ units if the fixture is placed in a Lekholm-Zarb type II bone (Lekholm and Zarb 1985); whereas a decrease of 4–9 or 5–11 ISQ units may be experienced if the fixture is placed in type III or type IV bone, respectively (Kang et al. 2011). Because of the significant decrease of implant stability, the use of fixtures with short pitch intervals seems to be beneficial, especially if the effective length is higher than 1 mm and if the implant is placed in type III or type IV quality bone (Kang et al. 2011). Although the placement of a fixture-abutment interface above the bone level may jeopardize osseointegration (especially in the case of low level quality bone), it has the advantage that the initial marginal bone loss (i.e. "saucerization" during the first year of load) seems to be significantly smaller than if the fixture-abutment interface is placed in the bone level or placed "submerged" below the bone level (Yi et al. 2010). In contrast, if the fixture-abutment interface is placed in the bone level or placed submerged below it (usually ca. 1 mm below), the initial stability of the implant seems to be higher (Meredith et al. 1997; Kang et al. 2011; Lekholm and Zarb 1985), but the initial bone loss (i.e. "saucerization" during the first year of load) seems to be significantly higher in both cases; this is especially true in the case of the submerged placement.

It is very likely that the primary reason for the premised increased bone loss in bone level or below the bone level placed fixtures is the development of the biological width around the fixture (Berglundh et al. 1991; Berglundh and Lindhe 1996; Yi et al. 2010), which results in a deeper-placed bone level (more pronounced "saucerization") if the implant fixture is placed deeper in the bone (Abrahamsson et al. 1996, 1999; Yi et al. 2010). Classic implant surgical techniques tend to place the fixture-abutment interface submerged below the bone level to minimize implant movement during the osseointegration process (Yi et al. 2010). However, deep positioning of the fixture inevitably leads to increased initial bone loss; therefore (based on the newly developed, highly osseointegrative fixture surfaces), the placement of a fixture on the bone level or in certain cases somewhat (ca. 1 mm) over the bone level may be preferred (Yi et al. 2010).

8.4.4. Vertical Over- and Under-Preparation

Vertical over- and under-preparation means that the implant site (the "hole" for fixture) is prepared shallower (under-prepared) or deeper (over-prepared) in comparison to the normal guidelines of the manufacturer (Moon et al. 2010). It is likely that moderate vertical over-preparation (i.e. up to 1 mm) has no significant influence on primary stability (Moon et al. 2010); but because of theoretical considerations in relation to osseointegration, it seems reasonable to avoid this kind of preparation. In contrast, moderate vertical under-preparation (i.e. 1 mm shallower than the site) may have significant influence on the primary stability of tapered (but not straight) screws in any (high or low level) quality of bone (Moon et al. 2010) and therefore may also improve osseointegration in most cases. However, if the under-preparation technique is used, it should be noted that the screw should be positioned as deeply as expected according to the standard protocol of the manufacturer (Moon et al. 2010). Further, it should be emphasized that if the standard protocol (normal guideline) of the manufacturer already utilizes the under-preparation technique, a further increase in the under-preparation needs to be considered very carefully, even if it may be advantageous in the case of low level bone quality.

8.4.5. The Timing of Implant Site Preparation

Although immediate implant placement (discussed in detail elsewhere) may be used with a high success rate if properly indicated (McNutt and Chou 2003; Khanifam et al. 2013), for more predictable results it is recommended that proper time be allowed for bone healing (and for the resolution of earlier pathologies associated with the extraction site) prior to proceeding with implant treatment (Nagaraj et al. 2010; Pagni et al. 2012; D'Addona et al. 2012; Khanifam et al. 2013). This may be especially important if there are significant pathologies affecting the hard and/or soft tissues in the area of the extracted tooth (D'Addona et al. 2012) and from an esthetic point of view in the case of incisor, canine, and premolar regions with a thin gingival biotype (Nagaraj et al. 2010). In the case of thick gingival biotype, the esthetic results may be more predictable (Nagaraj et al. 2010), and the immediate placement may be advantageous with regard to the preservation of the alveolar ridge (discussed in detail elsewhere). If there is no implant placed into the socket *immediately* (Type-1 implant), it may be advantageous to place an implant *early* into the extraction site during early stage healing (within 4–8 weeks; Type-2 implant) or during the "partial bone" stage (within 12–16 weeks; Type-3 implants). Early insertion (i.e. Type-2 and Type-3 implants) not only advantageously shortens the duration of the treatment, but it may also decrease the amount of bone resorption and the loss of the soft tissue profile (D'Addona et al. 2012). Further, bone augmentation around early inserted implants (i.e. Type-2 and Type-3 implants) may provide better hard tissue dimensions and less postoperative complications compared to *delayed* (6 months or more; Type-4) implants (Hammerle et al. 2004; Pagni et al. 2012; Sanz et al. 2012).

8.5. Immediate, Early, and Delayed Loading

8.5.1. Immediate Loading

The term "*immediate loading*" (Ledermann 1979) has been defined as the situation where the abutment and superstructure (i.e. crown, bridge, attachment with RPD [removable partial denture], etc.) is connected to the implant fixture within a period not longer than 48–72 hours after surgery and where there is occlusion with the teeth of the opposite jaw (Ledermann 1979; Cochran et al. 2004; Aguirre-Zorzano et al. 2011; Yoon et al. 2012). One-stage surgical procedures and immediate loading of implants have shown promising clinical results. The general success rate of immediately loaded implants is roughly 90%–95% (Romanos and

Nentwig 2006; Romanos et al. 2010). Low level bone quality (i.e. in the maxilla) may lead to a decrease in the success rate since the masticatory forces might give rise to micro-movements that may jeopardize osseointegration (Lindeboom et al. 2006; Romanos and Nentwig 2006; Aguirre-Zorzano et al. 2011). In contrast, immediate loading procedures for the rehabilitation of the edentulous mandible by means of either splinted (Ledermann 1979; Branemark et al. 1999; Randow et al. 1999; Gonzalez et al. 2006; Aguirre-Zorzano et al. 2011; Gfeller et al. 2011) or unsplinted (Buttel et al. 2012) implants seem to have a higher success rate. Importantly, if cementation is used (for fixation of crowns or bridges) for early loading, great care should be taken to remove all small cement remnants around the abutment and implant-supported crown, because the development of the implanto-gingival complex may suffer a loss if the cement residue keeps the soft tissues from attaching to the implant (Aguirre-Zorzano et al. 2011).

8.5.2. Non-Functional and Progressive Immediate Loading

The term *non-functional immediate loading* (also referred to as "immediate restoration" or "immediate provisionalization") means that the abutment and a provisorical superstructure (i.e. a provisorical fixed or removable denture) are placed on the implant fixture within a period not longer than 48(–72) hours after surgery; but the procedure is done without full occlusal contact with the teeth of the opposite jaw (Lindeboom et al. 2006; Garcia et al. 2008; Aguirre-Zorzano et al. 2011). Keeping the provisional restoration out of occlusion may prevent the overload of osseointegrating implant fixtures (Kan and Rungcharassaeng 2000; Hui et al. 2001; Aguirre-Zorzano et al. 2011), whereby an advantageous immediate esthetic result is achieved (Kan and Rungcharassaeng 2000; Hui et al. 2001; Aguirre-Zorzano et al. 2011; Aguirre-Zorzano et al. 2011). Importantly, initial bone loss around non-functionally loaded implants seems to be the same as the initial bone loss found around those of delayed loading (Aguirre-Zorzano et al. 2011). However, data have indicated that progressive functional loading performed through the serial alterations of the provisional restorations may increase bone mass and bone density around the implant fixture and may decrease initial crestal bone loss in comparison to delayed (conventional) loading protocols (Binon and Sullivan 1990; Appleton et al. 2005). These observations have resulted in the *progressive immediate loading* protocols, which may be considered a gradual transition from the non-functional immediate loading to full occlusion with the teeth of the opposite jaw. If provisional cementation is used either in the case of non-functional immediate loading or in the case of progressive immediate loading protocols, great care should be taken to remove small cement remnants around the abutment and the implant supporting provisional crown, because in the presence of such remnants the peri-implant soft tissues cannot attach to the implant and the development of the implanto-gingival complex may suffer a loss (Aguirre-Zorzano et al. 2011).

8.5.3. Early Loading

In accordance with the definition of immediate loading, "*early loading*" is defined as loading with a restoration being in contact with the opposing teeth and placed at least 48(–72) hours after the implant placement but not longer than three months afterward (Yoon et al. 2012). Although the time-related difference between "immediate" and "early" loading may seem rather unimportant, especially if we consider that a load applied right after 48(–72) hours would already not be categorized as "immediate" but as "early," it should be noted that a few hours' difference in time may correspond to highly significant biological differences in the very early stages of the osseointegration process. This may explain why early loading exhibits a significantly higher success rate when compared to immediate loading. The success rate of early loading is comparable to delayed (conventional) loading (Kim et al. 2009/b). Importantly, if cementation is used (for fixation of crowns or bridges) for early loading, great care should be taken to remove all small cement remnants around the abutment and implant-supported crown, because the development of the implanto-gingival complex may suffer a loss if the cement rests keep the soft tissues from attaching to the implant (Aguirre-Zorzano et al. 2011).

8.5.4. Delayed ("Conventional") Loading

In the case of "*delayed loading*" (also referred to as "conventional" loading), the recommended waiting time after surgery according to the original Branemark protocol is at least three months for the mandible and six months for the maxilla (Branemark et al. 1977). This is because disturbances of the osseointegration process (i.e. encapsulation by fibrous tissue) may occur if the implants are loaded immediately or too early (Branemark et al. 1977). Therefore, in the case of delayed loading, the prosthesis is attached in a second procedure that takes place after the conventional healing period of 3–6 months has passed (Yoon et al. 2012). Even today the classic delayed loading protocol can be considered the safest approach. However, over the past few decades, technological developments and continuous experimental and clinical research has provided us with improved protocols even if delayed loading will still be used (Aguirre-Zorzano et al. 2011).

8.6. Soft Tissue Surgery

8.6.1. Obtaining Adequate Keratinized Tissue

There is no consensus in the literature regarding the significance of keratinized mucosa in implant maintenance or on the relationship between the width of the keratinized mucosa and the health of peri-implant tissues (Park et al. 2010; Penarrocha et al. 2012). Although it is very likely that a lack of keratinized peri-implant tissue does not influence the long-term survival rate of oral implants (Park et al. 2010), the presence of an adequate band of keratinized tissue adjacent to the implant does reduce the risk of inflammation (Zarb and Schmitt 1990; Warrer et al. 1995), hyperplasia (Zarb and Schmitt 1990), and the retraction of the marginal peri-implant soft tissues (Adell et al. 1981; Zarb and Schmitt 1990). Further, the presence or reconstruction of an adequate band of keratinized tissue facilitates restorative procedures leading to improved esthetics (Block and Kent 1990; Buser et al. 1990;

Penarrocha et al. 2012) and enables patients to maintain good oral hygiene without irritation or discomfort during routine oral hygiene (Albrektsson et al. 1986).

Various techniques have been introduced to obtain an adequate amount of keratinized tissue (Park et al. 2010). Apically and/or laterally positioned partial-thickness flap techniques are basic tools used to preserve existing keratinized tissue (Langer and Sullivan 1989; Langer and Langer 1990; Lee et al. 2010/b; Park et al. 2010). Recently, apical/lateral positioning of partial thickness flaps fixed in their new position by means of implant-retained stents has also been used for this purpose (Park et al. 2010). If there is not enough keratinized tissue, free gingival grafts (FGG) may also be used (Langer and Sullivan 1989; Langer and Langer 1990; Park et al. 2010) in combination with an apically positioned flap (APF) (Lee et al. 2010/b). Similarly, the combination of an apically positioned flap and a free gingival graft can be used also in the case of shallow vestibules with minimal keratinized tissue (Landi and Sabatucci 2001; Lee et al. 2010/b). Considering the limitations on the amount of available donor tissue (Reiser et al. 1996), collagen matrix coverage may also be used as a soft tissue substitute with the aim of increasing keratinized tissue (Lee et al. 2010/b).

8.6.2. Reconstruction of the Inter-Implant Papilla

Various techniques for the reconstruction of the inter-implant papilla during second stage surgery (i.e. during the uncovering of the fixture) have also been introduced (Lee et al. 2010/a). These include the rotation of the pedicle flap to the mesial side of the healing abutment followed by a semilunar beveled incision (Palacci et al. 1995) or a horizontal incision creating a double-pedicle flap (Grossberg 2001); performing a divergent U-shaped incision opened toward the buccal side of the implant site, which creates a double-pedicle flap that is sutured over the de-epithelized papillae (Nemcovsky et al. 2000); undermining the papillae from their insertion to the bone followed by an insertion of connective tissue into the pouch-like tunnel (Azzi et al. 2002); making three interlacing “finger-like” incisions followed by the fixation of the “fingers” over the desired inter-implant papilla position by means of sutures (Misch et al. 2004); pulling the buccal flap coronally by means of a ramp mattress suture to obtain a papilla in the buccal area (Tinti and Benfenati 2002); or the plumping up of the soft tissue that formerly covered the implant by means of the healing abutment (i.e. without any sutures) following an I-shaped (Lee et al. 2010/a) or mesially opened U-shaped (Shahidi et al. 2008) incision.

8.6.3. Coverage of Mucosal Dehiscences

Mucosal dehiscences around implants/abutments caused by soft tissue recession may be covered with a coronally advanced flap (CAF) in combination with a subepithelial connective tissue graft (Burkhardt et al. 2008), as well as by means of subepithelial connective tissue grafts (SCTG) that are harvested from the palate and placed in a partial-thickness pouch constructed around the dehiscence (Hidaka and Ueno 2012). The procedure may be repeated if only the partial coverage of the dehiscence at issue occurred during the initial procedure (Hidaka and Ueno 2012).

8.7. Bone Augmentation

8.7.1. Donor Sites for an Autologous Bone Graft

Autologous bone is the gold standard of bone grafts/substitutes (Freilich and Sandor 2006; Neumann and Kevenhoerster 2009; Liu et al. 2010). The demand for other bone substitutes is generally justified by certain disadvantages of autologous bone, including the morbidity/scarring of the donor site, the prolongation of operation time, highly complex operative procedures, the limited individual shape modulation available, and their limited availability in cases of large defects (Neumann and Kevenhoerster 2009; Liu et al. 2010; Andersen et al. in press).

This is in opposition to the problems of non-autologous bone substitutes in terms of expenses, storage, biocompatibility, rejection, and product safety with regard to infectious diseases in the case of non-autologous bone products (Neumann and Kevenhoerster 2009).

Different donor sites (i.e. calvaria, rib, iliac ala, tibia, scapula, sternum) had already been described in the early 20th century and the procedure was referred to as "spongioplasty" (Neumann and Kevenhoerster 2009); these donor sites may also be used today for oral surgical purposes (Freilich and Sandor 2006; Clementini et al. 2009; Gherlone et al. 2009; Parbo et al. 2013). *Intraoral donor sites* are also certainly available (Freilich and Sandor 2006; Akintoye et al. 2008; Escoda-Francoli et al. 2010; Carlsen et al. 2013; Andersen et al. in press), and importantly, autologous bone grafts originating from intraoral (maxillary or mandibular) sources seem to exert superior osteogenic properties around oral implants when compared to autologous bone grafts of other origin (Akintoye et al. 2008). In general, three intraoral donor sites are considered: the mandibular symphysis region, mandibular ramus, and the maxillary tuberosity (Veis et al. 2004; Freilich and Sandor 2006; Clementini et al. 2009; Escoda-Francoli et al. 2010; Tang et al. 2010; Hernandez-Alfaro et al. 2011; D'Addona et al. 2012), of which the symphysis and the ramus are the preferred donor sites (Veis et al. 2004; Freilich and Sandor 2006; Escoda-Francoli et al. 2010; Tang et al. 2010; Hernandez-Alfaro et al. 2011; D'Addona et al. 2012).

Although the symphysis grafts are more accessible (Escoda-Francoli et al. 2010; Andersen et al. in press), the ramus grafts encounter fewer complications and morbidity (Verdugo et al. 2009; Tang et al. 2010; D'Addona et al. 2012), especially if the surgical technique in relation to the ramus includes an increase in the amount of access available to the mandibular body area and the use of a long-shafted bur (and/or trephine and/or tip of a piezoelectric surgical device) to create a groove instead of an inferior border osteotomy (Verdugo et al. 2009; Tang et al. 2010; D'Addona et al. 2012).

Autologous bone may also be collected during bone drilling for fixture installation by means of bone collectors (bone traps) as an alternative method for obtaining graft material to fill small bone imperfections such as fenestrations and dehiscences (Blay et al. 2003). Data indicate that if proper care is taken to prevent saliva contamination during the surgical procedure, autologous bone collected in this way may be used for bone augmentation if only small amounts of bone are required (Blay et al. 2003).

8.7.2. Augmentation Prior to Implant Placement

With the exception of frequently used "socket grafting" following tooth extraction (discussed elsewhere), usually "onlay" and/or "inlay" type grafts are used for the augmentation of bone prior to implant placement (Clementini et al. 2009; Tang et al. 2010; Perdijk et al. 2011). Data indicate that cortical block grafts perform the best in the maintenance of such onlay- and/or inlay-type grafting (Ozaki et al. 1999; Tang et al. 2010; D'Addona et al. 2012). Clinical experiences also indicate that autogenous onlay- and/or inlay-type cortical block grafts fixated with titanium screw(s) may be used without membranes (Cordaro et al. 2002; Levin et al. 2007; Hernandez-Alfaro et al. 2011; D'Addona et al. 2012), but in certain cases, it may be advantageous to also use membranes. In all other cases, including those in which block onlay grafts are combined with other grafts/substitutes (Tang et al. 2010; Hernandez-Alfaro et al. 2011), the use of either resorbable or nonresorbable membranes is advisable in terms of a guided bone regeneration technique.

8.7.3. Simultaneous Augmentation and Implant Placement

Simultaneous bone augmentation and implant placement may be needed if immediate implant placement will be done following tooth extraction (Wilson Jr. et al. 1998; Covani et al. 2003; Yun et al. 2011), if there is a bone defect/dehiscence in the planned implant site (Yeh and Hsu 2003; Kim et al. 2011), or if the sinus floor elevation will need to be created. Sinus floor elevation will be discussed later in this chapter, whereas immediate implant placement in relation to the esthetic maxillary region is discussed elsewhere. Thus, here only simultaneous bone augmentation with regard to the immediate placement of implant fixtures in the mandible and maxillary molar regions (Wilson Jr. et al. 1998; Yun et al. 2011), as well as the placement of fixtures in bone with a defect/dehiscence at the implant site (Yeh and Hsu 2003; Kim et al. 2011) will be introduced.

The immediate placement of an implant fixture into the extraction socket has been proposed to improve patient comfort and shorten treatment time if the alveolus remains intact (Yun et al. 2011; Khanifam et al. 2013). However, if an implant is placed immediately, there is often a wide gap between the walls of the extraction socket and the inserted fixture (Khanifam et al. 2013), as well as a wide soft tissue opening (Khanifam et al. 2013), especially in the case of the posterior maxilla but also in the posterior mandible. Although small peri-implant bone defects can be completely healed without using guided bone regeneration procedures (Covani et al. 2003; Yun et al. 2011; Khanifam et al. 2013), gaps around the inserted fixture exceeding 2 mm should be filled with bone graft/substitute (Wilson Jr. et al. 1998; Yun et al. 2011) and should be covered by means of resorbable or non-resorbable membranes within the guidelines of the GBR technique, followed by the primary closure of the flap over the augmented socket including the fixture with the healing screw (Yun et al. 2011). If it that there is insufficient soft tissue to completely cover the GBR site, the double-membrane GBR technique (Yun et al. 2011) may be used as follows: the fixture should be placed at least 1–2 mm beneath the top of the surrounding bony wall, the cover screw should be screwed in, and both the fixture and the bone graft/substitute should be covered by a collagen membrane. Thereafter the whole GBR site should be covered by a high-density polytetrafluoroethylene (dPTFE) membrane that is extended at least 4–5 mm over the surrounding bone (Yun et al. 2011). This latter dPTFE membrane does not require primary closure and can be left exposed for 4 weeks, after which it should be removed gently with forceps and without flap elevation (Yun et al. 2011). After 3–6 months the fixtures can be uncovered and either healing abutments can be inserted or the prosthetic rehabilitation can be started immediately with the insertion of a definitive abutment (Yun et al. 2011)

In the case of a bone defect/dehiscence in the planned implant site, the surgical process is rather similar (Yeh and Hsu 2003; Kim et al. 2011). Following crestal/paracrestal incision, full-thickness flaps should be elevated, the implant sites should be prepared, and the fixtures should be inserted and closed with healing screws (Yeh and Hsu 2003). After implant placement, the bone graft/substitute material should be placed in the bone defect/dehiscence area (Yeh and Hsu 2003), and the GBR site (including the fixtures with their healing screws) should be covered with a resorbable or non-resorbable membrane, followed by the primary closure of the flap over the screw and the augmented area (Kim et al. 2011). The augmented site should be allowed to heal for at least 3–6 months (Kim et al. 2011). Thereafter the fixtures can be uncovered and either healing abutments can be inserted or prosthetic rehabilitation can be started immediately with the insertion of a definitive abutment.

8.7.4. Augmentation in Relation to Peri-Implantitis

From a surgical view, peri-implantitis may be divided into two basic subgroups: marginal and periapical forms. The *periapical form* (also referred to as “retrograde peri-implantitis” or “implant periapical lesion”) is relatively rare. If there is no loss of implant stability (which would necessitate the removal of the implant), treatment protocols usually include curettage of the periapical bone lesion followed by irrigation with a saline solution (Ayangco and Sheridan 2001; Quirynen et al. 2005; Penarrocha-Diago et al. 2009, 2012/a) and decontamination of the implant surface with chlorhexidine (Ataullah et al. 2006; Penarrocha-Diago et al. 2009, 2012/a; Chan et al. 2011) or tetracycline pastes (Ayangco and Sheridan 2001; Balshi et al. 2007; Chan et al. 2011; Penarrocha-Diago et al. 2012/a); however there is no evidence of the efficacy of any of these items (Penarrocha-Diago et al. 2012/a). Bone substitutes accompanied or unaccompanied by resorbable membranes may also be used to achieve complete bone regeneration of the bone defect (Bretz et al. 1997; Quirynen et al. 2005; Tozum et al. 2006; Penarrocha-Diago et al. 2012/a). Sectioning the implant apex should also be considered if the total removal of the granular tissue cannot be otherwise assured (Ayangco and Sheridan 2001; Balshi et al. 2007; Dahlin et al. 2009; Penarrocha-Diago et al. 2012/a). It may be advantageous to reduce the functional load of the implant(s) under treatment as far as possible, at least during the primary healing period over the first few weeks.

In the case of the more usual *marginal form*, bone augmentation procedures are rather similar to those described above in relation to simultaneous augmentation and implant placement, with the differences being that in this case, the fixture should not be inserted because it has already been put in place, per se, and the fixtures are usually under a functional load because in spite of the peri-implantitis, a significant part of them are still osseointegrated (if this is not the case, they should be removed). Another important difference is that the walls of the bone defect should be scraped/curettaged and any bacterial biofilm (plaque) or calculus attached to the implant surface should be removed; the implant surface should be disinfected as well before the bone augmentation procedure (Bassetti et al. 2011; Marotti et al. 2013).

The effective decontamination of titanium surfaces is a crucial and rather difficult step in this case, which may be carried out through mechanical cleaning (i.e. dental curettes, ultrasonic scalers, air flow glycine-powdering) and/or by means of chemical procedures (i.e. citric acid, H_2O_2, chlorhexidine digluconate, EDTA), and may be supplemented with local or systemic antibiotics (Bassetti et al. 2011; Marotti et al. 2013). Moderately high level lasers and in particular photodynamic therapy carried out by means of low level lasers combined with a suitable photosensitizer dye may also be used efficiently (Takasaki et al. 2009; Marotti et al. 2013), as described in detail elsewhere. Air flow glycine-powdering may also be used efficiently (Bassetti et al. 2011) based on the phenomenon that the glycine powder is water soluble; therefore the rest of the powder can be resorbed without any problem in the peri-implant tissues (Bassetti et al. 2011).

Following the decontamination of the implant surface, the augmentation procedure within the frame of GBR should be carried out based on the same basic principles described above with regard to simultaneous augmentation and implant placement (Wilson Jr. et al. 1998; Covani et al. 2003; Bassetti et al. 2011; Kim et al. 2011; Yun et al. 2011), with the additional consideration that the functional load of the implant(s) under treatment should be reduced as far as possible at least during the primary healing period over the first few weeks (Bassetti et al. 2011).

8.8. Sinus Floor Elevation

8.8.1. General Considerations

In lateral maxillary rehabilitations an osseous ridge that is insufficient for inserting a dental implant in will often be found because of the combined effect of post-extraction bone resorption and maxillary sinus extension (Misch 1987; Grandi and Pacifici 2008). In general, four basic clinical situations can be characterized (Misch 1987) in this area in relation to bone availability for implant placement; they are as follows (Misch 1987; Grandi and Pacifici 2008): *Misch type class I*: bone availability is more than 12 mm, which makes it possible to insert fixtures of optimal dimensions according to the usual techniques; *Misch type class II*: bone availability is between 12 and 8 mm, with the consequence that either shorter fixtures should be used or sinus floor elevation should be carried out by means of noninvasive (i.e. osteotome based) sinus elevation techniques; *Misch type class III*: the available bone is between 8 and 5 mm, with the consequence that sinus floor elevation should be carried out to a greater extent, preferably by means of the lateral window approach followed by the insertion of fixtures at the same time (Tatum 1986; Misch 1987); and *Misch type class IV*: the available bone is less than 5 mm, with the consequence that either (ultra)short fixtures should be used (Huang et al. 2012) or the sinus floor should be elevated to a great extent. In this class, the fixture insertion should be either postponed until after graft integration (Misch 1987), or if fixtures are placed at the same time, the sinus implant stabilizer plates (SIS plates) should be used (Grandi and Pacifici 2008).

Besides bone availability, anatomical issues related to the sinus should also be considered before sinus floor elevation surgery is initiated. It should be considered that the lowest level of the alveolar wall (floor of the sinus) is usually about 1.25 cm below the level of the floor of the nasal cavity (Williams and Warwick 1980); therefore a sinus floor elevation that is to a greater extent over this level may lead to the obstruction of the natural ostium of the sinus to the middle meatus of the nose. It may be considered as a general rule that the sinus must not be lifted more than 2 cm to avoid occluding the sinusal ostium and should preferably not be lifted less than 12 mm to allow the placement of implants of a sufficient size to guarantee the adequate long-run stability of the implant and the implant-supported prosthesis (Hieu et al. 2010).

It should also be noted that in many cases, radiating septa of varying sizes spring from the floor in the intervals between the adjacent teeth (Williams and Warwick 1980), especially at the border region between the premolars and molars and between the second and third molars (Underwood 1910; Krennmair et al. 1997; Beretta et al. 2012). The so-called secondary septa may also arise from the irregular pneumatization of the sinus floor following tooth loss (Krennmair et al. 1997; Beretta et al. 2012). All these septa should be considered carefully, because they can complicate sinus elevation by hampering the inversion of the bone plate and the lifting of the sinus membrane (Pignataro et al. 2008; Beretta et al. 2012; Meleo et al. 2012). It should also be kept in mind that there is an extended and contiguous bony canal structure of the anterior and lateral wall of the maxillary sinus (Solar et al. 1999; Traxler et al. 1999; Sato et al. 2010; Yoshida et al. 2010) in many cases in the deeper regions of the lateral wall and in some cases rather near to the sinus floor (Yoshida et al. 2010). The location of these bony canal structures can be evaluated via CBCT (Sato et al. 2010; Yoshida et al. 2010) and should be considered before any sinus surgery to avoid laceration or damage of the posterior superior alveolar artery and nerve, which would lead to consequent bleeding and hemorrhage, vascular impairment, ischemia, or pain (Sato et al. 2010; Yoshida et al. 2010; Meleo et al. 2012).

There are two major techniques of sinus floor elevation: the osteotome technique and lateral window technique. Although the osteotome technique is considered more conservative, its main drawback is that the sinus floor elevation procedure must be performed "blindly" because it is impossible to visualize the sinus floor (Taschieri et al. 2012). In spite of this limitation, membrane perforation was reported to be less frequent when compared to the lateral window technique (Taschieri et al. 2012). The basic principles of both techniques will be introduced briefly below with respect to the classic approaches, which include the insertion of bone grafts/substitutes. However, the possibility of a graft-less procedure for both the osteotome (Taschieri et al. 2012) and lateral window technique (Riben and Thor 2012) was also considered as rather promising recently (Riben and Thor 2012; Taschieri et al. 2012).

8.8.2. The Osteotome Technique

For the osteotome technique (Summers 1994/a, b), a crestal incision (located in the edentulous area) is made and full-thickness buccal and palatal flaps are reflected. The site preparation process begins using N°1 and N°2 Summers-osteotomes, which are eventually supplemented with twist drilling (i.e. 2 mm diameter) if the bone is too dense for hand instrumentation (Jung et al. 2010/a). This initial preparation should be stopped roughly 1 mm below the floor of the sinus and the preparation site should be widened using N°2 and N°3 osteotomes (Zhou et al. 2008; Jung et al. 2010/a). Thereafter, the prepared bone graft/substitute material (in this case acting also as a "shock absorber") is placed into the implant site, and forced (together with the scraps of the bone in the prepared site) ahead of the tip of the osteotome (N°3) achieving the up-fracturing of the sinus floor and the elevation of the maxillary sinus membrane (Zhou et al. 2008; Jung et al. 2010/a). At this stage, the integrity of the sinus membrane should be confirmed (Jung et al. 2010/a) by means of a modified Valsalva maneuver (by attempting to exhale carefully through the nose while keeping it closed). If integrity is verified, filling up can be carried out with the necessary amount of bone graft/substitutes. During the filling up of the sinus floor, it should be always considered that the elevation of the sinus membrane should be created by the ("hydraulic") pressure of the forced blood and graft/substitute materials (De Vico et al. 2009); consequently, the osteotome never has to enter inside the sinus (De Vico et al. 2009). Upon completion of the filling up process, implant fixtures can be inserted; then the insertion of the healing screws and the closure of the flaps can commence (Zhou et al. 2008; Jung et al. 2010/a). The second surgical procedure and prosthetic rehabilitation (leading to the functional load) can be carried out roughly six (Zhou et al. 2008) or seven (Jung et al. 2010/a) months later.

8.8.3. The Lateral Window Technique

For the lateral window technique, a crestal incision (located in the edentulous area) is made in association with two (mesial and distal) vertical-releasing incisions (Grandi and Pacifici 2008; Hieu et al. 2010; Sanchez-Recio et al. 2010), and a full-thickness muco-periosteal flap is elevated (Grandi and Pacifici 2008; Hieu et al. 2010; Sanchez-Recio et al. 2010; Cha et al. 2011). Thereafter a buccal window is made at the lateral surface of the sinus wall using multiblade burs at first (Grandi and Pacifici 2008), followed by diamond burs (Grandi and Pacifici 2008; Hieu et al. 2010), and/or using a diamond round bur followed by a piezoelectric surgical device in the final phase (Cha et al. 2011), and/or using exclusively a piezoelectric surgical device (Vercellotti et al. 2001; Escoda-Francoli et al. 2010; Sanchez-Recio et al. 2010). Then the buccal window and the sinus membrane are raised with the usual manual tools (Grandi and Pacifici 2008; Cha et al. 2011; Hieu et al. 2010), alternating the surgical movements with pauses in order to verify the presence of synchronous sinus-membrane motion with respiratory actions (which refers to membrane integrity) (Grandi and Pacifici 2008). The sinus membrane may also be elevated through the use of special tips for the piezoelectric surgical device (Vercellotti et al. 2001; Escoda-Francoli et al. 2010; Sanchez-Recio et al. 2010).

If the needed volume is obtained and membrane integrity is verified, an initial filling up is carried out with an autologous bone graft and/or other bone substitutes (Grandi and Pacifici 2008). Thereafter, the implant fixtures are inserted in the alveolar bone and the initially filled bone graft/substitute (Grandi and Pacifici 2008). After the insertion of the fixtures (and their fixation with SIS plates if necessary), healing screws are screwed in; then the filling of the sinus floor with the bone graft/substitute is completed and the bone graft/substitute is covered with a resorbable (i.e. collagen) membrane (Grandi and Pacifici 2008; Hieu et al. 2010; Cha et al. 2011). Finally the flap is closed and sutures are applied using single and/or mattress stitches (Grandi and Pacifici 2008; Hieu et al. 2010; Cha et al. 2011). The second surgical procedure is usually carried out roughly eight (6–12) months later (Grandi and Pacifici 2008; Cha et al. 2011; Shigeshi et al. 2012). By means of a slightly palatal incision, a split-thickness flap is raised and a large band of keratinized gum is moved vestibular, cover screws (and the SIS plate if any) are removed, and after screwing in the healing abutments, the flap is closed and fixed with single-stitch sutures (Grandi and Pacifici 2008). The prosthetic treatment and functional loading can be started immediately (after the healing of the soft tissues around the healing abutment) in this case because the necessary healing period for fixtures inserted simultaneously with a sinus floor elevation is usually considered to be a period of 5–10 months after the insertion (Jung et al. 2010/b) is fulfilled.

If the fixtures were *not* inserted simultaneously, the filled bone graft/substitute is covered with a membrane and the flap is closed as described above (Grandi and Pacifici 2008; Cha et al. 2011). In this case, the fixtures are inserted later within the context of a second surgical procedure after a healing period of roughly 6–8 months (Hieu et al. 2010; Cha et al. 2011).

8.8.4. The Management of Sinus Membrane Perforation

Depending on the clinical situation, the anatomy of the sinus floor, previous phlogistic processes in the sinus, the surgical technique, and the experiences of the surgeon, the frequency of occurrence of a Schneiderian membrane perforation ranges roughly between 5%–44% (Vercellotti et al. 2001; Schwartz-Arad et al. 2004; Thor et al. 2007; Sanchez-Recio et al. 2010; Meleo et al. 2012). The frequency of the occurrence can be significantly reduced with the use of a piezoelectric surgical device (Wallace et al. 2007; Penarrocha-Diago et al. 2012/b), because in this case, perforation (if any) occurs primarily in the hand instrumentation phase but not during the preparation of the bone window (Wallace et al. 2007).

The occurrence of a perforation does not necessarily lead to serious complications (Branemark et al. 1984; Jung et al. 2007; Sanchez-Recio et al. 2010; Riben and Thor 2012). Most perforations are smaller than 5 mm and as such can be patched (following further detachment of the sinus membrane if necessary) with a collagen membrane that is in direct contact with the Schneiderian membrane (Hernandez-Alfaro et al. 2008; Sanchez-Recio et al. 2010; Meleo et al. 2012; Penarrocha-Diago et al. 2012/b); thereafter, the sinus floor elevation procedure and the insertion of fixtures can be continued immediately within the same sitting (Hernandez-Alfaro et al. 2008; Sanchez-Recio et al. 2010; Penarrocha-Diago et al. 2012/b). In the case of larger sinus membrane lesions, a resorbable or non-resorbable membrane should be applied above the bone window, the flaps should be closed properly, and the sinus floor elevation procedure should be postponed until after recovery (Biglioli et al. 2010).

With the osteotome technique, membrane perforation was reported to be less frequent in comparison to the lateral window technique (Taschieri et al. 2012). However, if membrane perforation occurs it may be difficult to evaluate the seriousness of the membrane perforation (and to manage it properly), because it is impossible to visualize the sinus floor (Taschieri et al. 2012). In such cases, either a shift to the lateral window technique (and the management of the perforation as described above) or the closure of the flaps and the repetition of the sinus floor elevation at a later point in time may be considered.

8.9. Other Techniques in Low Bone Availability

8.9.1. Alveolar Distraction Osteogenesis

Alveolar distraction osteogenesis is a "stretching-based" surgical technique that encourages the creation of new bone and soft tissue through the incremental lengthening of osseous segments (Walker 2005). It is particularly helpful in vertical ridge augmentation in both the mandible (Walker 2005; Perez-Sayans et al. in press) and the maxilla (Kanno et al. 2012; Perez-Sayans et al. in press). In the mandible, the alveolar distraction osteogenesis procedure usually targets the molar region (Walker 2005). In the case of the maxilla, the procedure may target either the molar/premolar region or the whole edentulous alveolar arch (Kanno et al. 2012; Perez-Sayans et al. in press) and may be combined with sinus floor elevation at the same time (Kanno et al. 2012). Most procedures are carried out under local anesthesia (Walker 2005), but for more advanced surgical interventions, general anesthesia may also be needed (Kanno et al. 2012).

In general, distraction osteogenesis involves five phases (Walker 2005; Kanno et al. 2012; Perez-Sayans et al. in press): an osteotomy (cut through) of a smaller or larger bony segment according to need (miniaturized distraction devices are also available), followed by the insertion of the distraction device (Walker 2005; Kanno et al. 2012; Perez-Sayans et al. in press); a latency or waiting period of roughly 5–7 days to allow resolution of inflammation and initial healing (Walker 2005; Perez-Sayans et al. in press); a distraction or callus manipulation period of roughly 8–10 days, with a distraction rate of 0.33 mm 3 times a day (Walker 2005) or 0.5 mm 1–2 times a day (Kanno et al. 2012; Perez-Sayans et al. in press) for a total distraction rate of 0.5–1 mm/day (Walker 2005; Kanno et al. 2005; Perez-Sayans et al. in press); a bone consolidation period of 3–4 months (Walker 2005; Kanno et al. 2005; Perez-Sayans et al. in press); and a second-stage surgery to remove the distraction device and to insert the implant fixtures (advantageously at the same time) at the end of the consolidation period (Walker 2005; Kanno et al. 2005; Perez-Sayans et al. in press).

For the surgical intervention, a deep-vestibular incision (ca. 5 mm to the junction of the attached gingiva and alveolar mucosa) is made with great attention paid to the mental foramen in the mandible as well as the retrotuberal region and pterygopalatine fossa in the maxilla (Walker 2005; Kanno et al. 2012). The osteotomy of the transport bone segment is carried out carefully with a bur and a reciprocating saw (Walker 2005; Kanno et al. 2012), supplemented by a spatula osteotome (Walker 2005) and/or piezosurgery (Kanno et al. 2012). The retraction device is fixed to both the intact bone and the osteotomy-separated "transport bone segment" by screws (Walker 2005; Kanno et al. 2012). During the whole surgical procedure, great care should be taken to protect the vascular pedicle and to leave soft tissue attachments to the transport bone segment (especially in the areas of flaring vertical osteotomy cuts) (Walker 2005; Kanno et al. 2012), because the vascularity (blood supply) of the transport segment is predominantly from the lingual/palatal periosteum (Walker 2005), at least during the latency/waiting period and the distraction phase, but also in the early consolidation period.

8.9.2. Alveolar Nerve Lateralization/Transposition

Dental implants are often placed in the posterior mandible. However, in many cases the bone has atrophied such that sufficiently long fixtures cannot be placed (Morrison et al. 2002; Del-Castillo-Pardo-de-Vera et al. 2008; Vasconselos et al. 2008). In that situation, a treatment option is to move the inferior alveolar nerve (IAN) laterally from its canal by either nerve lateralization or nerve transposition (Morrison et al. 2002; Del-Castillo-Pardo-de-Vera et al. 2008; Vasconselos et al. 2008). With *nerve lateralization*, the IAN is exposed and traction is used to deflect it laterally while the implants are being placed (advantageously with a bicortical anchorage), and the IAN is then left to fall back in against the fixtures (Morrison et al. 2002), following the positioning of a resorbable membrane between the nerve and the fixtures to prevent direct contact between the nerve and the fixtures (Del-Castillo-Pardo-de-Vera et al. 2008). There is no interference with the incisive nerve in this case (Morrison et al. 2002; Del-Castillo-Pardo-de-Vera et al. 2008). With *nerve transposition*, a corticotomy is done about the mental foramen, and the incisive nerve is transected (Morrison et al. 2002; Del-Castillo-Pardo-de-Vera et al. 2008; Vasconselos et al. 2008). Then, with the nerve fully lateralized, the dental implants are placed advantageously under direct visualization and with a bicortical anchorage (Morrison et al. 2002; Del-Castillo-Pardo-de-Vera et al. 2008; Vasconselos et al. 2008). Once the implants have been placed, the nerve is passively positioned against the implant following the positioning of a resorbable membrane between the nerve and the fixtures to prevent direct contact of the nerve with the fixtures. Because of the presence of the implants (that the nerve should go around), the emergence of the nerve becomes more distal (Morrison et al. 2002; Del-Castillo-Pardo-de-Vera et al. 2008; Vasconselos et al. 2008).

The inherent risk of both surgical procedures is damage to the IAN, with resultant neurosensory disturbance to the mental nerve (Morrison et al. 2002; Del-Castillo-Pardo-de-Vera et al. 2008; Vasconselos et al. 2008). The transposition of the IAN per se results in the loss of sensation in terms of its terminal incisive branch because it should be transected (Morrison et al. 2002; Del-Castillo-Pardo-de-Vera et al. 2008; Vasconselos et al. 2008), which has no consequence if the anterior mandible is edentulous, but may cause some disturbance to residual dental and periodontal sensibility in any remaining anterior teeth (Morrison et al. 2002). Both IAN lateralization and IAN transposition are delicate surgical interventions (Morrison et al. 2002; Del-Castillo-Pardo-de-Vera et al. 2008; Vasconselos et al. 2008). Although they may be carried out under local anesthesia (Del-Castillo-Pardo-de-Vera et al. 2008; Vasconselos et al. 2008), they are best performed under general anesthesia to eliminate patient movement and to maximize access (Morrison et al. 2002).

There are certain anatomical variations of the mandible that should be considered carefully. The presence of a double ("duplicated," "bifid") or in certain cases even a triple mandibular canal (Karamifar et al. 2009; Bogdan et al. 2006), anatomical variations of the mental foramen (Sawyer et al. 1998; Kaufman et al. 2000; Hanihara and Ishida 2001; Igarashi et al. 2004; Kulkarni et al. 2011; Silva Ramos Fernandes et al. 2011; Santos Jr. et al. 2013), and anatomical variations of the "*anterior loop*" of the mental canal (Arzouman et al. 1993; Williams and Warwick 1980; Neiva et al. 2004), as well as the presence of an accessory mental canal, especially distal to the mental foramen (Kulkarni et al. 2011), should be considered. The existence of such variations should be recognized and carefully evaluated by means of detailed radiologic examination prior to initiating alveolar nerve lateralization/transposition.

8.9.3. Tilted, Zygomatic, and Tuberal Implantation

The frontal and zygomatic processes, as well as the tuberal region, are important bony structures around the maxillary sinus. In certain cases, these bony structures may allow the insertion of angulated/tilted implants (Sorni et al. 2005; Koser et al. 2006; Galan-Gil et al. 2007; Branemark et al. 2004; De Vico et al. 2011). Although the insertion of such angulated/tilted implants into the premised maxillary processes and/or into the tuberal region is clearly not easy, the surgical technique has undergone considerable development in recent years (Sorni et al. 2005; Galan-Gil et al. 2007; De Vico et al. 2011). The insertion of implants into the premised bony structures may be of importance in the rehabilitation of patients with larger bony defects and/or with an extremely resorbed alveolar process (Branemark et al. 2004; Sorni et al. 2005; Galan-Gil et al. 2007; De Vico et al. 2011).

There is usually a rather compact cortical layer and a rather dense medullary bone in the *lower part of the frontal process* positioned between the nasal cavity and the maxillary sinus (Sorni et al. 2005) that may be used for the insertion of tilted/angulated implants in certain cases (Mattsson et al. 1999; Krekmanov et al. 2000; Sorni et al. 2005). Similarly, there is a rather compact bone structure of the zygomaticoalveolar crest along with the zygomatic process (Sorni et al. 2005), which may advantageously be utilized for the insertion of implants in certain cases (Krekmanov 2000; Balshi and Wolfinger 2002; Parel et al. 2001; Branemark et al. 2004) if there is no extension of the maxillary sinus into the zygomatic process.

The tuberal region comprises three bony structures: the maxillary tuberosity, the pyramidal process of the palatine bone, and the pterygoid process of the sphenoid bone (Williams and Warwick 1980; Sorni et al. 2005). In contrast to the maxillary tuberosity, the pyramidal process of the palatine bone and the anterior portion of the pterygoid process are composed of corticalized bone (Sorni et al. 2005); therefore the junction-region of the premised three bony structures (i.e. the maxillary tuberosity, pyramidal process, and pterygoid process) may be used for implant placement in certain cases (Graves 1994; Balshi et al. 1995; Fernandez and Fernandez 1997; Balshi and Wolfinger 1999; Nocini et al. 2000). However, an extremely careful surgical technique is needed if the implant is placed into this region, because there is a high risk of damaging branches of the maxillary artery (Fernandez and Fernandez 1997; Sorni et al. 2005) as well as the maxillary nerve. It should also be considered carefully that the pterygopalatine fossa is nearby; therefore, serious complications because of the dangerous spreading of the occasional infection through this fossa may also appear.

Although tilted implants are primarily used in the maxilla for the rehabilitation of patients with larger bony defects and/or with an extremely resorbed alveolar process (Sorni et al. 2005; Koser et al. 2006; Branemark et al. 2004; De Vico et al. 2011), in certain cases, it may also be advantageous to insert tilted implants in the interforaminal region of the distally atrophied mandible in order to improve chewing capacity in the molar regions and/or to decrease the size of the bilateral cantilever of the interforaminally placed, implant-supported fixed dentures (De Vico et al. 2011).

8.10. Virtual Implant Placement and Navigational Surgery

With the aid of CBCT images, a dentist can place implants virtually (VIP: virtual implant placement), and thereafter data can be sent to a CAD/CAM manufacturing facility, which can create a surgical guide, including metal cylinders that direct osteotomy drills into precise locations in the jaw as planned by the dentist (Howerton Jr. and Mora 2008; Pozzi et al. 2008; De Vico et al. 2012; Svensson et al. 2014). This workflow should include a rather sophisticated, high-quality radiological evaluation, including planning via virtual implant placement coupled with surgical template manufacturing by means of a highly developed manufacturing facility (Pedersen et al. 2014; Svensson et al. 2014). In the framework of prosthodontic-driven implant planning, fixed prostheses may also be planned virtually and manufactured in connection with the above-mentioned CAD/CAM surgical guide technology, which allows the dentist to place implants using a surgical guide and place a fixed prosthesis during the same dental visit (Howerton Jr. and Mora 2008; Pozzi et al. 2008; De Vico et al. 2012; Svensson et al. 2014). If the premised radiological evaluation, planning, and coupled manufacturing are properly done, the surgical template can be considered accurate (Huh et al. 2012), and the use of such an accurate template may then lead to a minimally invasive, precise, and safe surgical procedure (Svensson et al. 2014). However, it should be emphasized that the appearance of complications cannot be excluded if deviations appear because of inaccuracies during the procedure (Svensson et al. 2014).

The weak point of such procedures from a surgical point of view is that they rely on accuracy in transferring information derived from CBCT-based VIP data into surgery. Concretely, even if the template is accurate, it may be difficult to guarantee a close fit of the template with the hard and/or soft tissue surfaces in a proper and stable position in order to accurately transfer the preoperative VIP treatment plan into the real surgical implant placement (Frisardi et al. 2011). It should be considered that small deviations between the virtually planned and the real position of the surgical template may lead to rather significant deviation of the post-insertion positions of the implants, which may lead to irreversible damage to important anatomical structures, such as sensory nerves, the maxillary sinus floor, neighboring teeth, etc. (Frisardi et al. 2011). To overcome this problem, the surgical template may be supported/anchored by the remaining teeth (if any) via clasps. The template may also be stabilized by placing anchor pins in the bone through the template (and through the mucosa if the flap was not raised) (Serrano et al. 2008; De Vico et al. 2011, 2012). The template may also be stabilized by the dental surgeon pressing the template against the mucosa (similarly to how full dentures are stabilized by masticatory forces).

Further, real-time computer-assisted navigational surgery, allowing virtual direct vision of the drill tip related to the bone and other surrounding tissues (i.e. the sinus floor, alveolar nerve, neighboring teeth, etc.) in real time during the surgery may also be applied (Ng et al. 2005). In this case, navigation is made possible through a series of sensors attached to the rotary instruments, the surgical template, and to a cap fixed on the patient's head, all of which are coupled to the same data-analyzing system (Serrano et al. 2008). Data obtained are transferred immediately to the computer and enable the dental surgeon to see the real situation in CBCT images that are used as a map and provide the dental surgeon with a real-time representation of the surgical instruments in relation to the images of the patient (Serrano et al. 2008).

8.11. Removal of Implant Fixtures

Removal of implants may be needed if a fracture of the fixture occurs (Balshi 1996; Sanchez-Perez et al. 2010) and if advanced peri-implantitis or other serious peri-implant bone necrosis appears (Shin et al. 2010). *In the case of implant fracture*, three management options may be considered as follows (Sanchez-Perez et al. 2010). Complete removal of the fractured implant using explantation trephines (eventually followed by the insertion of a new, wider implant) should be considered first (Balshi 1996; Sanchez-Perez et al. 2010). Alternatively, removal of the coronal portion of the fractured implant with the purpose of placing a new prosthetic post may also be considered (Balshi 1996; Sanchez-Perez et al. 2010) if the percentage of bone contact is high and there is a sufficient remaining internal thread for adequate post retention (Balshi 1996; Sanchez-Perez et al. 2010). Finally, removal of the coronal portion of the fractured implant, leaving the remaining apical part integrated in the bone, is also an option, but only if the previously mentioned alternatives cannot be carried out (Sanchez-Perez et al. 2010).

In the case of advanced peri-implantitis, bone augmentation in the framework of GBR may initially be considered as described previously. If the prognosis of bone augmentation is not promising or is hopeless, complete removal of the fixture using elevators and/or explantation trephines should be considered. *In the case of serious peri-implant bone necrosis*, the fixtures should be removed completely using elevators and/or explantation trephines (Shin et al. 2010).

Conclusion

In this chapter the most important surgical aspects of implant dentistry, including principles of implant site preparation and implant placement, the timing of implant site preparation (i.e. immediate, early, and delayed implant placement), the timing of loading (i.e. immediate, early, and delayed loading), the type of loading (i.e. functional, nonfunctional, and progressive), the surgical management of various implant failures (i.e. peri-implantitis, fracture), several forms of bone augmentation, major techniques of sinus floor elevation (including management of sinus membrane perforation), and soft tissue surgery, as well as certain important related topics, like the assessment of bone quality and primary stability, were discussed. Besides these, several other surgical techniques, like alveolar distraction osteogenesis, alveolar nerve lateralization, alveolar nerve transposition, and the use of tilted, zygomatic, and tuberal implantation, as well as principles of virtual implant placement and navigational surgery were also introduced. The authors hope that this presentation of the most important related data helps the reader to be comfortable with the surgical aspects of implant dentistry.

References

Abrahamsson, I; Berglundh, T; Wennstrom, J; Lindhe, J. The peri-implant hard and soft tissues at different implant systems. A comparative study in the dog. *Clin Oral Implant Res*, 1996, 7, 212–219.

Abrahamsson, I; Berglundh, T; Moon, IS; Lindhe, J. Peri-implant tissues at submerged and non-submerged titanium implants. *J Clin Periodontol*, 1999, 26, 600–607.

Adell, R; Lekholm, U; Rockler, B; Branemark, PI. A 15-year study of osseointegrated implants in the treatment of the edentulous jaw. *Int J Oral Surg*, 1981, 10, 387–416.

Aguirre-Zorzano, LA; Rodriguez-Andres, C; Estefania-Fresco, R; Fernandez-Jimenez, A. Immediate temporary restoration of single-tooth implants: Prospective clinical study. *Med Oral Patol Cir Bucal*, 2011, 16, e794–e799.

Akintoye, SO; Giavis, P; Stefanik, D; Levin, L; Mante, FK. Comparative osteogenesis of maxilla and iliac crest human bone marrow stromal cells attached to oxidized titanium – a pilot study. *Clin Oral Implant Res*, 2008, 19, 1197–1201.

Albrektsson, T; Zarb, G; Worthington, P; Eriksson, AR. The long-term efficacy of currently used dental implants: a review and proposed criteria of success. *Int J Oral Maxillofac Implants*, 1986, 1, 11–25.

Albrektsson, T; Isidor, F. Consensus report of session V. In: Lang NP, Karring T, editors. *Proceedings of the 1st European Workshop on Periodontology*. London: Quintessence; 1993; 365–369.

Andersen, K; Norholt, SE; Knudsen, J; Kuseler, A; Jensen, J. Donor site morbidity after reconstruction of alveolar bone defects with mandibular symphyseal bone grafts in cleft patients – 111 consecutive patients. *Int J Oral Maxillofac Surg*, in press, DOI: 10.1016/j.ijom.2013.09.007.

Andres-Garcia, R; Vives, NG; Climent, FH; Palacin, AF; Santos, VR; Climent, MH; Bullon, P. In vitro evaluation of the influence of the cortical bone on the primary stability of two implant systems. *Med Oral Patol Oral Cir Bucal*, 2009, 14, E93–E97.

Appleton, RS; Nummikoski, PV; Pigno, MA; Cronin, RJ; Chung, KH. A radiographic assessment of progressive loading on bone around single osseointegrated implants in the posterior maxilla. *Clin Oral Implants Res*, 2005, 16, 161–167.

Arataki, T; Furuya, Y; Ito, T; Miyashita, Y; Shimamura, I; Yajima, Y. Pre-operative drilling simulation method for dental implant treatment. *Bull Tokyo Dent Coll*, 2007, 48, 27–35.

Arzouman, MJ; Otis, L; Kipnis, V; Levine, D. Observations of the anterior loop of the inferior alveolar canal. *Int J Oral Maxillofac Implants*, 1993, 8, 295–300.

Ataullah, K; Chee, LF; Peng, LL; Lung, HH. Management of retrograde peri-implantitis: A clinical case report. *J Oral Implantol*, 2006, 32, 308–312.

Ayangco, L; Sheridan, PJ. Development and treatment of retrograde peri-implantitis involving a site with a history of failed endodontic and apicoectomy procedures: a series of reports. *Int J Oral Maxillofac Implants*, 2011, 16, 412–417.

Azzi, R; Etienne, D; Takei, H; Fenech, P. Surgical thickening of the existing gingiva and reconstruction of interdental papillae around implant-supported restorations. *Int J Periodontics Restorative Dent*, 2002, 22, 71–77.

Balshi, TJ. An analysis and management of fractured implants: a clinical report. *Int J Oral Maxillofac Implants*, 1996, 11, 660–666.

Balshi, TJ; Lee, HY; Hernandez, RE. The use of pterygomaxillary implants in the partially edentulous patient: a preliminary report. *Int J Oral Maxillofac Implants*, 1995, 10, 89–98.

Balshi, TJ; Wolfinger, GJ. Analysis of 356 pterygomaxillary implants in edentulous arches for fixed prosthesis anchorage. *Int J Oral Maxillofac Implants*, 1999, 14, 398–406.

Balshi, TJ; Wolfinger, GJ. Treatment of congenital ectodermal dysplasia with zygomatic implants: a case report. *Int J Oral Maxillofac Implants*, 2002, 17, 277–281.

Balshi, SF; Wolfinger, GJ; Balshi, TJ. A retrospective evaluation of a treatment protocol for dental implant periapical lesions: long-term results of 39 implant apicoectomies. *Int J Oral Maxillofac Implants*, 2007, 22, 267–272.

Bassetti, R; Bassetti, M; Kremer, U; Mericske-Stern, R. Existiert das Kombinationssyndrom? Ein Fallbericht. *Schweiz Monatsschr Zahnmed*, 2010, 120, 771–778.

Bassetti, R; Bassetti, M; Enkling, N; Mericske-Stern, R. Behandlung einer fortgeschrittenen periimplantitis im unterkiefer. *Schweiz Monatsschr Zahnmed*, 2011, 121, 325–332.

Beretta, M; Cicciu, M; Bramanti, E; Maiorana, C. Schneider membrane elevation in presence of sinus septa: anatomic features and surgical management. *Int J Dentistry*, 2012, Article ID 261905. DOI: 10.1155/2012/261905.

Berglundh, T; Lindhe, J. Dimension of the periimplant mucosa. Biological width revisited. *J Clin Periodontol*, 1996, 23, 971–973.

Berglundh, T; Lindhe, J; Ericsson, I; Marinello, CP; Linjenberg, B; Thomsen, P. The soft tissue barrier at implants and teeth. *Clin Oral Implants Res*, 1991, 2, 81–90.

Biglioli F; Pedrazzoli, M; Colletti, G. Repair of a perforated sinus membrane with a palatal fibromucosal graft: a case report. *Minerva Stomatol*, 2010, 59, 299–302.

Binon, PP; Sullivan, DY. Provisional fixed restorations technique for osseointegrated implants. *J Calif Dent Assoc*, 1990, 18, 23–30.

Blay, A; Tunchel, S; Sendyk, WR. Viability of autologous bone graft obtained by using bone collectors: histological and microbiological study. *Pesqui Odontol Bras*, 2003, 17, 234–240.

Block, MS; Kent, JN. Factors associated with soft- and hard-tissue compromise of endosseous implants. *J Oral Maxillofac Surg*, 1990, 48, 1153–1160.

Bogdan, S; Pataky, L; Barabas, J; Nemeth, Z; Huszar, T; Szabo, G. Atypical courses of the mandibular canal: comparative examination of dry mandibles and x-rays. *J Craniofac Surg*, 2006, 17, 487–491.

Branemark, PI; Hansson, BO; Adell, R; Breine, U; Lidstrom, J; Hallen, O; Ohman, A. Osseointegrated implants in the treatment of the edentulous jaw. Experience from a 10-year period. *Scand J Plast Reconstr Surg*, 1977, 16(Suppl.), 1–132.

Branemark, PI; Adell, R; Albrektsson, T; Lekholm, U; Lindstrom, J; Rockler, B. An experimental and clinical study of osseointegrated implants penetrating the nasal cavity and maxillary sinus. *J Oral Maxillofac Surg*, 1984, 42, 497–505.

Branemark, PI; Engstrand, P; Ohrnell, LO; Grondahl, K; Nilsson, P; Hagberg, K; Darle, C; Lekholm, U. Branemark Novum: a new treatment concept for rehabilitation of the edentulous mandible. Preliminary results from a prospective clinical follow-up study. *Clin Implant Dent Relat Res*, 1999, 1, 2–16.

Branemark, PI; Grondahl, K; Ohrnell, LO; Nilsson, P; Petruson, B; Svensson, B; Engstrand, P; Nannmark, U. Zygoma fixture in the management of advanced atrophy of the maxilla: technique and long-term results. *Scan J Plast Reconstr Surg Hand Surg*, 2004, 38, 70–85.

Bretz, WA; Matuck, AN; de Oliveira, G; Moretti, AJ; Bretz, WA. Treatment of retrograde peri-implantitis: clinical report. *Implant Dent*, 1997, 6, 287–290.

Brkovic, BMB; Prasad, HS; Konandreas, G; Milan, R; Antunovic, D; Sandor, GKB; Rohrer, MD. Simple preservation of a maxillary extraction socket using beta-tricalcium phosphate with type I collagen: Preliminary clinical and histomorphometric observations. *J Can Dent Assoc*, 2008, 74, 523–528.

Burkhardt, R; Joss, A; Lang, NP. Soft tissue dehiscence coverage around endosseous implants: a prospective cohort study. *Clin Oral Implants Res*, 2008 19, 451–457.

Buser, D; Weber, HP; Lang, NP. Tissue integration of non-submerged implants. 1-year results of a prospective study with 100 ITI hollow-cylinder and hollow-screw implants. *Clin Oral Implants Res*, 1990, 1, 33–40.

Buttel, AE; Gratwohl, DA; Sendi, P; Marinello, CP. Immediate loading of two unsplinted mandibular implants in edentulous patients with an implant-retained overdenture: an observational study over two years. *Schweiz Monatsschr Zahnmed*, 2012, 122, 392–397.

Caneva, M; Botticelli, D; Salata, LA; Souza, SLS; Bressan, E; Lang, NP. Flap vs. "flapless" surgical approach at immediate implants: a histomorphometric study in dogs. *Clin Oral Implant Res*, 2010, 21, 1314–1319.

Carlsen, A; Gorst-Rasmussen, A; Jensen, T. Donor site morbidity associated with autogenous bone harvesting from the ascending mandibular ramus. *Implant Dent*, 2013, 22, 503–506.

Cha, JK; Park, JC; Jung, UW; Kim, CS; Cho, KS; Choi, SH. Case series of maxillary sinus augmentation with biphasic calcium phosphate: a clinical and radiographic study. *J Periodontal Implant Sci*, 2011, 41, 98–104.

Chan, HL; Wang, HL; Bashutski, J; Edwards, PC; Fu, JH; Oh, TJ. Retrograde peri-implantitis: A case report introducing an approach to its management. *J Periodontol*, 2011, 82, 1080–1088.

Clementini, M; Boniello, R; Gasparini, G; Moro, A; Pelo, S. Surgical treatment of severe atropic maxilla by means of multiple extraoral harvesting. ORAL & Implantology, 2009, 2, 4–10.

Cochran, DL; Morton, D; Weber, HP. Consensus statements and recommended clinical procedures regarding loading protocols for endosseus dental implants. *Int J Oral Maxillofac Implants*, 2004, 19 (Suppl), 109–113.

Cordaro, L; Amade, DS; Cordaro, M. Clinical results of alveolar ridge augmentation with mandibular block bone grafts in partially edentulous patients prior to implants placement. *Clin Oral Implants Res*, 2002, 13, 103–111.

Cox, JF; Zarb, GA. The longitudinal clinical efficacy of osseointegrated dental implants: a 3-year report. *Int J Oral Maxillofac Implants*, 1987, 2, 91–100.

Covani, U; Cornelini, R; Barone, A. Bucco-lingual bone remodeling around implants placed into immediate extraction socket: a case series. *J Periodontol*, 2003 74, 268–273.

D'Addona, A; Ghassemian, M; Raffaelli, L; Manicone, PF. Soft and hard tissue management in implant therapy – Part I: Surgical concepts. *Int J Biomaterials*, 2012, Article ID: 531202. DOI: 10.1155/2012/531202.

Dahlin, C; Nikfarid, H; Alsen, B; Kashani, H. Apical peri-implantitis: possible predisposing factors, case reports, and surgical treatment suggestions. *Clin Implant Dent Relat Res*, 2009, 11, 222–227.

de Carvalho Crusoe Silva, IM; de Feritas, DQ; Ambrosano, GMB; Boscolo, FN; Almeida, SM. Bone density: comparative evaluation of Hounsfield units in multislice and cone-beam computed tomography. *Braz Oral Res (Sao Paulo)*, 2012, 26, 550–556.

Del-Castillo-Pardo-de-Vera, JL; Chamorro-Pons, M; Cebrian-Carretero, JL. Repositioning of the inferior alveolar nerve in cases of severe mandibular atrophy. A clinical case. *Med Oral Patol Oral Cir Buccal*, 2008, 13, E778–E782.

De Vico, G; Bonino, M; Spinelli, D; Pozzi, A; Barlattani, A. Clinical indications, advantages and limits of the expansion-condensing osteotomes technique for the creation of implant bed. *ORAL & Implantology*, 2009, 2, 27–36.

De Vico, G; Bonino, M; Spinelli, D; Schiavetti, R; Sannino, G; Pozzi, A; Ottria, L. Rationale for tilted implants: FEA considerations and clinical reports. *ORAL & Implantology*, 2011, 4, 23–33.

De Vico, G; Spinelli, D; Bonino, M; Schiavetti, R; Pozzi, A; Ottria, L. Computer-assisted virtual treatment planning combined with flapless surgery and immediate loading in the rehabilitation of partial edentulies. *ORAL & Implantology*, 2012, 5, 3–10.

Escoda-Francoli, J; Rodriguez-Rodriguez, A; Berini-Aytes, L; Gay-Escoda, C. Application of ultrasound in bone surgery. Two case reports. *Med Oral Patol Oral Cir Bucal*, 2010, 15, e902–e905.

Farre-Pages, N; Auge-Castro, ML; Alaejos-Algarra, F; Mareque-Bueno, J; Ferres-Padro, E; Hernandez-Alfaro, F. Relation between bone density and primary implant stability. *Med Oral Patol Oral Cir Bucal*, 2011, 16, e62–e67.

Fernandez, J; Fernandez L. Placement of screw type implants in the pterygo-maxillary-pyramidal region: a surgical procedure and preliminary results. *Int J Oral Maxillofac Implants*, 1997, 12, 814–819.

Fickl, S; Zuhr, O; Wachtel, H; Bolz, W; Huerzeler, M. Tissue alterations after tooth extraction with and without surgical trauma: a volumetric study in the beagle dog. *J Clin Periodontol*, 2008, 35, 356–363.

Freilich, AM; Sandor, GKB. In-office iliac crest bone harvesting for peri-implant jaw reconstruction. *J Can Dent Assoc*, 2006, 72, 543–547.

Friberg, B; Sennerby, L; Roos, J; Lekholm, U. Identification of bone quality in conjunction with insertion of titanium implants. A pilot study in jaw autopsy specimen. *Clin Oral Implant Res*, 1995, 6, 213–219.

Frisardi, G; Chessa, G; Barone, S; Paoli, A; Razionale, A; Frisardi, F. Integration of 3D anatomical data obtained by CT imaging and 3D optical scanning for computer aided implant surgery. *BMC Medical Imaging*, 2011, 11, 5.

Galan-Gil, S; Penarroca-Diago, M; Balaguer-Martinez, J; Marti-Bowen, E. Rehabilitation of severely resorbed maxillae with zygomatic implants: an update. *Med Oral Patol Oral Cir Buccal*, 2007, 12, E216–E220.

Garcia, CC; Lopez, AB; Diago, MP. Immediately restored dental implants for partial-arch applications. A literature update. *Med Oral Patol Oral Cir Buccal*, 2008, 13, E451–455.

Gfeller, F; Zitmann, NU; Lambrecht, JT. Sofort belastete monotype Implantate im zahnlosen Unterkiefer. *Schweiz Monatsschr Zahnmed*, 2011, 121, 235–242.

Gherlone, EF; Vinci, R; D'Aversa, L. Autologus parietal grafts in preprosthetic surgery. *ORAL & Implantology*, 2009, 2, 2–13.

Glauser, R; Sennerby, L; Meredith, N; Ree, A; Lundgren, A; Gottlow, J; Hammerle, CH. Resonance frequency analysis of implants subjected to immediate or early functional occlusal loading. Successful vs. failing implants. *Clin Oral Implant Res*, 2004, 15, 428–434.

Gonzalez, JMM; Dorado, CB; Sanchez, JC; Caliz, FF; Turrion, AS. Evaluation of 80 implants subjected to immediate loading in edentulous mandibles after two years of follow-up. *Med Oral Patol Oral Cir Bucal*, 2006, 11, E165–E170.

Grandi, C; Pacifici, L. Two stage surgery in IV class of Misch with SIS device: A case report. *ORAL & Implantology*, 2008, 1, 131–136.

Graves, SL. The pterygoid plate implant: a solution for restoring the posterior maxilla. *Int J Periodontics Restorative Dent*, 1994, 14, 513–523.

Grossberg, DE. Interimplant papilla reconstruction: assessment of soft tissue changes and results of 12 consecutive cases. *J Periodontol*, 2001, 72, 958–962.

Hammerle, CHF; Chen, ST; Wilson Jr., TG. Consensus statements and recommended clinical procedures regarding the placement of implants in extraction sockets. *Int J Oral Maxillofac Implants*, 2004, 19, 26–28.

Hanihara, T; Ishida, H. Frequency variations of discrete cranial traits in major human populations. IV. Vessel and nerve related variations. *J Anat*, 2001, 199, 273–287.

Hernandez-Alfaro, F; Torradeflot, MM; Marti, C. Prevalence and management of Schneiderian membrane perforations during sinus-lift procedures. *Clin Oral Implant Res*, 2008, 19, 91–98.

Hernandez-Alfaro, F; Salvan-Garcia, E; Mareque-Bueno, J; Ferres-Padro, E. "Envelope" approach for onlay bone grafting: Preliminary surgical and prosthetic results. *Med Oral Patol Oral Cir Bucal*, 2011, 16, e45–e49.

Hidaka, T; Ueno, D. Mucosal dehiscence coverage for dental implant using sprit pouch technique: a two-stage approach. *J Periodontal Implant Sci*, 2012, 42, 105–109.

Hieu, PD; Chung, JH; Yim, SB; Hong, KS. A radiological study on the changes in height of grafting materials after sinus lift: a comparison between two types of xenogenic materials. *J Periodontal Implant Sci*, 2010, 40, 25–32.

Homolka, P; Beer, A; Birkfellner, W; Nowotny, R; Gahleitner, A; Tschabitscher, M; Bergmann, H. Bone mineral density measurement with dental quantitative CT prior to dental implant placement. *Radiology*, 2002, 224, 247–252.

Howerton Jr., WB; Mora, MA. Advancements in digital imaging: What is new and on the horizon? *Am J Dent Assoc*, 2008, 139(suppl 3), 20S–24S.

Huang, J. Risk factors and strategies of dental implants in the maxillary posterior without sufficient bone available. *West China J Stomatol*, 2012, 30, 1–9.

Huh, YJ; Choi, BR; Huh, KH; Yi, WJ; Heo, MS; Lee, SS; Choi, SC. In-vitro study on the accuracy of a simple-design CT-guided stent for dental implants. *Imaging Sci Dent*, 2012, 42, 139–146.

Hui, E; Chow, J; Li, D; Liu, J; Wat, P; Law, H. Immediate provisional for single-tooth implant placement with Branemark system: preliminary report. *Clin Implant Dent Relat Res*, 2001, 3, 79–86.

Igarashi, C; Kobayashi, K; Yamamoto, A; Morita, Y; Tanaka, M. Double mental foramina of the mandible on computed tomography images: a case report. *Oral Radiol*, 2004, 20, 68–71.

Ihde, S; Kopp, S; Maier, T. Comparison of implant survival with implants placed in acceptable and compromised bone: a literature review. *J Maxillofac Oral surg*, 2009, 8, 1–7.

Irinakis, T. Rationale for socket preservation after extraction of a single-rooted tooth when planning for future implant placement. *J Can Dent Assoc*, 2006, 72, 917–922.

Jemt, T; Lekholm, U; Grondahl, K. 3-year follow up study of early single implant restorations ad modum Branemark. *Int J Periodontics Restorative Dent*, 1990, 10, 340–349.

Johansson, P; Strid, KG. Assessment of bone quality from placement resistance during implant surgery. *Int J Oral Maxillofac Implants*, 1994, 9, 279–288.

Jung, JH; Choi, BH; Jeong, SM; Li, J; Lee, SH; Lee, HJ. A retrospective study of the effects on sinus complications of exposing dental implants to the maxillary sinus cavity. *Oral Surg Oral Med Oral Pathol Oral Radiol Endodontol*, 2007, 103, 623–625.

Jung, JH; Choi, SH; Cho, KS; Kim, CS. Bone-added osteotome sinus floor elevation with simultaneous placement of non-submerged sand blasted with large grit and acid etched implants: a 5-year radiographic evaluation. *J Periodontal Implant Sci*, 2010/a, 40, 69–75.

Jung, UW; Hong, JY; Lee, JS; Kim, CS; Cho, KS; Choi, SH. A hybrid technique for sinus floor elevation in the severely resorbed posterior maxilla. *J Periodontal Implant Sci*, 2010/b, 40, 76–85.

Kan, JY; Rungcharassaeng, K. Immediate placement and provisonalization of maxillary anterior single implants: a surgical and prosthodontic rationale. *Pract Periodontics Aesthet Dent*, 2000, 12, 817–824.

Kang, IH; Kim, CW; Lim, YJ; Kim, MJ. A comparative study on the initial stability of different implants placed above the bone level using resonance frequency analysis. *J Adv Prosthod*, 2011, 3, 190–195.

Khanifam, P; Pullisaar, H; Leknes, K. Dental implant placement in fresh extraction sockets. *Danish Dent J*, 2013, 117, 1002–1007.

Kanno, T; Mitsugi, M; Paeng, JY; Sukegawa, S; Furuki, Y; Ohwada, H; Nariai, Y; Ishibashi, H; Katsuyama, H; Sekine, J. Simultaneous sinus lifting and alveolar distraction of a severely atrophic posterior maxilla for oral rehabilitation with dental implants. *Int J Dentistry*, 2012, Article ID: 471320. DOI: 10.1155/2012/471320.

Karamifar, K; Shahidi, S; Tondari, A. Bilateral bifid mandibular canal: Report of two cases. *Ind J Dent Res*, 2009, 20, 235–237.

Kaufman, E; Serman, NJ; Wang, PD. Bilateral mandibular accessory foramina and canals: a case report and review of the literature. *Dentomaxillofac Radiol*, 2000, 29, 170–75.

Kim, JM; Kim, SJ; Han, I; Shin, SW; Ryu, JJ. A comparison of the implant stability among various implant systems: clinical study. *J Adv Prosthodont*, 2009, 1, 31–36.

Kim, JH; Kim, JK; Yi, YJ; Yun, PY; Lee, HJ; Kim, MJ; Yeo, IS. Results of immediate loading for implant restoration in partially edentulous patients: a 6-month preliminary prospective study using SinusQuick™ EB implant system. *J Adv Prosthodont*, 2009, 1, 136–139.

Kim, D; Kang, T; Gober, D; Orlich, C. A liquid membrane as a barrier membrane for guided bone regeneration. *ISRN Dentistry*, 2011, Article ID: 468282. DOI: 10.5402/2011/468282.

Koser, LR; Campos, PSF; Mendes, CMC. Length determination of zygomatic implants using tridimensional computed tomography. *Braz Oral Res*, 2006, 20, 331–336.

Krekmanov, L; Kahn, M; Rangert, B; Lindstrom, H. Tilting of posterior mandibular and maxillary implants for improved prosthesis support. *Int J Oral Maxillofac Implants*, 2000, 15, 405–414.

Krennmair, G; Ulm, C; Lugmayr, H. Maxillary sinus septa: incidence, morphology and clinical implications. *J Cranio-Maxillo-Facial Surg*, 1997, 25, 261–265.

Kulkarni, S; Kumar, S; Kamath, S; Thakur, S. Accidental identification of accessory mental nerve and foramen during implant surgery. *J Indian Soc Periodontol*, 2011, 15, 70–73.

Landi, L; Sabatucci, D. Plastic surgery at the time of membrane removal around mandibular endosseous implants: a modified technique for implant uncovering. *Int J Periodontics Restorative Dent*, 2001, 21, 280–287.

Langer, B; Langer, L. Overlapped flap: a surgical modification for implant fixture installation. *Int J Periodontics Restorative Dent*, 1990, 10, 208–215.

Langer, B; Sullivan, DY. Osseointegration: its impact on the interrelationship of periodontics and restorative dentistry: Part I. *Int J Periodontics Restorative Dent*, 1989, 9, 84–105.

Ledermann, P. Bar-prosthetic management of the edentulous mandible by means of plasma-coated implantation with titanium screws. *Deutsche Zahnarztl Z*, 1979, 34, 907–911.

Lee, EK; Herr, Y; Kwon, YH; Shin, SI; Lee, DY; Chung, JH. I-shaped incisions for papilla reconstruction in second stage implant surgery. *J Periodontal Implant Sci*, 2010/a, 40, 139–143.

Lee, KH; Kim, BO; Jang, HS. Clinical evaluation of a collagen matrix to enhance the width of keratinized gingiva around dental implants. *J Periodontal Implant Sci*, 2010/b, 40, 96–101.

Lekholm, U; Zarb, GA. Patient selection and preparation. In: Branemark PI, Zarb GA, Albrektsson, T, editors. *Tissue integrated prostheses. Osseointegration in clinical dentistry.* Chicago: Quintessence Publishing Company, 1985, 199–209.

Levin, L; Nitzan, D; Schwartz-Arad, D. Success of dental implants placed in intraoral block bone grafts. *J Periodontol*, 2007, 78, 18–21.

Lindeboom, JA; Frenken, JW; Dubois, L; Frank, M; Abbink, I; Kroon, FH. Immediate loading versus immediate provisionalization of maxillary single-tooth replacements: a prospective randomized study with BioComp implants. *J Oral Maxilofac Surg*, 2006, 64, 936–942.

Liu, H; Webster, TJ. Mechanical properties of dispersed ceramic nanoparticles in polymer composites for orthopedic applications. *Int J Nanomedicine*, 2010, 5, 299–313.

Madrigal, C; Ortega, R; Meniz, C; Lopez-Quiles, J. Study of available bone for interforaminal implant treatment using cone-beam computed tomography. *Med Oral Patol Oral Cir Bucal*, 2008, 13, E307–E312.

Marotti, J; Tortamano, P; Cai, S; Ribeiro, MS; Franco, JEM; de Campos, TT. Decontamination of dental implant surfaces by means of photodynamic therapy. *Lasers Med Sci*, 2013, 28, 303–309.

Martinez, H; Davarpanah, M; Missika, P; Celletti, R; Lazzara, R. Optimal implant stabilization in low density bone. *Clin Oral Implants Res*, 2001, 12, 423–432.

Mattsson, T; Kondell, PA; Gynther, GW; Fredholm, U; Bolin, A. Implant treatment without bone grafting in severely resorbed edentulous maxillae. *Int J Oral Maxillofac Surg*, 1999, 57, 281–287.

McCracken, MS; Aponte-Wesson, R; O'Neal, SJ; Rajdev, K. Low-cost implant overdenture option for patients treated in a predoctoral dental school curriculum. *J Dent Education*, 2006, 70, 662–666.

McNutt, MD; Chou, CH. Current trends in immediate osseous dental implant case selection criteria. *J Dent Education*, 2003, 67, 850–859.

Meleo, D; Mangione, F; Corbi, S; Pacifici, L. Management of the Schneiderian membrane perforation during the maxillary sinus elevation procedure: a case report. *Annali di Stomatologia*, 2012, 3, 24–30.

Meredith, N; Alleyne, D; Cawley, P. Quantitative determination of the stability of the implant-tissue interface using resonance frequency analysis. *Clin Oral Implant Res*, 1996, 7, 261–267.

Meredith, N; Book, K; Friberg, B; Jemt T; Sennerby, L; Resonance frequency measurements of implant stability in vivo. A cross-sectional and longitudinal study of resonance frequency measurements on implants in the edentulous and partially dentate maxilla. *Clin Oral Implants Res*, 1997, 8, 226–233.

Misch, CE. Maxillary sinus augmentation for endosteal implants: organized alternative treatment plans. *Int J Oral Implantol*, 1987, 4, 49–58.

Misch, CE. Density of bone: effect on treatment plans, surgical approach, healing, and progressive bone loading. *Int J Oral Implantol*, 1990, 6, 23–31.

Misch, CE; Al-Shammari, KF; Wang, HL. Creation of interimplant papillae through a split-finger technique. *Implant Dent*, 2004, 13, 20–27.

Moon, SH; Um, HS; Lee, JK; Chang, BS; Lee, MK. The effect of implant shape and bone preparation on primary stability. *J Periodontal Implant Sci*, 2010, 40, 239–243.

Morrison, A; Chiarot, M; Kirby, S. Mental nerve function after inferior alveolar nerve transposition for placement of dental implants. *J Can Dent Assoc*, 2002, 68, 46–50.

Nagaraj, KR; Savadi, RC; Savadi, AR; Parashanth Reddy, GT; Srilakshmi, J; Dayalan, M; John, J. Gingival biotype – Prosthodontic perspective. *Ind J Prosthodontic Soc*, 2010, 10, 27–30.

Neiva, RF; Gapski, R; Wang, HL. Morphometric analysis of implant-related anatomy in Caucasian skulls. *J Periodontol*, 2004, 75, 1061–1067.

Nemcovsky, CE; Moses, O; Artzi, Z. Interproximal papillae reconstruction in maxillary implants. *J Periodontol*, 2000, 71, 308–314.

Neumann, A; Kevenhoerster, K. Biomaterials for craniofacial reconstruction. *GMS Curr Top Otorhinolaryngol Head Neck Surg*, 2009, 8, Doc08. DOI: 10.3205/ cto000060.

Ng, FC; Ho, KH; Wexler, A. Computer-assisted navigational surgery enhances safety in dental implantology. *Ann Acad Med Singapore*, 2005, 34, 383–388.

Nocini, PF. Albanese, M; Fior A; De Santis, D. Implant placement in the maxillary tuberosity: the Summers' technique performed with modified osteotomes. *Clin Oral Impl Res*, 2000, 11, 273–278.

Olive, J; Aparicio, C. Periotest method as a measure of osseointegrated oral implant stability. *Int J Oral Maxillofac Implants*, 1990, 5, 390–400.

O'Sullivan, D; Sennerby, L; Meredith, N. Measurements comparing the initial stability of five designs of dental implants: a human cadaver study. *Clin Implant Dent Relat Res*, 2000, 2, 85–92.

O'Sullivan, D; Sennerby, L; Meredith, N. Influence of implant taper on the primary and secondary stability of osseointegrated titanium implants. *Clin Oral Implants Res*, 2004, 15, 474–480.

Ozaki, W; Buchman, SR; Goldsteinand, SA; Fyhrie, DP. A comparative analysis of the microarchitecture of cortical membranous and cortical endochondral onlay bone grafts in the craniofacial skeleton. *Plast Reconstr Surg*, 1999, 104, 139–147.

Palacci, P. Papilla regeneration technique. In: Palacci P, Ericsson I, Engstrand P, Ranger B, editors. *Optimal implant positioning & soft tissue management for Branemark system.* Chicago: Quintessence Pub. Co., 1995, 59–70.

Pagni, G; Pellegrini, G; Giannobile, WV; Rasperini, G. Postextraction alveolar ridge preservation: Biological basis and treatments. *Int J Dentistry*, 2012, Article ID: 151030. DOI: 10.1155/2012/151030.

Parbo, N; Murra, N; Andersen, K; Buhl, J; Kiil, B; Norholt, SE. Outcome of partial mandibular reconstruction with fibula grafts and implant-supported prostheses. *Int J Oral Maxillofac Surg*, 2013, 42, 1403–1408.

Parel, SM; Branemark, PI; Ohrnell, LO; Sensson, B. Remote implant anchorage for the rehabilitation of maxillary defects. *J Prosthet Dent*, 2001, 86, 377–381.

Park, JC; Yang, KB; Choi, Y; Kim, YT; Jung, UW; Kim, CS; Cho, KS; Chai, JK; Kim, CK; Choi, SH. A simple approach to preserve keratinized mucosa around implant using a prefabricated implant retained stent: a report of two cases. *J Periodontal Implant Sci*, 2010, 40, 194–200.

Park, JC; Hwang, JW; Lee, JS; Jung, UW; Choi, SH; Cho, KS; Chai, JK; Kim, CS. Development of the implant surgical technique and assessment rating system. *J Periodontal Implant Sci*, 2012, 42, 25–29.

Pedersen, TK; Dalstra, M; Cattaneo, P; Blomlof, J; Buhl, J; Norholt, SE. Use of digital dental cast and 3D models in orthodontics, orthognathic and reconstructive surgery. *Danish Dent J*, 2014, 118, 14–19.

Perez-Sayans, M; Leon-Camacho, MA; Sozoma-Martin, JM; Fernandez-Gonzalez, B; Blanes-Vazquez-Gundin, S; Gandara-Rey, JM; Garcia-Garcia, A. Dental implants placed on bone subjected to vertical alveolar distraction show the same performance as those placed on primitive bone. *Med Oral Patol Oral Cir Bucal*, In press, DOI: 104317/medoral.18545.

Penarrocha, MA; Vina, JA; Maestre, L; Penarrocha, D; Balaguer, J. Guided implant surgery with modification of the technique involving the raising of a semicircular miniflap: A preliminary study. *Med Oral Patol Oral Cir Bucal*, 2012, 17, e775–e780.

Penarrocha-Diago, M; Boronat-Lopez, A; Garcia-Mira, B. Inflammatory implant periapical lesion: etiology, diagnosis, and treatment-presentation of 7 cases. *J Oral Maxillofac Surg*, 2009, 67, 168–173.

Penarrocha-Diago, M; Maestre-Ferrin, L; Cervera-Ballester, J; Penarrocha-Oltra, D. Implant periapical lesion: diagnosis and treatment. *Med Oral Patol Oral Cir Bucal*, 2012/a, 17, e1023–e1027.

Penarrocha-Diago, MA; Penarrocha-Diago, M; Sanchez-Recio, C; Penarrocha-Oltra, D; Romero-Millan, J. Osteotomy in direct sinus lift. A comparative study of the rotary technique and ultrasound. *Med Oral Patol Oral Cir Bucal*, 2012/b, 17, e457–e461.

Perdijk, FBT; Meijer, GJ; Bronkhorst, EM; Koole, R. Implants in the severely resorbed mandibles: whether or not to augment? What is the clinician's preference? *Oral Maxillofac Surg*, 2011, 15, 225–231.

Pignataro, L; Mantovani, M; Torretta, S; Felisati, G; Sambataro, G. ENT assessment in the integrated management of candidate for (maxillary) sinus lift. *Acta Otorhinolaryngologica Italica*, 2008, 28, 110–119.

Pozzi, A; Gargari, M; Barlattani, A. CAD/CAM technologies in the surgical and prosthetic treatment of the edentulous patient with biomymetic individualized approach. *ORAL & Implantology*, 2008, 1, 2–14.

Quirynen, M; Vogels, R; Alsaadi, G; Naert, I; Jacobs, R; van Steenberghe, D. Predisposing conditions for retrograde peri-implantitis, and treatment suggestions. *Clin Oral Implant Res*, 2005, 16, 599–608.

Rambla-Ferrer, J; Penarrocha-Diago, M; Guarinos-Carbo, J; Analysis of the use of expansion osteotomes for the creation of implant beds. Technical contributions and review of the literature. *Med Oral Patol Oral Cir Bucal*, 2006, 11, E267–E271.

Randow, K; Ericsson, I; Nilner, K; Petersson, A; Glantz, PO. Immediate functional loading of Branemark dental implants. An 18-month clinical follow-up study. *Clin Oral Implants Res*, 1999, 10, 8–15.

Reiser, G; Brun, J; Mahan, P; Larkin, L. The subepithelial connective tissue graft palatal donor site: Anatomic considerations for surgeons. *Int J Periodontics Restorative Dent*, 1996, 16, 130–137.

Riben, C; Thor, A. The maxillary sinus membrane elevation procedure: Augmentation of bone around dental implants without grafts – A review of a surgical technique. *Int J Dentistry*, 2012, Article ID 105483. DOI: 10.1155/2012/105483.

Romanos, GE; Nentwig, GH. Immediate versus delayed functional loading of implants in the posterior mandible: a 2-year prospective clinical study of 12 consecutive cases. *Int J Periodontics Restorative Dent*, 2006, 26, 459–469.

Romanos, G; Froum, S; Hery, C; Cho, SC; Tarnow, D. Survival rate of immediately vs. delayed loaded implants: analysis of the current literature. *J Oral Implantol*, 2010, 36, 315–324.

Sanchez-Perez, A; Moya-Villaescusa, MJ; Jornet-Garcia, A; Gomez, S. Etiology, risk factors and management of implant fractures. *Med Oral Patol Oral Cir Bucal*, 2010, 15, e504–e508.

Sanchez-Recio, C; Penarrocha-Diago, M; Penarrocha-Diago, M; Penarrocha-Oltra, D. Maxillary sinus lift performed using ultrasound. Evaluation of 21 patients. *Med Oral Patol Oral Cir Bucal*, 2010, 15, e371–e374.

Santos Jr., O; Pinheiro, LR; Umetsubo, OS; Sales, MAO; Cavalcanti, MGP. Assessment of open source software for CBCT in detecting additional mental foramina. *Braz Oral Res (Sao Paulo)*, 2013, 27, 128–135.

Sanz, I; Garzia-Gargallo, M; Herrera, D; Martin, C; Figuero, E; Sanz, M. Surgical protocols for early implant placement in post-extraction sockets: a systematic review. *Clin Oral Implants Res*, 2012, 23, 67–79.

Sato, I; Kawai, T; Yoshida, S; Miwa, Y; Imura, K; Asaumi, R; Sunohara, M; Yosue, T. Observing the bony canal structure of the human maxillary sinus in Japanese cadavers using cone beam CT. *Okajimas Folia Anat Jpn*, 2010, 87, 123–128.

Sawyer, DR; Kiely, ML; Pyle, MA. The frequency of accessory mental foramina in four ethnic groups. *Arch Oral Biol*, 1998, 43, 417–420.

Schwartz-Arad, D; Herzberg, R; Dolev, E. The prevalence of surgical complications of the sinus graft procedure and their impact on implant survival. *J Periodontol*, 2004, 75, 511–516.

Serrano, MR; Estela, SA; Diago, MP; Diago, MP. Software applied to oral implantology: Update. *Med Oral Patol Cir Bucal*, 2008, 13, E661–E665.

Shahidi, P; Jacobson, Z; Dibart, S; Pourati, J; Nunn, ME; Barouch, K; Van Dyke, TE. Efficacy of a new papilla generation technique in implant dentistry: a preliminary study. *Int J Oral Maxillofac Implants*, 2008, 23, 926–934.

Shigeshi, H; Takechi, M; Nishimura, M; Takamoto, M; Minami, M; Ohta, K; Kamata, N. Clinical evaluation of novel interconnected porous hydroxyapatite ceramics (IP-CHA) in a maxillary sinus floor augmentation procedure. *Dent Materials J*, 2012, 31, 54–60.

Shin, EY; Kwon, YH; Herr, Y; Shin, SI; Chung, JH. Implant failure associated with oral bisphosphonate-related osteonecrosis of the jaw. *J Periodontal Implant Sci*, 2010, 40, 90–95.

Silva Ramos Fernandes, L; Capelozza, A; Rubira-Bullen, I. Absence and hypoplasia of the mental foramen detected in CBCT images: a case report. *Surg Radiol Anat*, 2011, 33, 731–734.

Solar, P; Geyerhofer, U; Traxler, H; Windisch, A; Ulm, C; Watzek, G. Blood supply to the maxillary sinus relevant to sinus floor elevation procedures. *Clin Oral Impl Res*, 1999, 10, 34–44.

Sorni, M; Guarinos, J; Penarrocha, M. Implants in anatomical buttresses of the upper jaw. *Med Oral Patol Oral Cir Bucal*, 2005, 10, 163–168.

Summers, RB. A new concept in maxillary implant surgery: the osteotome technique. *Compendium*, 1994, 15, 152–158.

Summers, RB. The osteotome technique: Part 3 – Less invasive methods of elevating the sinus floor. *Compendium*, 1994, 15, 698–704.

Svensson, KG; Trulsson, M; Hultin, M. Computer aided implant treatment. *Danish Dent J*, 2014, 118, 22–29.

Takasaki, AA; Aoki, A; Mizutani, K; Schwarz, F; Sculean, A; Wang, CY; Koshy, G; Romanos, G; Ishikawa, I; Izumi, Y. Application of antimicrobial photodynamic therapy in periodontal and peri-implant diseases. *Periodontol*, 2009, 51, 109–140.

Tan, WL; Wong, TLT; Wong, MCM; Lang, NP. A systemic review of post-extractional alveolar hard and soft tissue dimensional changes in humans. *Clin Oral Implants Res*, 2012, 23, 1–21.

Tang, ZH; LV, H; Cao, MX; Wu, MJ. Clinical effects of ridge augmentation with the half-columnar shaped mandibular bone block for the placement of dental implants. *J Peking Univ (Health Sci)*, 2010, 42, 94–97.

Taschieri, S; Corbella, S; Saita, M; Tsesis, I; Del Fabbro, M. Osteotome-mediated sinus lift without grafting material: A review of literature and a technique proposal. *Int J Dentistry*, 2012, Article ID 849093. DOI: 10.1155/2012/849093.

Tatum, H. Maxillary and sinus implants reconstruction. *Dent Clin North Am*, 1986, 30, 107–119.

Thor, A; Sennerby, L; Hirsch, JM; Rasmusson, L. Bone formation at the maxillary sinus floor following simultaneous elevation of the mucosal lining and implant installation without graft material: an evaluation of 20 patients treated with 44 Astra Tech implants. *J Oral Maxillofac Surg*, 2007, 65, 64–72.

Tinti, C; Benfenati, SP. The ramp mattress suture: a new suturing technique combined with a surgical procedure to obtain papillae between implants in the buccal area. *Int J Periodontics Restorative Dent*, 2002, 22, 63–69.

Tozum, TF; Sencimen, M; Otakoglu, K; Ozdemir, A; Aydin, OC; Keles, M. Diagnosis and treatment of a large periapical implant lesion associated with adjacent natural tooth: a case report. *Oral Surg Oral Med Oral Pathol Oral Radiol Endod*, 2006, 101, 132–138.

Traxler, H; Windisch, A; Geyerhofer, U; Surd, R; Solar, P; Firbas, W. Arterial blood supply of the maxillary sinus. *Clin Anat*, 1999, 12, 417–421.

Turkyilmaz, I; McGlumphy, EA. Influence of bone density on implant stability parameters and implant success: a retrospective clinical study. *BMC Oral Health*, 2008, 8, 32.

Underwood, AS. An inquiry into the anatomy and pathology of the maxillary sinus. *Journal of Anatomy and Physiology*, 1910, 44, 354–369.

Vasconselos, JA, Avila, GB; Ribeiro, JC; Dias, SC; Pereira, LJ. Inferior alveolar nerve transposition with involvement of the mental foramen for implant placement. *Med Oral Patol Oral Cir Buccal*, 2008, 13, E722–E725.

Veis, AA; Tsirlis, AT; Parisis, NA. Effect of autogenous harvest site location on the outcome of ridge augmentation for implant dehiscences. *Int J Periodontics Restorative Dent*, 2004, 24, 155–163.

Vercellotti, T; De Paoli, S; Nevins, M; The piezoelectric bony window osteotomy and sinus membrane elevation: introduction of a new technique for simplification of the sinus augmentation procedure. *Int J Periodontics Restorative Dent*, 2001, 21, 561–567.

Verdugo, F; Simonian, K; Nowzari, H. Periodontal biotype influence on the volume maintenance of onlay grafts. *J Periodontol*, 2009, 80, 816–823.

Walker, DA. Mandibular distraction osteogenesis for endosseous dental implants. *J Can Dent Assoc*, 2005, 71, 171–175.

Wallace, SS; Mazor, Z; Froum, SJ; Cho, SO; Tarnow, DP. Schneiderian membrane perforation rate during sinus elevation using piezosurgery: clinical results of 100 consecutive cases. *Int J Periodontics Restorative Dent*, 2007, 27, 413–419.

Wang K; Li, DH; Zhou, JX; Zhang, CJ; Liu, BL; Li YL. Influence of bicortical anchorage on the natural frequencies of dental implants. *West China J Stomatol*, 2006, 24, 86–88.

Warrer, K; Buser, D; Lang, NP; Karring, T. Plaque-induced peri-implantitis in the presence or absence of keratinized mucosa. An experimental study in monkeys. *Clin Oral Implant Res*, 1995, 6, 131–138.

Williams, PL; Warwick, R. (Ed-in-chiefs). *Gray's Anatomy*. Thirty-sixth edition. Edinburgh-London-Melbourne-New York: Churchill Livingstone, 1980, 316–319, 340, 342, 257–259.

Wilson Jr., TG; Schrenk, R; Buser, D; Cochran, D. Implants placed in immediate extraction sites: a report of histologic and histometric analyses of human biopsies. *Int J Oral Maxillofac Implants*, 1998, 13, 333–341.

Yeh, HC; Hsu, KW. Guided bone regeneration for fenestration defects in dental implants. *Chang Gung Med J*, 2003, 26, 684–689.

Yi, JM; Lee, JK; Um, HS; Chang, BS; Lee, MK. Marginal bony changes in relation to different vertical positions of dental implants. *J Periodontal Implant Sci*, 2010, 40, 244–248.

Yoon, HG; Heo, SJ; Koak, JY; Kim, SK; Lee, SY. Effect of bone quality and implant surgical technique on implant stability quotient (ISQ) value. *J Adv Prosthodont*, 2011, 3, 10–15.

Yoon, JH; Park, YB; Cho, Y; Kim, CS; Choi, SH; Moon, HS; Lee, KW; Shim, JS. Development of implant loading device for animal study about various loading protocol: a pilot study. *J Adv Prosthodont*, 2012, 4, 227–234.

Yoshida, S; Kawai, T; Asaumi, R; Miwa, Y; Imura, K; Koseki, H; Sunohara, M; Yosue, T; Sato, I. Evaluation of the blood and nerve supply patterns in the molar region of the maxillary sinus in Japanese cadavers. *Okajimas Folia Anat Jpn*, 2010, 87, 129–133.

Yun, JH; Jun, CM; Oh, NS. Secondary closure of an extraction socket using the double-membrane guided bone regeneration technique with immediate implant placement. *J Periodontal Implant Sci*, 2011, 41, 253–258.

Zarb, GA; Schmitt, A. The longitudinal clinical effectiveness of osseointegrated dental implants: the Toronto study. Part III: Problems and complications encountered. *J Prosthet Dent*, 1990, 64, 185–194.

Zhou, L; Xu, SL; Xu, ST; Huang, JS; Song, GB; Zhang, XY. Clinical application of maxillary sinus lift with Summers osteotome. *West China J Stomatol*, 2008, 26, 296–298.

Chapter 9

Abutment

Abstract

The abutment is an important part of most implant systems. It is positioned between the fixture and the denture, and this "mesostructure" position makes it possible to connect dentures to fixtures and to modify the long axis of the implant-abutment-denture complex using an angled abutment. Abutments may be classified as healing or definitive. Healing abutments may be used right after the insertion of implant fixtures in the case of a one-stage surgery or after establishing the mini-flap access at the uncovering stage of two-stage surgery. Definitive abutments may be used either in all premised healing phases, if no healing abutment was used, or after the healing phase following the removal of the healing abutments. Abutments may also be classified based on major fabrication methods, such as industrially manufactured stock abutments, individually cast metal abutments, and CAD-CAM-milled individual abutments. Stock abutments exhibit durability and a fit accuracy superior to individually fabricated abutments. However, their finish line is located according to average values, which might not necessarily coincide with the existing gingival/mucosal contour. To overcome this limitation, individually fabricated abutments may be used. In general, metallic and ceramic (zirconia) abutments may be used. The mechanical properties of metallic abutments seem to be somewhat better; however, a typical esthetic limitation of metallic abutments is the grayish coloration of the mucous tissues, especially in the case of a thin gingival biotype. To overcome this problem, ceramic (i.e. zirconia) abutments or metal abutments with porcelain fused to the metal coverage may be used in the esthetic zone. The disadvantage of the abutment is the appearance of two (i.e. the fixture-abutment and the abutment-denture) interfaces, from which at least one could be discounted if the abutment was not used. On the other hand, the use of an abutment clearly increases the plasticity and adaptability of the whole implant system, and creative use of the abutment, together with provisional restorations, is a rather efficient tool for soft tissue modeling (contouring, profiling), which is crucial for obtaining proper soft tissue esthetics in many cases.

9.1. Introduction

The abutment is an important part of most implant systems. It is positioned between the fixture and the denture, and this "mesostructure" position (i.e. between the fixture as "infrastructure" and the denture as "suprastructure") makes it possible to connect dentures to fixtures and to modify the long axis of the implant-abutment-denture complex using an angled abutment that fits with a correct prosthetic emergence profile (Cardelli et al. 2009; Manicone et al. 2012).

Abutments may be classified as healing or definitive. If a healing abutment is used, it should certainly be replaced with a definitive abutment after the healing phase. Healing abutments may be used right after the insertion of implant fixtures in the case of one-stage surgery or after establishing mini-flap access at the uncovering stage of two-stage surgery. Accordingly, a definitive abutment may be used either in all the premised healing phases, if no healing abutment was used, or after the healing phase following removal of the healing abutment.

Abutments may also be classified based on the major fabrication method, such as industrially manufactured straight/angled stock abutments (slightly modifiable chair-side), individually cast metal abutments, or CAD-CAM-milled individual metal/zirconia abutments (Manicone et al. 2012). Stock abutments are available as commercially pure titanium, titanium alloys, and zirconia, and are provided by all implant suppliers (Apicella et al. 2010; Abduo and Lyons 2013). Stock abutments exhibit durability and a fit accuracy superior to individually fabricated abutments. However, their finish line is located according to average values, which might not necessarily coincide with the existing gingival/mucosal contour (Apicella et al. 2010; Abduo and Lyons 2013). To overcome this limitation, individually fabricated abutments may be used; however, in this case, an impression should be taken. An impression may be taken either following the removal of the healing abutment or in the absence of a healing abutment, right after the insertion of the fixture (one-stage surgery) or after establishing mini-flap access at the uncovering stage of two-stage surgery (Manicone et al. 2012; Abduo and Lyons 2013).

In general, both metallic and ceramic (zirconia) abutments may be used. The mechanical properties of metallic abutments seem to be somewhat better; however, a typical esthetic limitation of metallic abutments is the grayish coloration of the mucous tissues, especially in the case of patients with a thin gingival biotype (Abduo and Lyons 2013). To overcome this problem, ceramic (i.e. zirconia) abutments (Abduo and Lyons 2013) or metal abutments with porcelain fused to the metal coverage (Jaime et al. 2007), fabricated industrially or individually, may be used advantageously in the esthetic zone.

9.2. Fixation of an Abutment

The fixture-abutment connection is usually established by means of a screw screwed into the fixture through the abutment. The fixture-abutment interface can be either internal (i.e. the fixture serves as the matrix and the abutment as the patrix) or external (i.e. the fixture serves as the patrix and the abutment as the matrix), and currently there are many types of geometry used in both cases (Manicone et al. 2012). Proper fixation of the abutment is crucial because abutment screw loosening is one of the most common complications (Laney et al. 1994; Jemt and Pettersson 1993; Kang et al. 1996; Kim and Shin 2013). A major factor behind screw loosening may be inappropriate tightening torque (Jorneus et al. 1992). In general, a tightening torque of 20–35 Ncm (the higher the better) may be considered, but in this respect, the manufacturer's recommendation and the clinical situation should be considered first. Besides inappropriate tightening force, other possible reasons for screw loosening are fatigue, a settling effect, vibrating micromovement, and excessive bending (Lazzara et al. 1996; Kim and Shin 2013). Although the fabrication method of the abutment (i.e. stock, casted, or CAD-CAM-milled) seems to not be a major factor in this regard (Kim and Shin 2013), the quality (i.e. precision, material, and shape) of the abutment surely exerts an influence on the screw-loosening phenomenon.

Although screw fixation is the original and most commonly used method to connect an abutment to an implant, screw loosening and screw fracture are the major disadvantages of this method (Laney et al. 1994; Jemt and Pettersson 1993; Kang et al. 1996; Moon et al. 2009; Kim and Shin 2013). A locking taper connection (also referred to as a "Morse taper") has been introduced as an alternative. This fixation does not utilize any screw. Locking taper systems utilize a 1–2 degree tapered patrix that fits into a mirror-image-shaped matrix (Moon et al. 2009). Although the tapered surfaces appear to be smooth, they are not absolutely smooth at the microscale level. Therefore, the retention of the locking taper connection is primarily based on frictional resistance (Moon et al. 2009). The high frictional force is due to the high-contact pressure caused by the relative slip between the two tapered surfaces (Moon et al. 2009), similar to the case of *Morse taper systems*, which are frequently used in numerous industrial fields even today. Because of the high forces, the surface oxide layers break down and the asperities fuse, leading to an additional cold-welding phenomenon (Moon et al. 2009) that further increases retention. A major disadvantage of the locking taper system is that it makes it difficult to place the abutment precisely, and there is a risk that the abutment will sink (Moon et al. 2009).

9.3. Fixture-Abutment Interface

Currently, particular attention has been given to the fixture-abutment interface, because research suggests that bacterial colonization and plaque formation may occur in the microgap of this interface, which may cause soft/hard tissue inflammation and bone resorption (Manicone et al. 2012). Considering that the size of this microgap is usually roughly between 5–12 μm, though ranging between 1–50 μm (Kano et al. 2007; Tsuge et al. 2008; Silva-Neto et al. 2012; Abduo and Lyons 2013), and the size of oral bacteria may be roughly between 0.5–5 μm, up to 10 μm (Silva-Neto et al. 2012) at most, there is a real risk of bacterial colonization and microfilm accumulation. Therefore, the abutment should fit as accurately as possible on the fixture, which implies simultaneous and even contact of all fitting surfaces at the fixture-abutment interface (Abduo and Lyons 2013). In the case of a stock abutment, the width of the microgap can be reduced to 5–6 μm (Kano et al. 2007) or below, whereas in the case of individually cast abutments, roughly double the width (i.e. 11–12 μm or below) can be considered (Kano et al. 2007; Abduo and Lyons 2013). The fit accuracy of individually cast abutments may be improved significantly by means of cast rectifiers (Jaime et al. 2007). The fit accuracy of CAD-CAM-milled individual abutments can in general be considered to lie between the values of stock and individually cast abutments (Abduo and Lyons 2013); however, there may be significant differences in terms of the precision between different CAD/CAM systems (von Steyern et al. 2014).

9.4. Platform Switching

To prevent inflammation-induced bone resorption because of the bacterial colonization of the microgap at the fixture-abutment interface, the concept of platform switching has been introduced (Lazzara and Porter 2006) to preserve bone around the heads of wider-diameter implants (Lazzara and Porter 2006; Lopez-Mari et al. 2009; Serrano-Sanchez et al. 2011; Yun et al. 2011; Manicone et al. 2012). In platform switching, the diameter of the abutment is smaller than that of the fixture (Lazzara and Porter 2006), and it is widely accepted today that bone resorption can be reduced in this way (Hermann et al. 2007; Lopez-Mari et al. 2009; Atieh et al. 2010; Canullo et al. 2009, 2010, 2011; Serrano-Sanchez et al. 2011; Yun et al. 2011; Manicone et al. 2012). It is also likely that the degree of marginal bone resorption is inversely related to the extent of the fixture-abutment mismatch (Canullo et al. 2010).

It is also likely that platform switching preserves the marginal bone from mechanical stress overloading by means of a notable shift of mechanical stress from the bone-fixture interface toward the fixture-abutment interface (Maeda et al. 2007; Rodriguez-Ciurana et al. 2009; Canullo et al. 2011). Thus, in this case, the greatest amount of stress concentration is mostly localized on the interface between the fixture and the abutment (Maeda et al. 2007; Rodriguez-Ciurana et al. 2009) rather than on the fixture-bone interface (Canullo et al. 2011). This important biomechanical phenomenon is also likely to contribute to the advantageous effect of platform switching on the maintenance of the marginal bone if the load of the implant system is really high. On the other hand, it should also be mentioned that *slightly* increased mechanical stress of the marginal bone may be advantageous for its maintenance (Kwon et al. 2010; Lee et al. 2012).

9.5. Soft-Tissue Modeling

The creation of a properly contoured restoration with a natural gingival emergence profile that harmonizes with the gingival profile of the adjacent teeth is very important for esthetically successful implant therapy (Son and Jang 2011). For efficient soft tissue modeling (contouring, profiling), surgical, anatomical, and prosthetic factors should be considered from the initial to the final stages of treatment (Son and Jang 2011; Manicone et al. 2012). From a *surgical viewpoint* (besides general surgical considerations discussed elsewhere), it is important to mention that abutments (whether healing or definitive) should be placed immediately (i.e. stock abutments) or as soon as possible (i.e. individually fabricated abutments) after the insertion of implant fixtures (one-stage surgery) or after establishing mini-flap access at the uncovering stage (two-stage surgery), thereby allowing the healing of soft tissue around an ideal profile (Manicone et al. 2012). From an *anatomical viewpoint*, the most important prerequisite is an adequate blood supply to the marginal gingiva to ensure the responsiveness of the soft tissue to the prosthetic stimuli (Manicone et al. 2012); a thick gingival biotype may be considered more advantageous in this respect (Sorni-Broker et al. 2009; Nagaraj et al. 2010; Si et al. 2012). It should be also considered from this perspective that it is easier to obtain an optimal gingival contour around implant restorations placed next to an adjacent natural tooth (Kim et al. 2009), whereas a greater thickness of buccal supra-implant mucosa is needed for implant restorations without a neighboring natural tooth to achieve a favorable level and contour of the buccal/labial gingival margin (Kim et al. 2009). From a *prosthetic viewpoint*, accurately connected and positioned healing/definitive abutments and well-designed provisional/definitive denture components (fixed denture or attachment for RPD) are crucial (Manicone et al. 2012). An accurate impression technique, together with the maintenance of the soft tissue profile to prevent the peri-implant soft tissue from collapsing while the impression is poured and the definitive denture is fabricated (Attard and Barzilay 2003), is also crucial.

Soft tissue modeling (contouring, profiling) is usually obtained by means of a healing abutment and/or a provisional fixed denture placed on a healing or definitive abutment (Son and Jang 2011; Maiorana et al. 2012). If larger alterations of the gingival contour are needed, the contour should be changed gradually. In this case, a stock healing abutment with a gradually relined provisional restoration may be useful (Son and Jang 2011). Alternatively, a series of individually fabricated healing abutments with a gradually changed contour can be used.

The treatment takes roughly a month if all the necessary conditions are satisfied (Son and Jang 2011), and the contour of the provisional restoration should be relined (or the individual abutments should be changed) two to three times during this time to achieve the desired emergence profile. It is likely that a few dis/reconnections of the healing (or definitive) abutment and/or provisional restoration will not jeopardize optimal mucosal attachment (Abrahamsson et al. 2003; Manicone et al. 2012). However, a larger number of dis/reconnections is likely to compromise the integrity of the implanto-gingival complex (Abrahamsson et al. 1997), leading to marginal bone loss and the consequent apical shift of the implanto-gingival complex (Abrahamsson et al. 1997; Manicone et al. 2012).

If the desired gingival emergence profile is achieved, a further stabilization period of six weeks is recommended before the final impression is taken for fabrication of the definitive individual abutment and/or definitive fixed restoration (Son and Jang 2011). In the case of optimal definitive prosthodontic restoration, the interproximal papilla level (and the gingival contour in general) may further improve after insertion of the definitive restoration (Si et al. 2012) within a few months, especially around single-implant restorations in cases of thick gingival biotype (Si et al. 2012) and if the general and interproximal oral hygiene are perfect.

Importantly, great care should be taken regarding proper oral hygiene during and after the whole soft-tissue modeling (contouring, profiling) process. Thus, periodic examination of the patient is also crucial in this respect (Son and Jang 2011). Accordingly, for cement-retained restorations, great care should certainly be taken to remove all small cement remnants around the abutment and the supported provisional or definitive restoration (Son and Jang 2011).

9.6. Abutment-Denture Interface

The denture (fixed denture or attachment for RPD) should exhibit an accurate fit on the abutment, which implies simultaneous and even contact of all the fitting surfaces (Abduo and Lyons 2013). Fit accuracy is highly important because it reduces the width of the microgap (and the consequent decrease of bacterial accumulation) and also achieves "passive fitting" (well, accurately fitting) of the restoration to the abutment, which does not jeopardize osseointegration of the fixture due to plastic distortion-induced elastic forces appearing in the denture following insertion (Kano et al. 2004).

The highest fit accuracy can be achieved using stock (premade) metal cylinder frameworks, usually made of noble (i.e. gold or silver-palladium) alloys. Such premade cylinders can be covered by porcelain fused to the metal after being reshaped by means of (over)casting (Moraes et al. 2005) in the dental laboratory using alloys of a molding temperature below that of the premade framework (Kano et al. 2004). Besides being reshaped, premade cylinders can also be connected to each other by means of (over)casting (i.e. not in single tooth restorations but in larger dentures like bridges, bar retainers for RPD, etc.) (Kano et al. 2004).

Using such stock (premade) metal cylinder frameworks, the width of the microgap between the abutment and the restoration ranges roughly between 4–15 μm (Kano et al. 2004), whereas in the case of individually cast noble metal restorations, the width of the gap can be roughly double that amount. Importantly, the width of the gap can be significantly (even four to five times) higher if non-noble metal alloys like nickel-chromium and cobalt-chromium (Kano et al. 2004; Castillo-de-Oyague et al. 2012) or titanium (Castillo-de-Oyague et al. 2012) are used in the individual casting of the metal framework of restorations. The fit accuracy of CAD-CAM-milled individual dentures can in general be considered as being between the values of stock (premade) metal cylinders and individually cast abutments (Abduo and Lyons 2013).

In the case of cement-retained restorations, an ideal abutment geometry is required to provide proper retention of the denture (Abduo and Lyons 2013). Because of esthetic reasons (and also to facilitate removal of cementation material), the finish line should be closely related to the soft tissue contour and follow the mucosal outline (Abduo and Lyons 2013). Importantly, the quality of the luting agents (both temporary and definitive) also significantly influences the final position, fit accuracy, and retention of the inserted fixed dentures (Pan and Lin 2005; Castillo-de-Oyague et al. 2012). It should also be emphasized that great care should be taken to remove all small cement remnants around the abutment and supported provisional or definitive restoration to obtain optimal soft tissue conditions (Son and Jang 2011). Depending on the implant system, the restoration may also be fixed by means of a screw.

Conclusion

The abutment is a highly important part of most implant systems. Positioned between the fixture and the denture, the abutment makes it possible to connect the two and to modify the long axis of the implant-abutment-denture complex if needed (Cardelli et al. 2009; Manicone et al. 2012). The disadvantage of an abutment is the appearance of two (i.e. the fixture-abutment and the abutment-denture) interfaces, from which at least one could be discounted if an abutment was not used. On the other hand, using an abutment clearly increases the plasticity and adaptability of the whole implant system. Further, creative use of an abutment, together with provisional restorations, is a rather efficient tool for soft tissue modeling (contouring, profiling), which is crucial for obtaining proper soft tissue esthetics in many cases.

References

Abduo, J; Lyons, K. Rationale for the use of CAD/CAM technology in implant prosthodontics. *Int J Dentistry*, 2012, Article ID: 768121. DOI: 10.1155/2013/768121.

Abrahamsson, I; Berglungh, T; Lindhe, J. The mucosal barrier following abutment dis/reconnection an experimental study in dogs. *J Clin Periodontol*, 1997, 24, 568–572.

Abrahamsson, I; Berglundh, T; Sekino, S; Lindhe, J. Tissue reactions to abutment shift: an experimental study in dogs. *Clin Implant Dent Related Res*, 2003, 5, 82–88.

Apicella, D; Veltri, M; Chieffi, N; Polimeni, A; Giovannetti, A; Ferrari, M. Implant adaptation of stock abutments versus CAD/CAM abutments: a radiographic and scanning electron microscopy study. *Annali di Stomatol*, 2010, 1, 9–13.

Atieh, MA; Ibrahim, HM; Atieh, AH. Platform switching for marginal bone preservation around dental implants: a systematic review and meta-analysis. *J Periodontol*, 2010, 81, 1350–1366.

Attard, N; Barzilay, I. A modified impression technique for accurate registration of peri-implant soft tissues. *J Can Dent Assoc*, 2003, 69, 80–83.

Canullo, L; Iurlaro, G; Iannello, G. Double-blind randomized controlled trial study on post-extraction immediately restored implants using the switching platform concept: soft tissue response. Preliminary report. *Clin Oral Implant Res*, 2009, 20, 414–420.

Canullo, L; Fedele, GR; Iannello, G; Jepsen, S. Platform switching and marginal bone-level alterations: the results of a randomized-controlled trial. *Clin Oral Implant Res*, 2010, 21, 115–121.

Canullo, L; Pace, F; Coelho, P; Sciubba, E; Vozza, I. The influence of platform switching on the biomechanical aspects of the implant-abutment system. A three dimensional finite element study. *Med Oral Patol Oral Cir Bucal*, 2011, 16, e852–e856.

Cardelli, P; Montani, M; Gallio, M; Biancolini, M; Brutti, C; Barlattani, A. Angulated abutments and periimplant stress: F.E.M. analysis. *ORAL & Implantology*, 2009, 2, 3–10.

Castillo-de-Oyague, R; Sanchez-Turrioun, A; Lopez-Lozano, JF; Albaladejo, A; Torres-Lagares, D; Montero, J; Suarez-Garcia, MJ. Vertical misfit of laser-sintered and vacuum cast implant-supported crown copings luted with definitive temporary luting agents. *Med Oral Patol Oral Cir Bucal*, 2012, 17, e610–e617.

Hermann, F; Lerner, H; Palti, A. Factors influencing the preservation of the periimplant marginal bone. *Implant Dent*, 2007, 16, 165–175.

Jaime, APG; de Vasconcellos, DK; Mesquita, AMM; Kimpara, ET; Bottino, MA. Effect of cast rectifiers on the marginal fit of UCLA abutments. *J Appl Oral Sci*, 2007, 15, 169–174.

Jemt, T; Pettersson, P. A 3-years follow-up study on single implant treatment. *J Dent*, 1993, 21, 203–208.

Jorneus, L; Jemt, T; Carlsson, L. Loads and designs of screw joints for single crowns supported by osseointegrated implants. *Int J Oral Maxillofac Implants*, 1992, 7, 353–359.

Kang, YM; Lim, JH; Cho, IH. A study on the abutment screw loosening of dental implants. *J Korean Acad Prosthodont*, 1996, 34, 1–14.

Kano, SC; Bonfante, G; Hussne, R; Siqueria, AF. Use of base metal casting alloys for implant framework: marginal accuracy analysis. *J Appl Oral Sci*, 2004, 12, 337–343.

Kano, SC; Binon, PP; Curtis, DA. A classification system to measure the implant-abutment micrograp. *Int J Oral Maxillofac Implants*, 2007, 22, 879–885.

Kim, YB; Shim, JS; Han, CH; Kim SJ. The level of buccal gingival margin around single and two adjacent implant restorations: a preliminary result. *J Adv Prosthodont*, 2009, 1, 140–144.

Kim, ES; Shin, SY. Influence of the implant abutment types and the dynamic loading on initial screw loosening. *J Adv Prosthodont*, 2013, 5, 21–28.

Kwon, MJ; Yeo, IS; Kim, YK; Yi, YJ; Yang, JH. Use of separate single-tooth implant restorations to replace two or more consecutive posterior teeth: a prospective cohort study for up to 1 year. *J Adv Prosthodont*, 2010, 2, 54–57.

Laney, WR; Jemt, T; Harris, D; Henry, PJ; Krogh, PH; Polizzi, G; Zarb, GA; Herrmann, I. Osseointegrated implants for single-tooth replacement: progress report from a multicenter prospective study after 3 years. *Int J Oral Maxillofac Implants.* 1994, 9, 49–54.

Lazzara, R; Siddiqui, AA; Binon, P; Feldman, SA; Weiner, R; Phillips, R; Gonshor, A. Retrospective multicenter analysis of 3i endosseous dental implants placed over a five-year period. *Clin Oral Implans Res*, 1996, 7, 73–83.

Lazzara, RJ; Porter, SS. Platform switching: a new concept in implant dentistry for controlling postrestorative crestal bone levels. *Int J Periodontics Restorative Dent*. 2006, 26, 9–17.

Lee, KJ; Kim, YG; Park, JW; Lee, JM; Suh, JY. Influence of crown-to-implant ratio on periimplant marginal bone loss in the posterior region: a five-year retrospective study. *J Periodontal Implant Sci*, 2012, 42, 231–236.

Lopez-Mari, L; Calvo-Guirado, JL; Martin-Castellote, B; Gomez-Moreno, G; Lopez-Mari, M. Implant platform switching concept: an updated review. *Med Oral Patol Oral Cir Bucal*, 2009, 14, e450–e454.

Maeda, Y; Miura, J; Taki, I; Sogo, M. Biomechanical analysis on platform switching: is there any biomechanical rationale? *Clin Oral Implant Res*, 2007, 18, 581–584.

Maiorana, C; Speroni, S; Herford, AS; Cicciu, M. Slow orthodontic teeth extrusion to enhance hard and soft periodontal tissue quality before implant positioning in aesthetic area. *The Open Dentistry J*, 2012, 6, 137–142.

Manicone, PF; Raffaelli, L; Gassemian, M; D'Addona, A. Soft and hard tissue management in implant therapy – Part II: Prosthetic concepts. *Int J Biomaterials*, 2012, Article ID: 356817. DOI: 10.1155/2012/356817.

Moraes, LMC; Rossetti, PHO; Rossetti, LMN; Pedreira, APRdV; do Valle, AL; Bonachella, WCB. Marginal fit at cylinder-abutment interface before and after overcasting procedure. *J Appl Oral Sci*, 2005, 13, 366–371.

Moon, SJ; Kim, HJ; Son, MK; Chung, CH. Sinking and fit of abutment of locking taper implant systems. *J Adv Prosthodont*, 2009, 1, 97–101.

Nagaraj, KR; Savadi, RC; Savadi, AR; Reddy, GTP; Srilakshmi, J; Dayalan, M; John, J. Gingival biotype – Prosthodontic perspective. *J Indian Prosthodontic Soc*, 2010, 10, 27–30.

Pan, YH; Lin, CK. The effect of luting agents on the retention of dental implant-supported crowns. *Chang Gung Med J*, 2005, 28, 403–410.

Rodriguez-Ciurana, X; Vela-Nebot, X; Segala-Torres, M; Rodado-Alonso, C; Mendez-Blanco, V; Mata-Bugueroles, M. Biomechanical repercussions of bone resorption related to biological width: a finite element analysis of three implant-abutment configurations. *Int J Periodontics Restorative Dent*, 2009, 29, 479–487.

Serrano-Sanchez, P; Calvo-Guirado, JL; Manzanera-Pastor, E; Lorrio-Castro, C; Bretones-Lopez, P; Perez-Llanes, JA. The influence of platform switching in dental implants. A literature review. *Med Oral Patol Oral Cir Bucal*, 2011, 16, e400–e405.

Si, MS; Zhuang, LF; Huang, X; Gu, YX; Chou, CH; Lai, HC. Papillae alterations around single-implant restorations in the anterior maxillae: thick versus thin mucosa. *Int J Oral Sci*, 2012, 4, 94–100.

Silva-Neto, JP; Prudente, MS; Carneiro, TdA; Nobilo, MA; Penatti, MP; Neves, FD. Micro-leakage at the implant-abutment interface with different tightening torques in vitro. *J Appl Oral Sci*, 2012 20, 581–587.

Son, MK; Jang, HS. Gingival recontouring by provisional implant restoration for optimal emergence profile: report of two cases. *J Periodontal Implant Sci*, 2011, 41, 302–308.

Sorni-Broker, M; Penarrocha-Diago, M; Penarrocha-Diago, M. Factors that influence the position of the peri-implant soft tissues: A review. *Med Oral Patol Oral Cir Buccal*, 2009, 14, e475–e479.

Tsuge, T; Hagiwara, Y; Matsumura, H. Marginal fit and microgaps of implant-abutment interface with internal anti-rotation configuration. *Dental Materials Journal*, 2008, 27, 29–34.

von Steyern, PV; Ekstrand, K; Svanborg, P; Ortorp, A. Modern digital technologies for producing prosthetic constructions. *Danish Dent J*, 2014, 118, 104–113.

Yun, HJ; Park, JC; Yun, JH; Jung, UW; Kim, CS; Choi, SH; Cho, KS. A short-term clinical study of marginal bone level change around microthreaded and platform-switched implants. *J Periodontal Implant Sci*, 2011, 41, 211–217.

CHAPTER 10

MAINTENANCE CARE

Abstract

The survival rate of intraoral implants can be considered to be rather high (in *non*-complex cases), usually between 96%–100% in both the short and long run. Besides available bone, surgical technique, bone quality, and osseointegration processes, the outcome of dental implant therapy also strongly depends on factors like the vertical positioning of the fixture, the shape and surface properties of the neck of the fixture, and the fixture-abutment interface, as well as the "crown-to-implant" ratio and the mechanical stress exposure of the peri-implant bone during the masticatory function. Besides these, patients who have undergone implant therapy should also receive adequate maintenance care, including regular recalls and proper personal and professional oral hygiene (avoiding fluoride corrosion), as well as immediate and adequate therapeutic intervention (if needed) to reach a favorable outcome. Although the success of an implant has been defined as less than 1.5 mm of marginal bone loss during the first year after functional loading and less than 0.2 mm annual bone loss thereafter, with optimal maintenance care, a marginal bone loss of roughly 1.1 mm during the first year and 0.1 mm per year (or less) thereafter may be considered a satisfactory outcome.

10.1. Introduction

The survival rate of intraoral implants can be considered to be rather high (in *non*-complex cases), usually between 96%–100% in both the short run, 6–12 months, (Kemppainen et al. 1997; Norton 2004; Kim et al. 2011) and the long run, three years or more (Barona-Dorado et al. 2009; Shibuya et al. 2009). Although the premised results are rather satisfactory, patients who have undergone implant therapy should receive individualized, systematic, and continuous maintenance care of their peri-implant tissues to reach the premised favorable outcome (Todescan et al. 2012). Regular recalls, proper personal and professional oral hygiene, and immediate adequate therapeutic intervention (if needed) are considered cornerstones of ideal maintenance care.

10.2. Recall

Maintenance care should include regular recalls. These recalls should include evaluation of implants, peri-implant tissues, dentures (including occlusion), other oral health conditions, and general health conditions (Todescan et al. 2012), as well as the evaluation and reinforcement of personal oral hygiene, together with professional removal of plaque and calculus (Todescan et al. 2012). Recalls should also include radiologic evaluation of the bone level if clinical signs suggest the presence of peri-implantitis (Todescan et al. 2012). Radiography may also be performed on a regular basis at six months and one year after the insertion and at least every two years thereafter, and an attempt should be made to standardize the radiographic technique (Fernandez-Formoso et al. 2011). Besides the daily oral hygienic care carried out by the patient (Mok et al. 2007), a regular recall for professional maintenance care every three months seems advisable, at least during the first year after the implantation (Hong et al. 2010; Todescan et al. 2012). Thereafter, the response of peri-implant tissues should be assessed and an appropriate frequency of recall should be determined (Todescan et al. 2012).

Patients at higher risk for peri-implantitis should be identified and monitored closely (Todescan et al. 2012). Sites of pre-existing chronic periodontitis may act as reservoirs for periopathogens that can spread to colonize the implant (Todescan et al. 2012); therefore, periodontitis patients (especially those with aggressive periodontitis) should be considered as high-risk individuals (Todescan et al. 2012). Other patients potentially at high risk are those with diabetes mellitus if they have poor metabolic control (Elsubeihi and Zarb 2002; Todescan et al. 2012). Patients with poor plaque control (Todescan et al. 2012) or who smoke (Elsubeihi and Zarb 2002; Todescan et al. 2012) should also be considered high-risk.

10.3. Professional Oral Hygiene

Good oral hygiene is one of the prerequisites for the long-term success of oral implants, whereas compromised oral hygiene resulting in bacterial biofilm (plaque) accumulation is a major risk factor that can contribute to implant failure (Unursaikhan et al. 2012). Besides the personal oral hygiene carried out by the patient, professional oral hygiene is also highly recommended. Common mechanical instruments widely used for professional oral hygiene and periodontal therapy may roughen titanium implant surfaces (Mengel et al. 2004; Todescan et al. 2012; Unursaikhan et al. 2012). Consequently, routine prophylactic/oral hygienic procedures using such instruments might cause damage to implant surfaces over time, leading to changes in surface topography that can increase the potential for plaque accumulation (Mengel et al. 2004; Unursaikhan et al. 2012). Therefore, the use of appropriate instruments to clean implant surfaces with minimal changes being made in the process is critical for the successful maintenance of dental implants (Mengel et al. 2004; Unursaikhan et al. 2012). There are various appropriate instruments available for such purposes, such as Teflon-coated and plastic curettes, special metal curettes (made of a metal softer than titanium to avoid damaging the implant surface), air flow glycine-powdering, and specially designed ultrasonic systems with newly developed metal scaler tips that are softer than titanium (Todescan et al. 2012; Unursaikhan et al. 2012).

10.4. Marginal Bone Loss

Although the success of an implant has been defined as less than 1.5 mm of marginal bone loss during the first year after functional loading (insertion of the prosthesis) and less than 0.2 mm annual bone loss thereafter (Albrektsson and Isidor 1993), with optimal maintenance care, a marginal bone loss of roughly 1.1 mm (0.9–1.6 mm) during the first year (Adell et al. 1981; Gfeller et al. 2011; Borgonovo et al. 2012; Todescan et al. 2012) and 0.1 mm per year (or less) thereafter may be considered proper (Borgonovo et al. 2012; Todescan et al. 2012; Gelb et al. 2013). The premised values of marginal bone loss should not be considered pathological; however, this more or less "naturally occurring" marginal bone loss around implant fixtures certainly should also be minimized as much as possible.

Surgical techniques and vertical positioning of the fixture may strongly influence initial bone loss. Data indicate that marginal bone loss is the highest around submerged fixtures (with a fixture-abutment interface below bone level), whereas it is lowest in the case of fixtures having their fixture-abutment interface above bone level (Yi et al. 2010). Besides initial bone loss caused by damage during the surgical procedure, the primary reason for increased marginal bone loss during the first year in the case of fixtures with submerged fixture-abutment interfaces may be that bacterial products from bacteria (colonizing the microgap of the fixture-abutment interface) cause upregulation of proinflammatory cytokines in peri-implant tissues/cells (i.e. peri-implant macrophages, mesenchymal cells, fibroblasts), resulting in osteoclast formation and the recruitment of resorptively active osteoclasts, which ultimately ends with bone resorption (Ujiie et al. 2012). This kind of rapid bone resorption continues until a "biological width" arises between the microgap and the most coronal bone-to-implant contact (BIC) (Leonardo et al. 2008).

Another important factor of marginal bone loss is the mechanical stress on the peri-implant marginal bone. Besides masticatory forces, another important factor of mechanical stress on the peri-implant bone is the "crown-to-implant" (C/I) ratio (Lee et al. 2012), which is the ratio of the length of the *osseointegrated* part of the fixture and the height of all other parts (i.e. height of the *not*-osseointegrated part of the fixture + abutment + denture) of the implant system (Lee et al. 2012). Interestingly, recent data indicate that implants with a (moderately) higher crown-to-implant ratio show *less* peri-implant marginal bone loss than implants with a low ($x \leq 1$) C/I ratio (Lee et al. 2012). An explanation for this interesting finding may be that a *moderately* increased stress concentration in the case of somewhat shorter fixtures at the bone crest caused by masticatory forces may stimulate bone formation around the implant fixture at the top of the crestal bone that is in contact with the implant (Lee et al. 2012). The premised expectable advantageous effect of moderately increased stress on the marginal peri-implant bone may also explain the unique finding that there was just a minimal initial marginal bone loss followed by a (small amount of) bone *gain* around *non*-splinted single-implant restorations replacing posterior teeth exposed to high masticatory forces in a study (Kwon et al. 2010). On the other hand, it should be emphasized that a *highly* increased stress concentration on the peri-implant marginal bone may lead to bone loss, and therefore should certainly be avoided.

The shape and surface properties of the neck of the fixture seem to be other important determinants of peri-implant marginal bone loss (Aloy-Prosper et al. 2011). With respect to shape, a microthreaded neck of the fixture (Aloy-Prosper et al. 2011; Yun et al. 2011), together with a platform-switched implant abutment interface (Yun et al. 2011), seem to constitute the most advantageous approach. With respect to the surface properties of the neck of the fixture, a roughened surface seems to be more advantageous than a smooth one, especially if the roughened surface is combined with a microthreaded shape (Aloy-Prosper et al. 2011).

10.5. Peri-Implantitis

Peri-implant disease can be classified into two major groups: peri-implant mucositis and peri-implantitis (Lindhe et al. 2008). Major clinical manifestations of peri-implant disease include gingival bleeding, pus secretion, swelling, and bone loss (Schmidlin et al. 2012). Both peri-implant mucositis and peri-implantitis are of infectious origin, caused by the development of bacterial biofilm (Mombelli et al. 1987; Leonhardt et al. 1999; Lindhe et al. 2008; Unursaikhan et al. 2012) with a similar spectrum of pathogens to that of periodontal inflammation (Mombelli et al. 1987; Sakka and Coulthard 2011; Schmidlin et al. 2012). Therefore, it is of primary importance to keep the bacterial load below the individual's threshold for disease through the mechanical removal of bacterial biofilm and the adjunctive use of chemical agents and laser applications (Unursaikhan et al. 2012).

It should be considered in this respect that peri-implant mucositis may be reversible and cured/managed by nonsurgical therapy (Lang at al. 2011; Sakka and Coulthard 2011), whereas the management of peri-implantitis is rather problematic, and roughly every fourth implant with peri-implantitis may be lost despite repeated treatment (Leonhardt et al. 2003). Therefore, both prevention and proper treatment of peri-implantitis (including prevention and treatment of peri-implant mucositis) is very important (Unursaikhan et al. 2012).

For both the prevention and treatment of peri-implantitis, the principal objective is the complete removal of bacterial biofilm, including calcified plaque, from implant surfaces (Unursaikhan et al. 2012). For preventive purposes, regular recalls together with common professional oral hygiene treatments are crucial. For the treatment of peri-implantitis, effective decontamination of titanium surfaces may be carried out by mechanical cleaning (e.g. dental curettes, ultrasonic scalers, air flow glycine-powdering) and/or by means of chemical procedures (e.g. citric acid, H_2O_2, chlorhexidine digluconate, EDTA), and these treatments may be supplemented by local or systemic antibiotics (Bassetti et al. 2011; Marotti et al. 2013). Moderately high level lasers and especially photodynamic therapy using low level lasers combined with a suitable photosensitizer dye may also be used efficiently (Takasaki et al. 2009; Marotti et al. 2013) in the framework of proper surgical treatment as described in detail elsewhere.

10.6. Fluoride Corrosion

Corrosion is a result of electrochemical reactions that occur between a metal and the surrounding environment (Roselino Ribeiro et al. 2007). Titanium (cpTi) and titanium alloys form a highly-protective oxide film on their surface that imparts excellent corrosion resistance (Yamazoe et al. 2007). However, the premised resistance may be significantly reduced in a fluoride-containing environment, since such an environment may destroy the oxide film, thereby decreasing the resistance of cpTi and titanium alloys to corrosion (Yamazoe et al. 2007). Data indicate that the phenomenon of fluoride corrosion strongly depends on both fluoride ion concentration and pH (Nakagawa et al. 1999; Yamazoe et al. 2007), because in acidic environments, fluoride ions form hydrofluoric acid, and a concentration of hydrofluoric acid over 30 ppm may result in the destruction of the oxide film on titanium surfaces (Nakagawa et al. 1999). The use of fluoridated gels and solutions containing high levels of fluoride as a prophylactic tool has been widespread due to its great caries-preventive effect (Roselino Ribeiro et al. 2007); consequently the damaging action of these substances on titanium surfaces is a rather important subject that has been investigated in several studies in recent years (Roselino Ribeiro et al. 2007). Evidence of fluoride corrosion through pitting on titanium (cpTi) surfaces was demonstrated, which may indicate the harmfulness of fluoride contamination to the mechanical properties of titanium implant structures (Roselino Ribeiro et al. 2007). Importantly, the surfaces of titanium alloys containing 0.5 wt% platinum seem to *not* be affected (or at least much less so) in fluoride-containing environments (Yamazoe et al. 2007).

Because of the premised dependence of fluoride corrosion on fluoride ion concentration and pH (Nakagawa et al. 1999; Yamazoe et al. 2007), great care should be taken to avoid direct contamination of titanium alloys by fluoridated gels/solutions containing high levels of fluoride. Similarly, the maintenance of a neutral (slightly alkaline) pH during and following fluoride application is also very important.

Conclusion

Besides available bone, surgical technique, bone quality, and osseointegration processes, the outcome of dental implant therapy also strongly depends on factors like the vertical positioning of the fixture (Yi et al. 2010), the shape and surface properties of the neck of the fixture, and the fixture-abutment interface (Aloy-Prosper et al. 2011; Yun et al. 2011), as well as the "crown-to-implant" ratio (Lee et al. 2012) and the mechanical stress exposure of the peri-implant bone during masticatory function (Lee et al. 2012). Besides these factors, patients who have undergone implant therapy should also receive adequate maintenance care (Todescan et al. 2012), including regular recalls and proper personal and professional oral hygiene (avoiding fluoride corrosion), as well as immediate and adequate therapeutic intervention (if needed) to reach a favorable outcome (Todescan et al. 2012). Although the success of an implant has been defined as less than 1.5 mm of marginal bone loss during the first year after functional loading (insertion of the prosthesis) and less than 0.2 mm annual bone loss thereafter (Albrektsson and Isidor 1993), with optimal maintenance care, a marginal bone loss of roughly 1.1 mm during the first year (Borgonovo et al. 2012; Todescan et al. 2012) and 0.1 mm per year thereafter may be considered (Borgonovo et al. 2012; Todescan et al. 2012; Gelb et al. 2013) a satisfactory outcome.

References

Adell, R; Lekholm, U; Rockler, B; Branemark, PI. A 15-year study of osseointegrated implants in the treatment of edentulous jaw. *Int J Oral Surg*, 1981, 10, 387–416.

Albrektsson, T; Isidor, F. Consensus report of session V. In: Lang NP, Karring T, editors. *Proceedings of the 1st European Workshop on Periodontology*. London: Quintessence, 1993, 365–369.

Aloy-Prosper, A; Maestre-Ferrin, L; Penarrocha-Oltra, D; Penarrocha-Diago, M. Marginal bone loss in relation to the implant neck surface: An update. *Med Oral Patol Oral Cir Bucal*, 2011, 16, e365–e368.

Barona-Dorado, C; Martinez-Rodriguez, N; Torres-Lear, F; Martinez-Gonzalez, JM. Observational study of 67 wide platform implants treated with avantblast surface. Results at three year. *Med Oral Patol Oral Cir Bucal*, 2009, 14, E183–E187.

Bassetti, R; Bassetti, M; Enkling, N; Mericske-Stern, R. Behandlung einer fortgeschrittenen periimplantitis im unterkiefer. *Schweiz Monatsschr Zahnmed*, 2011, 121, 325–332.

Borgonovo, AE; Fabbri, A; Vavassori, V; Censi, R; Maiorana, C. Multiple teeth replacement with endosseous one-piece yttrium-stabilized zirconia dental implants. *Med Oral Pathol Oral Cir Bucal*, 2012, 17, e981–e987.

Elsubeihi, ES; Zarb, GA. Implant prosthodontics in medically challenged patients: The University of Toronto experience. *J Can Dent Assoc*, 2002, 68, 103–108.

Fernandez-Formoso, N; Rilo, B; Mora, MJ; Martinez-Silva, I; Santana, U. A paralleling technique modification to determine the bone crest level around dental implants. *Dentomaxillofac Radiol*, 2011, 40, 385–389.

Gelb, D; McAllister, B; Nummikoski, P; Del Fabbro, M. Clinical and radiographic evaluation of Branemark implants with an anodized surface following seven-to-eight years functional loading. *Int J Dent*, 2013, Article ID: 583567. DOI: 10.1155/2013/ 583567.

Gfeller, F; Zitzmann, NU; Lambrecht, JT. Sofort belastete MonoType-Implantate im zahnlosen Unterkiefer. *Schweiz Monatsschr Zahnmed*, 2011, 121, 235–242.

Hong, JS; Yeo, IS; Kim, SH; Lee, JB; Han, JS; Yang, JH. Implants and all-ceramic restorations in a patient treated for aggressive periodontitis: a case report. *J Adv Prosthod*, 2010, 2, 97–101.

Kemppainen, P; Eskola, S; Ylipaavalniemi, P. A comparative prospective clinical study of two single-tooth implants: a preliminary report of 102 implants. *J Prosthet Dent*, 1997, 77, 382–387.

Kim, JS; Sohn, JY; Park, JC; Jung, UW; Kim, CS; Lee, JH; Shim, JS; Lee, KW; Choi, SH. Cumulative survival rate of Astra Tech implants: a retrospective analysis. *J Periodont Implant Sci*, 2011, 41, 86–91.

Kwon, MJ; Yeo, IS; Kim, YK; Yi, YJ; Yang, JH. Use of separate single-tooth implant restorations to replace two or more consecutive posterior teeth: a prospective cohort study for up to 1 year. *J Adv Prosthodont*, 2010, 2, 54–57.

Lang, NP; Berglundh, T. Group 4 of the Seventh European Workshop on Periodontology. Periimplant diseases: where are we now? Consensus of the Seventh European Workshop on Periodontology. *J Clin Periodontol*, 2011, 38, (Suppl. 11) 178–181.

Lee, KJ; Kim, YG; Park, JW; Lee, JM; Suh, JY. Influence of crown-to-implant ratio on periimplant marginal bone loss in the posterior region: a five-year retrospective study. *J Periodontal Implant Sci*, 2012, 42, 231–236.

Leonardo, MR; Borges, ATN; Martins-Junior, W; de Queiroz, AM; Assed, S. Vertical alveolar crest bone maintenance around implants in two-stage surgery: An in situ study in dogs. *Braz Dent J*, 2008, 19, 103–108.

Leonhardt, A; Renvert, S; Dahlen, G. Microbial findings at failing implants. *Clin Oral Implants Res*, 1999, 10, 339–345.

Leonhardt, A; Dahlen, G; Renvert, S. Five-year clinical, microbiological, and radiological outcome following treatment of peri-implantitis in man. *J Periodontol*, 2003, 74, 1415–22.

Lindhe, J; Meyle, J; Group D of the Sixth European Workshop on Periodontology. Peri-implant diseases: Consensus report of the Sixth European Workshop on Periodontology. *J Clin Periodontol*, 2008, 35 (Suppl. 8), 282–5.

Marotti, J; Tortamano, P; Cai, S; Ribeiro, MS; Franco, JEM; de Campos, TT. Decontamination of dental implant surfaces by means of photodynamic therapy. *Lasers Med Sci*, 2013, 28, 303–309.

Mengel, R; Meer, C; Flores-de-Jacoby, L. The treatment of uncoated and titanium nitride-coated abutments with different instruments. *Int J Oral Maxillofac Implants*, 2004, 19, 232–238.

Mok, J; Emami, E; Kobayashi, T; Feine, JS. An overdenture hygiene brochure for your implant overdenture patients. *J Can Dent Assoc*, 2007, 73, 713.

Mombelli, A; van Oosten, MA; Schurch, Jr. E; Land, NP. The microbiota associated with successful or failing osseointegrated titanium implants. *Oral Microbiol Immunol*, 1987, 2, 145–151.

Nakagawa, M; Matsuya, S; Shiraishi, T; Ohta, M. Effect of fluoride concentration and pH on corrosion behavior of titanium for dental use. *J Dent Res*, 1999, 78, 1568–1572.

Norton, MR. A short-term clinical evaluation of immediately restored maxillary TiOblast single-tooth implants. *Int J Oral Maxillofac Implants*, 2004, 19, 274–281.

Roselino Ribeiro, AL; Noriega, JR; Dametto, FR; Vaz, LG. Compressive fatigue in titanium dental implants submitted to fluoride ions action. *J Appl Oral Sci*, 2007, 15, 299–304.

Sakka, S; Coulthard, P. Implant failure: Etiology and complications. *Med Oral Patol Oral Cir Bucal*, 2011, 16, e42–e44.

Schmidlin, PR; Sahrmann, P; Ramel, C; Imfeld, T; Muller, J; Roos, M; Jung, RE. Peri-implantitis prevalence and treatment in implant-oriented private practices: A cross-sectional postal and internet survey. *Schweiz Monatsschr Zahnmed*, 2012, 122, 1136–1144.

Shibuya, Y; Kobayashi, M; Takeuchi, J; Asai, T; Murata, M; Umeda, M; Komori, T. Analysis of 472 Branemark System TiUnite implants: A retrospective study. *Kobe J Med Sci*, 2009, 55, E73–E81.

Takasaki, AA; Aoki, A; Mizutani, K; Schwarz, F; Sculean, A; Wang, CY; Koshy, G; Romanos, G; Ishikawa, I; Izumi, Y. Application of antimicrobial photodynamic therapy in periodontal and peri-implant diseases. *Periodontol*, 2009, 51, 109–140.

Todescan, S; Lavigne, S; Kelekis-Cholakis, A. Guidance for the maintenance care of dental implants: Clinical review. *J Can Dent Assoc*, 2012, 78, c107.

Ujiie, Y; Todescan, R; Davies, JE. Peri-implant crestal bone loss: A putative mechanism. *Int J Dent*, 2012, Article ID: 742439. DOI: 10.1155/2012/742439.

Unursaikhan, O; Lee, JS; Cha, JK; Park, JC; Jung, UW; Kim, CS; Cho, KS; Choi, SH. Comparative evaluation of roughness of titanium surfaces treated by different hygiene instruments. *J Periodont Implant Sci*, 2012, 42, 88–94.

Yamazoe, J; Nakagawa, M; Matono, Y; Takeuchi, A; Ishikawa, K. The development of Ti alloys for dental implant with high corrosion resistance and mechanical strength. *Dental Materials J*, 2007, 26, 260–267.

Yi, JM; Lee, JK; Um, HS; Chang, BS; Lee, MK. Marginal bony changes in relation to different vertical positions of dental implants. *J Periodontal Implant Sci*, 2010, 40, 244–248.

Yun, HJ; Park, JC; Yun, JH; Jung, UW; Kim, CS; Choi, SH; Cho, KS. A short-term clinical study of marginal bone level change around microthreaded and platform-switched implants. *J Periodontal Implant Sci*, 2011, 41, 211–217.

CHAPTER 11

SHORT, NARROW AND MINI-IMPLANTS

Abstract

Implant dentistry may utilize several special-sized implant systems, such as short, narrow, or mini-implants. Short implants are manufactured for use in atrophic regions of the jaws and may be considered as possible alternatives to bone augmentation, sinus floor elevation, or other advanced surgical procedures. Narrow-diameter implants are potential solutions for specific clinical situations, such as reduced interradicular bone, a thin alveolar crest, and the replacement of teeth with small cervical diameters. Mini-implants are manufactured primarily for orthodontic purposes. Temporary placement of orthodontic mini-implants is widely used to maximize anchorage during orthodontic treatment. The survival rate and marginal bone loss values of short implants are comparable to (or may be even better than) those of longer implants. Similarly, results for narrow implants are also rather good and comparable to those of regular-diameter implants. Orthodontic mini-implants serve as temporary skeletal anchorage devices and are excellent alternatives to conventional orthodontic intraoral or extraoral anchorages. All these data clearly indicate that special-sized implants are qualified for regular use in dentistry.

11.1. Introduction

Implant dentistry may utilize several special-sized implant systems, such as short, narrow, or mini-implants. Short implants are manufactured for use in atrophic regions of the jaws (Esposito et al. 2011, 2012; Huang 2012; Karthikeyan et al. 2012; Lops et al. 2012; Neldam and Pinholt 2012) and may be considered as possible alternatives to bone augmentation, sinus floor elevation, or other advanced surgical procedures (Huang 2012; Lops et al. 2012; Karthikeyan et al. 2012; Neldam and Pinholt 2012). Narrow-diameter implants are potential solutions for specific clinical situations, such as reduced interradicular bone, a thin alveolar crest, and the replacement of teeth with small cervical diameters (Franco et al. 2009; Sleiter et al. 2009; Balaji et al. 2010; Mohamed et al. 2012). Mini-implants are manufactured primarily for orthodontic purposes. Temporary placement of orthodontic mini-implants is widely used to maximize anchorage during orthodontic treatment (Nojima et al.

2001; Ismail and Johal 2002; Tinsley et al. 2004; Lai et al. 2010; Miyazawa et al. 2010; Park et al. 2012).

11.2. Short Implants

Short implants are manufactured for use in atrophic regions of the jaws (Esposito et al. 2011, 2012; Huang 2012; Karthikeyan et al. 2012; Lops et al. 2012; Neldam and Pinholt 2012) and may be considered as possible alternatives to bone augmentation, sinus floor elevation, or other advanced surgical procedures like alveolar distraction osteogenesis or alveolar nerve lateralization/transposition (Huang 2012; Lops et al. 2012; Karthikeyan et al. 2012; Neldam and Pinholt 2012). Although implants shorter than 8 mm are considered to be "short" (Lops et al. 2012; Neldam and Pinholt 2012), there are also 5–6 mm implants available for such purposes.

With the exception of 7–8 mm long versions, also available with a diameter of roughly 3–3.5 mm (or larger), short implants usually have a diameter of at least 4–5 mm, but in many cases their diameters are 5–6 mm. Because of the premised geometry, their use is especially advantageous in the posterior maxilla and mandible, but they may also be used in the premolar regions in many cases. Importantly, the survival rate and marginal bone loss values of short implants are comparable to (or may be even better than) those of longer implants (Esposito et al. 2011, 2012; Karthikeyan et al. 2012; Lops et al. 2012). Surgical insertion of short fixtures is based on the same principles developed for regular-sized implants. For the insertion of fixtures, ordinary tools are used and the procedure is relatively easy and safe.

If short implants are used, the "crown-to-implant" ratio should be considered carefully, because this ratio is necessarily rather high in most cases. A moderately high C/I ratio may lead to an increased stress concentration in the case of short fixtures at the bone crest that is experiencing masticatory forces (Lee et al. 2012). A *moderately* increased stress concentration may stimulate bone formation around a short implant fixture at the top of the crestal bone in contact with the implant (Lee et al. 2012), which may explain the interesting finding that the marginal bone loss values of short implants are comparable to (or even better than) those of longer implants (Esposito et al. 2011, 2012; Lops et al. 2012; Karthikeyan et al. 2012; Lops et al. 2012). On the other hand, it should be emphasized that a *highly* increased stress concentration on the peri-implant marginal bone may lead to bone loss. Therefore, an overload of short implant fixtures with high span or cantilever bridges (etc.) should certainly be avoided.

11.3. Narrow Implants

Narrow diameter implants (NDIs) are potential solutions for specific clinical situations, such as reduced interradicular bone, a thin alveolar crest, or the replacement of teeth with small cervical diameters (Franco et al. 2009; Sleiter et al. 2009; Balaji et al. 2010; Mohamed et al. 2012). In general, an implant (fixture) is considered "narrow" if its diameter is less than 3.75 mm (Franco et al. 2009). Although most narrow diameter implant systems include both a fixture and an abutment (Franco et al. 2009; Sleiter et al. 2011), there are also "single-piece" systems in which the fixture and the abutment are built together (Mohamed et al. 2009; Talreja et al. 2013). The premised single-piece systems may have the advantage that there is no problem with the fixture/abutment microgap because there is no fixture-abutment interface. On the other hand, certain advantageous functions of the abutment (e.g. the modification of the long axis of the implant-abutment-denture complex, soft-tissue modeling by means of healing abutment) are missing in these systems.

Guidelines developed for surgical insertion and prosthetic restoration of regular-sized fixtures (regular diameter implant, RDI) can be applied also to narrow diameter implants (Franco et al. 2009; Sleiter et al. 2009; El-Sheikh et al. 2012; Mohamed et al. 2012). Although concerns may arise from the fact that the reduced diameter means a reduction of osseointegrated bone-to-implant contact surface and may also increase the risk of implant fracture (Franco et al. 2009), the available data in the literature indicate rather good short- and long-term results (Vigolo et al. 2004; Comfort et al. 2005; Degidi et al. 2008; Franco et al. 2009; Balaji et al. 2010; El-Sheikh et al. 2012) that are comparable to those of regular diameter implants. Because of the decreased bone-to-implant surface, delayed load (Sleiter et al. 2011; El-Sheikh et al. 2012; Mohamed et al. 2012) and perhaps two-stage surgery (at least in the non-esthetic zone) are reasonable tactics to employ in order to avoid disturbing the osseointegration process.

11.4. Mini-Implants

Mini-implants are manufactured primarily for orthodontic purposes. Temporary placement of orthodontic mini-implants (OMI) is widely used to maximize anchorage during orthodontic treatment (Nojima et al. 2001; Ismail and Johal 2002; Tinsley et al. 2004; Lai et al. 2010; Miyazawa et al. 2010; Park et al. 2012). Although both mini-plate type (Cornelis et al. 2008; Takaki et al. 2010) and mini-screw type orthodontic mini-implants are available (Ishii et al. 2004; Cornelis et al. 2008; Takaki et al. 2010), in most cases, mini-screw type mini-implants are used because of their easy and minimally invasive implantation technique (Ishii et al. 2004; Cornelis et al. 2008). OMIs serve as temporary skeletal anchorage devices (TSAD) and are excellent alternatives to conventional orthodontic intraoral or extraoral (headgear) anchorages (Nojima et al. 2001; Ma et al. 2008; Bratu et al. 2011; Lee and Kim 2011; Koyama et al. 2011). Orthodontic mini-screws may also be used efficiently in preprosthetic orthodontics for the intrusion of elongated molar teeth (Bratu et al. 2011; Fabian et al. 2012).

These kinds of implants are usually placed in the bone of the maxillary palatine process (Nojima et al. 2001; Ismail and Johal 2002; Tinsley et al. 2004) or in the interalveolar septum between teeth (Ishii et al. 2004; Ismail and Johal 2002) of either the maxillae or the mandible. However, OMIs may also be inserted into other places, like the maxillary tuberosity, retromolar torus, and mental region (Ishii et al. 2004).

Although the use of OMIs can be considered safe, there are some risks of injury to the roots of the teeth and perforation of the nasal cavity or maxillary sinus during their insertion (Ishii et al. 2004; Miyazawa et al. 2010). Although the safety of insertion may be secured based on the clinician's experience in certain cases (Ishii et al. 2004; Dumitrache and Grenard 2010), for the highest degree of safety, CBCT can be used efficiently to determine optimal sites for the placement of palatal and/or approximal anchorage implants (Ishii et al. 2004; Dumitrache and Grenard 2010; Lai et al. 2010; Miyazawa et al. 2010). Further, CBCT- and VIP-based surgical guides (similar to that of implant placement for prosthodontic purposes) are also available for the safe insertion of orthodontic mini-implants (Tinsley et al. 2004; Cousley and Parberry 2005; Miyazawa et al. 2010), as introduced in detail elsewhere.

In the case of the maxillary palatine process, most orthodontic implants are placed either in the midline and 6–12 mm posterior to the incisive foramen, or in an ovoid area located on both sides of the midline 3–9 mm lateral from the midline and 3–9 mm posterior from the papillary coronal plane (Lai et al. 2010). Taking into consideration the anatomical conditions (bone height and density, discussed in more detail elsewhere), the median-palatal suture at least 6 mm posterior to the incisive foramen appears to be the most suitable for implantation, even if very short implants will be used (Lai et al. 2010). However, it should be considered that the median-palatal suture seems to be an important center of maxillary growth and development (Lai et al. 2010); therefore, for children and adolescents, palatal implantation, especially into the median-palatal suture, should be evaluated carefully (Lai et al. 2010).

Conclusion

The survival rate and marginal bone loss values of short implants are comparable to (or may be even better than) those of longer implants (Esposito et al. 2011, 2012; Karthikeyan et al. 2012; Lops et al. 2012). Similarly, results for narrow implants are also rather good and comparable to those of regular-diameter implants (Vigolo et al. 2004; Comfort et al. 2005; Degidi et al. 2008; Franco et al. 2009; Balaji et al. 2010; El-Sheikh et al. 2012). Orthodontic mini-implants serve as temporary skeletal anchorage devices and are excellent alternatives to conventional orthodontic intraoral or extraoral (headgear) anchorages (Nojima et al. 2001; Ma et al. 2008; Bratu et al. 2011; Lee and Kim 2011; Koyama et al. 2011). All these data clearly indicate that special-sized implants are qualified for regular use in dentistry.

References

Balaji, A; Mohamed, JB; Kathiresan, R. A pilot study of mini implants as treatment option for prosthetic rehabilitation of ridges with sub-optimal bone volume. *J Maxillofac Oral Surg*, 2010, 9, 334–338.

Bratu, CD; Pop, RV; Pop, SI; Bratu, EA. Adjusting dento-aveolar morphology with orthodontic mini-implants (miniscrews). A clinical case report. *Rom J Morphol Embriol*, 2011, 52, 1133–1137.

Comfort, MB; Chu, FC; Chai, J; Wat, PY; Chow, TW. A 5-year prospective study on small diameter screw-shaped oral implants. *J Oral Rehabil*, 2005, 32, 341–345.

Cornelis, MA; Scheffler, NR; Nyssen-Behets, C; De Clerk, HJ; Tulloch, JFC. Patients' and orthodontists' perceptions of miniplates used for temporary skeletal anchorage: A prospective study. *Am J Orthod Dentofacial Orthop*, 2008, 133, 18–24.

Cousley, RRJ; Parberry, DJ. Combined cephalometric and stent planning for palatal implants. *J Orthodontics*, 2005, 32, 20–25.

Degidi, M; Piattelli, A; Carinci, F. Clinical outcome of narrow diameter implants: a retrospective study of 510 implants. *J Periodontol*, 2008, 79, 1–6.

Dumitrache, M; Grenard, A. La cartographie des sites anatomiques mini-implantaires au niveau de la premiere molaire maxillaire a l'aide bu NewTom 3G®. *Orthod Fr*, 2010, 81, 287–299.

El-Sheikh, AM; Shihabuddin, OF; Ghoraba, SMF. Two versus three narrow-diameter implants with locator attachments supporting mandibular overdentures: A two-year prospective study. *Int J Dentistry*, 2012, Article ID: 285684. DOI: 10.1155/2012/285684.

Esposito, M; Cannizarro, G; Soardi, E; Pellegrino, G; Pistilli, R; Felice, P. A 3-year post-loading report of a randomized controlled trial on the rehabilitation of posterior atrophic mandibles: short implants or longer implants in vertically augmented bone? *Eur J Oral Implantol*, 2011, 4, 301–311.

Esposito, M; Cannizaro, G; Soardi, E; Pistilli, R; Piatelli, M; Corvino, V; Felice, P. Posterior atrophic jaws rehabilitated with prostheses supported by 6 mm-long, 4 mm-wide implants or by longer implants in augmented bone. Preliminary results from a pilot randomized controlled trial. *Eur J Oral Implantol*, 2012, 5, 19–33.

Fabian, TK; Beck, A; Rencz, B; Fejerdy, P; Hermann, P; Fabian, G. Orthodontics for patients of prosthetic dentistry. Possibilities and complications of psychosomatic origin. In: Fabian TK, Fejerdy P, Hermann P, editors. *Dentures. Types, benefits and potential complications.* New York: Nova Science Publishers, 2012, 15–26.

Franco, M; Viscioni, A; Rigo, L; Guidi, R; Zollino, I; Avantaggiato, A; Carinci, F. Clinical outcome of narrow diameter implants inserted into allografts. *J Appl Oral Sci*, 2009, 17, 301–306.

Huang, J. Risk factors and strategies of dental implants in the maxillary posterior without sufficient bone available. *West China J Stomatol*, 2012, 30, 1–9.

Ishii, T; Nojima, K; Nishii, Y; Takaki, T; Yamaguchi, H. Evaluation of the implantation position of mini-screws for orthodontic treatment in the maxillary molar area by a micro CT. *Bull Tokyo Dent Coll*, 2004, 45, 165–172.

Ismail, SFH, Johal, AS. The role of implants in orthodontics. *J Orthodontics*, 2002, 29, 239–245.

Karthikeyan, I; Desai, SR; Singh, R. Short implants: A systematic review. *J Indian Soc Periodontol*, 2012, 16, 302–312.

Koyama, I; Iino, S; Abe, Y; Takano-Yamamoto, T; Miyawaki, S. Differences between sliding mechanics with implant anchorage and straight-pull headgear and intermaxillary elastics in adults with bimaxillary protrusion. *Eur J Orthodontics*, 2011, 33, 126–131.

Lai, RF; Zou, H; Kong, WD; Lin W. Applied anatomic site study of palatal anchorage implants using cone beam computed tomography. *Int J Oral Sci*, 2010, 2, 98–104.

Lee, AY; Kim, YH. Comparison of movement of the upper dentition according to anchorage method: Orthodontic mini-implant versus conventional anchorage reinforcement in Class I malocclusion. *ISRN Dentistry*, 2011, Article ID: 321206. DOI: 10.5402/2011/321206.

Lee, KJ; Kim, YG; Park, JW; Lee, JM; Suh, JY. Influence of crown-to-implant ratio on periimplant marginal bone loss in the posterior region: a five-year retrospective study. *J Periodontal Implant Sci*, 2012, 42, 231–236.

Lops, D; Bressan, E; Pisoni, G; Cea, N; Corazza, B; Romeo, E. Short implants in partially edentulous maxillae and mandibles: A 10 to 20 years retrospective evaluation. *Int J Dentistry*, 2012, Article ID: 351793. DOI: 10.1155/2012/351793.

Ma, J; Wang, L; Zhang, W; Chen, W; Zhao, C; Smales, RJ. Comparative evaluation of micro-implant and headgear anchorage used with a pre-adjusted appliance system. *Eur J Orthodontics*, 2008, 30, 283–287.

Miyazawa, K; Kawaguchi, M; Tabuchi, M; Goto, S. Accurate pre-surgical determination for self-drilling miniscrew implant placement using surgical guides and cone-beam computed tomography. *Eur J Orthodontics*, 2010, 32, 735–740.

Mohamed, JB; Sudarsan, S; Arun, KV; Shivakumar, B. Rehabilitation using single stage implants. *J Indian Soc Periodontol*, 2009, 13, 32–40.

Mohamed, JB; Alam, MN; Salman, A; Chandrasekaran, SC. Narrow diameter implant in posterior region. *J Indian Soc Periodontol*, 2012, 16, 610–613.

Neldam, CA; Pinholt, EM. State of the art of short dental implants: A systematic review of the literature. *Clin Implant Dent Relat Res*, 2012, 14, 622–632.

Nojima, K; Komatsu, K; Isshiki, Y; Ikumoto, H; Hanai, J; Saito, C. The use of an osseointegrated implant for orthodontic anchorage to a class II div 1 malocclusion. *Bull Tokyo Dent Coll*, 2001, 42, 177–183.

Park, HM; Kim, BH; Yang, IH; Baek, SH. Preliminary three-dimensional analysis of tooth movement and arch dimension change of the maxillary dentition in Class II division 1 malocclusion treated with first premolar extraction: conventional anchorage vs. mini-implant anchorage. *Korean J Orthod*, 2012, 42, 280–290.

Sleiter, R; Klimek, K; Jenni, S. Frontzahnkronen auf CAD/CAM-individualisierten Implantataufbauten. Stand der Technik und Fallbeispiel. *Schweiz Monatsschr Zahnmed*, 2011, 121, 1055–1063.

Takaki, T; Tamura, N; Yamamoto, M; Takano, N; Shibahara, T; Yasumura, T; Nishii, Y; Sueishi, K. Clinical study of temporary anchorage devices for orthodontic treatment – Stability of micro/mini-screws and mini-plates: Experience with 455 cases. *Bull Tokyo Dent Coll*, 2010, 51, 151–163.

Talreja, PS; Gayathri, GV; Mehta, DS. Treatment of an early failing implant by guided bone regeneration using resorbable collagen membrane and bioactive glass. *J Indian Soc Periodontol*, 2013, 17, 131–136.

Tinsley, D; O'Dwyer, JJ; Benson, PE; Doyle, PT; Sandler, J. Orthodontic palatal implants? Clinical technique. *J Orthodontics*, 2004, 31, 3–8.

Vigolo, P; Givani, A; Majzoub, Z; Cordioli, G. Clinical evaluation of small-diameter implants in single-tooth and multiple-implant restorations: a 7-year retrospective study. *Int J Oral Maxillofac Implants*, 2004, 19, 703–709.

CHAPTER 12

PSYCHOSOMATIC CONSIDERATIONS

Abstract

Psychogenic complications are a complex and rising problem in dentistry. Even though a dental treatment may have been carried out properly, there is no assurance that the patient will be satisfied with the therapy. A normative evaluation by the dentist and a subjective evaluation by the patient related to the dental treatment may be rather different. Therefore, factors unrelated to operative/technological dental skills, but that contribute to the success of dental treatments can be very important in certain cases. It is no wonder that there is an increasing amount of available related scientific data in the literature. However, these data are rather divergent, sometimes even contradictory, and there are numerous scientific questions without any available data to answer them. This chapter is a short introduction to the most important clinical aspects of prevention, diagnosis, and treatment possibilities for these psychogenic phenomena, which may appear in relation to dental treatments, including implant dentistry. Several other relevant subject areas, such as the peculiarities of orofacial psychogenic manifestations, basic principles of communication, and the patient-dentist interrelationship, will also be mentioned briefly in this chapter.

12.1. Introduction

The orofacial region is an area of human privacy and is of special personal relevance with overproportional cortical representation; it is an area that appears to be particularly predisposed for a large number of different functional and somatoform psychosomatic disorders (Kreyer 2000; Fabian and Fejerdy 2010; Fabian et al. 2012). Oral psychogenic manifestations are based on the unique psychological and depth psychological function of the mouth and teeth during infancy (breasting), sexuality, aggressiveness, and communication (Fabian and Fabian 2000; Fabian et al. 2000, 2007, 2012; Fabian and Fejerdy 2010). Also of great importance is the symbolic value of the mouth, teeth, tongue, and face (Fabian and Fabian 2000; Fabian et al. 2000, 2007, 2012). The mouth (including the teeth and tongue) also serves as a primary zone of interaction with the environment, and as such, can have far-reaching emotional significance (Ament and Ament 1970; Benson 2000). It is surely tremendously important in a baby's life as an organ through which to receive nourishment, as an organ of pleasure, as an organ of contact with the mother, as an organ of testing, learning, and understanding, and as an organ of social signaling (Ament and Ament 1970). The mouth should also be considered as a highly charged erotogenic region from childhood (Ament and Ament 1970; Benson 2000; Fabian and Fejerdy 2010; Fabian et al. 2012). Tooth loss may profoundly affect the psychosocial well-being of patients, even those who are apparently coping well with dentures (Fiske et al. 1998; Allen and McMillan 2003), and complete edentulousness can be a serious life event (Bergendal 1989; Trulsson et al. 2002; Fabian and Fejerdy 2010; Fabian et al. 2012).

12.2. Prevention of Psychogenic Manifestations

12.2.1. General Considerations

Besides high quality preparative dental skills and technical background, the cornerstones of prevention are screening of patients at risk, proper treatment planning, and proper communication with the patient, as well as prevention of dental fear and prevention of treatment-induced pain (Fabian and Fejerdy 2010; Fabian et al. 2012). Besides these, the *unconscious* wishes of patients related to both dental treatment and their dentist should also be considered (Fabian and Fabian 2000; Fabian et al. 2007, 2012; Fabian and Fejerdy 2010). In contrast to conscious wishes, understanding unconscious wishes (e.g. to look younger, to stop the appearance of aging, to be loved by their dentist, etc.) may be more challenging, but it is similarly important for preventing the manifestation of symptoms (Fabian and Fabian 2000; Fabian et al. 2007, 2012; Fabian and Fejerdy 2010). It may occur that the patient's unconscious wishes may not harmonize with the reality and possibilities of treatment (Fabian and Fejerdy 2010; Fabian et al. 2012). It is a matter of considerable significance that the clinician carefully weigh the option of non-treatment in such cases (Stein 1983; Fabian and Fabian 2000; Fabian et al. 2007, 2012; Fabian and Fejerdy 2010).

12.2.2. Communication with the Patient

Communication with the patient is a key factor in prevention. There are three major facets of proper and efficient patient-dentist communication: (1) a good interpersonal relationship and mutual trust, (2) the exchange of information, and (3) making treatment-related decisions (Fabian and Fejerdy 2010; Fabian et al. 2012). *A good interpersonal relationship* and *mutual trust* can be created with friendliness, genuineness, readiness to help, empathy, respect, and warmth, as well as by eliciting feelings, paraphrasing, and reflecting (Fabian and Fejerdy 2010; Fabian et al. 2012). *Exchange of information* consists of information giving and seeking; to meet their needs, dentists and patients alternate between giving and seeking information (Fabian and Fejerdy 2010; Fabian et al. 2012). Patients need to know the cause of their disorder as well as what the treatment possibilities and possible treatment outcomes are. Patients also need to know that the dentist accepts them and takes them seriously. The dentist needs information to establish the right diagnosis and treatment plan. For such purposes, listening to what the patient says and also what he/she is unable to say is crucial (Fabian and Fejerdy 2010; Fabian et al. 2012). *Treatment-related decision-making* should be based on mutuality, because not only the dentist but also the patient is responsible for his/her health (Fabian and Fejerdy 2010; Fabian et al. 2012). The dentist should avoid hiding behind the facade of professional authority and should share the problem and problem solving with the patient (Freeman 1999/a, b; Lechner and Roessler 2001).

12.3. Diagnosis of Psychogenic Manifestations

The most important diagnostic tool for such purposes is collecting the patient's detailed history and careful evaluation of *all* relevant *psychosocial*, *medical*, and *dental* anamnestic data, including his/her understanding in the context of a *biopsychosocial model* of orofacial disorders (Ross et al. 1953; Engel 1977; Barsby 1994; Pertes 1998; Green and Laskin 2000; Dworkin and Sherman 2006; Fabian and Fejerdy 2010; Fabian et al. 2012). Although a history of symptoms that are inconsistent with the physical findings and a history of a *precipitating life event* after which the symptom first appeared (Muller-Fahlbusch and Sone 1982; Brodine and Hartshorn 2004; Dworkin and Sherman 2006) are hallmarks of psychogenic cases (Muller-Fahlbusch and Sone 1982; Brodine and Hartshorn 2004), a clear-cut diagnosis and proper differential diagnosis could be rather difficult. Therefore, *the diagnosis of psychogenic symptoms is a presumptive one in many cases* (Fabian and Fejerdy 2010; Fabian et al. 2012).

Since psychogenic symptoms may mimic a great variety of (most) somatic symptoms, to assess whether a symptom is of *psychogenic origin* or not, the next five characteristics of psychogenic symptoms (Marxkors and Muller-Fahlbusch 1981) can be considered: (1) well-marked divergence between symptoms and clinical findings, (2) unsuccessful previous somatic treatments, (3) fluctuation of symptoms, (4) conspicuous emotional involvement of the patient in the dental problem, and (5) the presumable relationship between the symptoms and the psychosocial history (Marxkors and Muller-Fahlbusch 1981). Symptoms that meet at least four of the above five criteria are very likely to be of psychogenic origin (Fabian and Fejerdy 2010; Fabian et al. 2012).

12.4. Treatment Possibilities

The majority of patients with psychogenic symptoms refuse to accept the psychological nature of their symptoms (Ross et al. 1953; Schwichtenberg and Doering 2008). Therefore, a simple referral to a psychiatrist and/or psychotherapist would not solve the problem in most cases. Consequently, initial psychosomatic therapy (IPT) is needed prior to definitive therapy, which is within the scope of the dental professional's duty (Moulton et al. 1957; Pomp 1974). The most important goals of the premised initial psychosomatic therapy are avoidance of further useless invasive dental treatment (Brodine and Hartshorn 2004; Reeves and Merrill 2007; Baad-Hansen 2008), as well as the obtainment of a decrease of (recovery from) symptoms and the motivation of patients to participate in definitive psychosomatic therapy, which is the highest level of care for patients with psychogenic symptoms (Fabian and Fejerdy 2010; Fabian et al. 2012).

Gradual escalation of therapy and the avoidance of irreversible forms of treatment are "cornerstones" of initial psychosomatic therapy (Laskin and Block 1986), which utilizes several placebo and/or palliative methods (e.g. physiotherapies, medication, medicinal herb therapy, diet therapy, complementary and alternative medicine, CAM therapy, etc.) combined with certain psychotherapeutic approaches and the administration of any mind-body therapies, which are the "basic therapeutics" for psychosomatic disorders (Iversen 1989; Binder and Bider 1989; Krause 1983, 1994, 2000; Fabian 2012; Beck et al. 2012; Fabian et al. 2012).

In contrast to initial therapy, definitive psychosomatic therapy (DPT) is the highest level of care for patients with psychogenic symptoms, utilizing any available dental, medical, and psychotherapeutical treatment possibilities in an evidence-based manner (Fabian and Fejerdy 2010; Fabian et al. 2012). Definitive psychosomatic therapy should be carried out by *specialized dental professionals* as members of a specialized *psychosomatic team* including *experienced dentists and other medical and psychotherapeutical professionals* (Fabian and Fejerdy 2010; Fabian et al. 2012). Definitive psychosomatic therapy should be offered for patients being refractory to the initial psychosomatic therapy, and for patients responding to it but without a stable treatment outcome in a long run (i.e. patients with frequent relapses).

Conclusion

Even though a dental treatment may have been carried out properly, there is no assurance that the patient will be satisfied with the therapy (Mazurat and Mazurat 2003/a, b). A normative evaluation by the dentist and a subjective evaluation by the patient related to the dental treatment may be rather different (Lechner and Roessler 2001). Therefore, factors unrelated to operative/technological dental skills, but that contribute to the success of dental treatments, are becoming more and more important in the field of implant dentistry.

References

Allen, PF; McMillan, AS. A review of the functional and psychosocial outcomes of edentulousness treated with complete replacement dentures. *J Can Dent Assoc*, 2003, 69, 662.

Ament, P; Ament, A. Body image in dentistry. *J Prosthet Dent*, 1970, 24, 362–366.

Baad-Hansen, L. Atypical odontalgia - pathophysiology and clinical management. *J Oral Rehabil*, 2008, 35, 1–11.

Barsby, MJ. The use of hypnosis in the management of "gagging" and intolerance to dentures. *Br Dent J*, 1994, 176, 97–102.

Beck, A; Varga, G; Hermann, P; Fabian, G; Fejerdy, P; Fabian, TK. Methods for the treatment denture induced psychogenic symptoms. In: Fabian TK, Fejerdy P, Hermann P, editors. *Dentures. Types, benefits and potential complications.* New York: Nova Science Publishers, 2012, 165–197.

Benson, PE. Suggestion can help. *Ann R Australas Coll Dent Surg*, 2000, 15, 284–285.

Bergendal, B. The relative importance of tooth loss and denture wearing in Swedish adults. *Community Dent Health*, 1989, 6, 103–111.

Binder, H; Binder, K. *Autogenes Training, Basispsychotherapeutikum*. Köln: Deutscher Arzteverlag, 1989.

Brodine, AL; Hartshorn, MA. Recognition and management of somatoform disorders. *J Prosthet Dent*, 2004, 91, 268–273.

Dworkin, SF; Sherman J. Chronic orofacial pain: biobehavioral perspectives. In: Mostofsky DI, Forgione AG, Giddon, DB editors. *Behavioral dentistry*. Ames (Iowa): Blackwell Munksgaard, 2006, 99–113.

Engel, G. The need for a new medical model: a challenge for biomedicine. *Science*, 1977, 196, 129–136.

Fabian, TK; Fabian, G. Dental stress. In: Fink G, editor in chief. *Encyclopedia of Stress*. Vol. 1. San Diego: Academic Press, 2000, 657–659.

Fabian, TK; Vertes, G; Toth, Zs. Some depth-psychological aspects of the psychogenic symptoms of the orofacial tissues. *Fogorv Szle*, 2000, 93, 262–267.

Fabian, TK; Fabian, G; Fejerdy, P. Dental Stress. In: Fink G, editor in chief. *Encyclopedia of Stress. 2-nd enlarged edition*, Vol. 1. Oxford: Academic Press, 2007, 733–736.

Fabian, TK; Fejerdy P. *Psychogenic denture intolerance. Theoretical background, prevention and treatment possibilities*. New York: Nova Science Publishers, 2010.

Fabian, TK; Beck, A; Gotai, L; Hermann, P; Fejerdy, P. Psychogenic complications of making dentures. Theoretical background, prevention and treatment possibilities. In: Fabian TK, Fejerdy P, Hermann P, editors. *Dentures. Types, benefits and potential complications*. New York: Nova Science Publishers, 2012, 199–241.

Fiske, J; Davis, DM; Frances, C; Gelbier, S. The emotional effects of tooth loss in edentulous people. *Brit Dent J*, 1998, 184, 90–93.

Freeman, R. Strategies for motivating the non-compliant patient. *Brit Dent J*, 1999/a, 187, 307–312.

Freeman, R. A psychodynamic understanding of the dentist-patient interaction. *Brit Dent J*, 1999/b, 186, 503–505.

Green, CS; Laskin, DM. Temporomandibular disorders: Moving from a dentally based to a medically based model. *J Dent Res*, 2000, 79, 1736–1739.

Iversen, G. Geleitwort. In: Binder H, Binder K editors. *Autogenes Training, Basispsychotherapeutikum*. Köln: Deutscher Arzteverlag; 1989.

Krause, WR. Grundlagen der Biofeedback-Therapie und ihre therapeutischen Anwendungsmoglichkeiten. *Z arztl Fortbild*, 1983, 77, 493–494.

Krause, WR. Hypnose und Autogenes Training (Selbsthypnose) in der Rehabilitation. Erganzung in: Schultz, JH. *Hypnose-Technik. Praktische Anleitung zum Hypnotisieren fur Arzte*. 9. Auflage - bearbeitet und erganzt von G. Iversen und W.-R. Krause. Stuttgart - Jena - New York: Gustav Fischer Verlag; 1994. 71–79.

Krause, WR. Hypnose und Autogenes Training. *Mitteldeutsch Hausarzt*, 2000, 2, 20–22.

Kreyer, G. Psychosomatics of the orofacial system. *Wien Med Wochenschr*, 2000, 150, 213–216.

Laskin, DM; Block, S. Diagnosis and treatment of myofacial pain-dysfunction (MPD) syndrome. *J Prosthet Dent*, 1986, 56, 75–85.

Lechner, SK; Roessler, D. Strategies for complete denture success: beyond technical excellence. *Compend Contin Educ Dent*, 2001, 22, 553–559.

Marxkors, R; Muller-Fahlbusch, H. Zur Diagnose psychosomatischer Storungen in der zahnarztlich-prothetischen Praxis. *Dtsch Zahnarztl Z*. 1981, 36, 787–790.

Mazurat, NM; Mazurat, RD. Discuss before fabricating: Communicating the realities of partial denture therapy. Part I: Patient expectations. *J Can Dent Assoc*, 2003/a, 69, 90–94.

Mazurat, NM; Mazurat, RD. Discuss before fabricating: Communicating the realities of partial denture therapy. Part II: Clinical outcomes. *J Can Dent Assoc*, 2003/b, 69, 90–94.

Moulton, R; Ewen, S; Thieman, W. Emotional factors in periodontal disease. *Oral Surg Oral Med Oral Pathol*, 1957, 5, 833–860.

Muller-Fahlbusch, H; Sone, K. Praprotetische Psychagogik. *Dtsch Zahnarztl Z*, 1982, 37, 703–707.

Pertes, RA. Differential diagnosis of orofacial pain. *Mt Sinai J Med*, 1998 65, 348–354.

Pomp, AM. Psychotherapy for the myofascial pain-dysfunction syndrome: a study of factors coinciding with symptom remission. *J Am Dent Assoc*, 1974, 89, 629–632.

Reeves 2nd, JL; Merrill, RL. Diagnostic and treatment challenges in occlusal dysesthesia. *J Calif Dent Assoc*, 2007, 35, 198–207.

Ross, GL; Bentley, HJ; Greene Jr., GW. The psychosomatic concept in dentistry. *Psychosom Med*, 1953, 15, 168–173.

Schwichtenberg, J; Doering, S. Success of referral in a psychosomatic-psychotherapeutic outpatient unit of a dental school. *Z Psychosom Med Psychother*, 2008, 54, 285–292.

Stein, RS. Mutual protective complex of dental restorations. In: Laney WR, Gibilisco JA editors. *Diagnosis and treatment of prosthodontics*. Philadelphia: Lea & Febiger, 1983, 306–326.

Trulsson, U; Engstrand, P; Berggren, U; Nannmark, U; Branemark, PI. Edentulousness and oral rehabilitation: experiences from the patients' perspective. *Eur J Oral Sci*, 2002, 110, 417–424.

Chapter 13

Medicamentous Therapy

Abstract

Medicamentous therapy is an important supplementary modality of implant dentistry. Medication is primarily utilized for the management of pain and inflammation, including antibiotic treatment if needed. Antibiotics may also be administered for preventive purposes in the case of cardiac conditions associated with the highest risk of an adverse outcome from infective endocarditis and in the case of patients with total joint replacement. In certain cases, medicamentous therapy may also be used for the management of fear of the surgical intervention, for the management of muscle spasms, and for the management of allergic reactions. Although medication is an important supplementary modality of implant dentistry, there are various medical (and/or dental) contraindications, possible side effects, and adverse effects, as well as possible dangerous interactions that should be considered. Utilizing pharmacological databases and *up-to-date* pharmacological and clinical knowledge, dentists should be familiar with both the benefits and potential hazards before prescribing any medication. In this chapter, the most important aspects of medicamentous therapy from the viewpoint of implant dentistry will be introduced.

13.1. Introduction

Medicamentous therapy is an important supplementary modality of implant dentistry. Medication is primarily utilized for the management of pain and inflammation (Fabian and Fejerdy 2010; Beck et al. 2012; Bakke et al. 2013), including antibiotic treatment if needed (Bowen-Antolin et al. 2007; Khoury et al. 2008; Hong et al. 2010; Larsen et al. 2013). Antibiotics may also be administered for preventive purposes in the case of cardiac conditions associated with the highest risk of an adverse outcome from infective endocarditis (Wilson et al. 2008) and in the case of patients with total joint replacement (Kuong et al. 2009). Besides these, medicamentous therapy may also be used for the management of fear of the surgical intervention (Lu 1994; Fabian and Fabian 2000; Fabian et al. 2007; Fabian and Fejerdy 2010; Gonzalez-Lemonnier et al. 2010, 2011; Hillerup and Risby 2013), for the management of muscle spasms (Fabian and Fejerdy 2010; Beck et al. 2012), and for the management of allergic reactions (Hansen and West 1997; Fabian and Fejerdy 2010; Rasmussen et al. 2013) in certain cases. In this chapter, the most important aspects of medicamentous therapy from the viewpoint of implant dentistry will be introduced.

13.2. Management of Pain and Inflammation

Based on the lowest risk of side effects, pain killers should be preferred first if postoperative pain appears with the absence of significant inflammatory reaction (Bakke et al. 2013). Paracetamol is well tolerated and may be the first choice in these cases (Bakke et al. 2013). However, it should be noted that even a modest overdosage of the drug may result in life-threatening intoxication (Bakke et al. 2013). Paracetamol may be advantageously supplemented with light opioids like codeine and tramadol (Bakke et al. 2013), but it should be recognized that these drugs are potentially addictive (Bakke et al. 2013).

If both the pain and significant inflammatory reaction appear non-steroidal, anti-inflammatory drugs (NSAIDs), for example ibuprophen or naproxen, can be used (Fabian and Fejerdy 2010; Beck et al. 2012; Bakke et al. 2013). Further, it should also be noted that most postoperatively appearing pain symptoms are (at least partially) of inflammatory origin, even if there is no clinically significant inflammatory reaction (Fabian and Fejerdy 2010). Therefore, the administration of NSAIDs (together with or instead of pain killers) may also be indicated if great pain is experienced without clinically significant signs of inflammation (Fabian and Fejerdy 2010; Beck et al. 2012). However, if NSAIDs are used, possible cardiovascular and gastrointestinal side effects should be considered carefully (Bakke et al. 2013). It should also be recognized that the administration of NSAIDs during the early postoperative period may negatively influence early osseointegration processes (Kalyvas and Tarenidou 2008) even if the premised negative influence seems to be temporary and does not affect the final outcome of the osseointegration processes (Kalyvas and Tarenidou 2008).

In certain cases, anticonvulsant drugs may also be used to manage the greatest pain caused by nerve injury (if any). The use of anticonvulsant drugs is especially reasonable for neuropathic pain such as neuralgia of several origins (Derra and Egle 2003; Grond and Lehman 2003; Sarlani et al. 2005/a; Fabian and Fejerdy 2010; Beck et al. 2012); although they may also be used for the treatment of severe atypical facial pain and atypical odontalgia (Benoliel et al. 1997; Derra and Egle 2003; Grond and Lehman 2003; Sarlani et al. 2005/b; Fabian and Fejerdy 2010; Beck et al. 2012). In general, carbamazepine, clonazepam, or gabapentin may be used (Derra and Egle 2003; Grond and Lehman 2003; Sarlani et al. 2005/a; Fabian and Fejerdy 2010; Beck et al. 2012). In the orofacial region, carbamazepine seems to be significantly more efficient than other anticonvulsant drugs (Derra and Egle 2003; Grond and Lehman 2003) with the exception of herpetic and postherpetic neuralgia, in which case gabapentin can also be offered (Sarlani et al. 2005/a).

13.3. Use of Antibiotics

The current guidelines of the American Heart Association (AHA) and the American Dental Association (ADA) for the prevention of infective endocarditis (IE) were released and published in 2008 (Wilson et al. 2008). These guidelines recommend antibiotic prophylaxis in the case of patients with underlying cardiac conditions associated with the *highest risk of adverse outcome* from infective endocarditis (Wilson et al. 2008). The cardiac conditions associated with the highest risk of adverse outcome from infective endocarditis for which prophylaxis with dental procedures is reasonable are (Wilson et al. 2008): *prosthetic cardiac valve or prosthetic material used for cardiac valve repair; previous infective endocarditis; unrepaired cyanotic congenital heart disease (CHD), including palliative shunts and conduits; completely repaired congenital heart defect with prosthetic material or device, whether placed by surgery or by catheter intervention (but during the first six months after the procedure only); repaired CHD with residual defects at the site or adjacent to the site of a prosthetic patch or prosthetic device (which inhibit endothelialization); and cardiac transplantation recipients who develop cardiac valvulopathy* (Wilson et al. 2008). For patients with such conditions, *prophylaxis is recommended for all dental procedures* that involve the manipulation of gingival tissue or the periapical region of the teeth or the perforation of the oral mucosa (Wilson et al. 2008), *with the exception* of routine anesthetic injections through non-infected tissue, taking dental radiographs, the placement of removable prosthodontic or orthodontic appliances, the adjustment of orthodontic appliances, the placement of orthodontic brackets, shedding of primary teeth, and bleeding from trauma to the lips or oral mucosa (Wilson et al. 2008). For the prevention of infective endocarditis in the premised cases, oral administration of 2 g amoxicillin (or in case of penicillin allergy, 600 mg clindamycin) one hour prior to surgery is recommended (Wilson et al. 2008). In general, the same recommendations are used in most European countries (Larsen et al. 2013) and may also be used worldwide.

Similar to the prevention of infectious endocarditis, in the case of patients with total joint replacement, it is also recommended that 2 g amoxicillin (or in case of penicillin allergy, 600 mg clindamycin) be administered orally one hour prior to surgery (Kuong et al. 2009). An earlier recommendation from the American Academy/Association of Orthopaedic Surgeons (AAOS) considered antibiotic prevention as mandatory in all cases of total joint replacement (Kuong et al. 2009). However, the newest guideline released by the AAOS together with the American Dental Association suggests that the practitioner might consider discontinuing the practice of routinely prescribing prophylactic antibiotics for patients with total joint replacement (AAOS and ADA 2012; Rethman et al. 2012). Several societies in Europe (Kuong et al. 2009) and worldwide (Kuong et al. 2009) usually recommend antibiotic prophylaxis in the case of patients considered at *increased risk for infection*, including joint replacement done within the past two years, previous infection of a prosthetic joint, inflammatory arthritis, type 1 diabetes mellitus, hemophilia, immunosuppression, and a history of previous or current malignancy (Kuong et al. 2009).

In contrast to the use of antibiotics for prevention in relation to infective endocarditis (with a widely accepted guideline), and total joint replacement (with more or less clear guidelines), there is still debate concerning the use of antibiotic prophylaxis before invasive dental procedures for patients at risk of acquiring a distant site infection other than endocarditis (Lockhart et al. 2002). There may be increased risk of acquiring a distant site infection (DSI) in various health conditions, for example, in patients with lupus erythematosus, poorly controlled diabetes mellitus, dialysis catheters and shunts, a cardiac pacemaker, ventriculoperitoneal shunts, prosthetic vascular grafts, orthopedic implants, or chemotherapy-induced neutropenia (Lockhart et al. 2002) or other strongly compromised health conditions. However, there is no consensus on whether there is a need for antibiotic prophylaxis in these cases (Lockhart et al. 2002). As long as there is no clear evidence available, it is advisable that the dentist consult with the medical professional responsible for the management of patients with such conditions before surgery.

Oral administration of 2 g amoxicillin prior to surgery (Larsen et al. 2013), followed by 500 mg amoxicillin three times a day for the first postoperative week (Khoury et al. 2008) may also be advantageous in preventing complications in relation to implant placement and osseointegration (Larsen et al. 2013; Khoury et al. 2008); however, the evidence of the usefulness (if any) of this treatment is rather limited (Larsen et al. 2013; Khoury et al. 2008). In the case of acute bacterial inflammation following surgery, either oral administration of 250 mg amoxicillin together with 125 mg clavulanic acid three times a day for 3–7 days (Bowen-Antolin et al. 2007; Hong et al. 2010) or oral administration of 1 MIE penicillin V together with 500 mg metronidazol three times a day for 3(–7) days may be the first choice (Larsen et al. 2013). In the case of penicillin allergy, 300 mg clindamycin 3(–4) times a day for 3(–7) days can be administered orally (Larsen et al. 2013). In more severe cases, culture and sensitivity tests of bacteria followed by targeted antibiotic treatment eventually supplemented by incision, drainage, and removal of graft material (if any) may also be needed (Hong et al. 2010).

13.4. Management of Fear

Anxiolytics (especially short-acting benzodiazepines such as midazolam or triazolam) may be used advantageously for the prevention and management of fear of the surgical intervention and/or other dental fears (Lu 1994; Fabian and Fabian 2000; Fabian et al. 2007; Fabian and Fejerdy 2010; Gonzalez-Lemonnier et al. 2010, 2011; Hillerup and Risby 2013). Anxyolitics, (i.e. benzodiazepines like midazolam and triazolam) can be administered intraorally or sublingually as premedication or intravenously for conscious sedation during surgery (Fabian and Fabian 2000; Fabian et al. 2007; Fabian and Fejerdy 2010; Gonzalez-Lemonnier et al. 2010, 2011; Hillerup and Risby 2013). Intravenous conscious sedation should be carried out by an anesthetist and with monitoring of hemodynamic and ventilatory changes (Gonzalez-Lemonnier et al. 2010, 2011; Wakita et al. 2012) because of possible serious complications, especially respiratory depression and upper airway obstruction (Gonzalez-Lemonnier et al. 2010, 2011; Wakita et al. 2012). Although optimal sedation was also reported using a combination of midazolam and dexmedetomidine (Wakita et al. 2012), usually a combination of midazolam and propofol is used for such purposes (Gonzalez-Lemonnier et al. 2010, 2011; Wakita et al. 2012).

13.5. Management of Muscle Spasm

In certain cases, painful muscle spasms may also appear, especially following more complex surgeries and/or extended prosthetic rehabilitation. A spasm produces pain that in turn produces more spasms in many cases (Laskin and Block 1986; Fabian and Fejerdy 2010). Thus, muscle relaxants may be used to interrupt this *vicious cycle*, especially when used in conjunction with a pain-relieving medication (Laskin and Block 1986; Fabian and

Fejerdy 2010; Beck et al. 2012). Importantly, certain anxiolytics (especially benzodiazepines) also possess significant myorelaxant properties (Chaco 1973; Laskin and Block 1986; Dahlstrom 1989, 1992). Since the tranquilizing (anxiolytic) properties themselves may also be beneficial in relieving muscle tension (Laskin and Block 1986; Fabian and Fejerdy 2010; Beck et al. 2012), benzodiazepines are the drugs most often prescribed as muscle relaxants (Laskin and Block 1986; Dahlstrom 1992). Again, benzodiazepines should also be taken in conjunction with an analgesic for the best effect (Laskin and Block 1986; Fabian and Fejerdy 2010; Beck et al. 2012). Interestingly, drugs with only muscle relaxant properties (i.e. without any anxiolytic effects) do not seem to be as successful as benzodiazepines for the treatment of muscle spasm-induced pain (Laskin and Block 1986).

For most severe muscle spasms, local anesthetics may also be used (Clark 1981; Sarlani et al. 2005/a; Fabian and Fejerdy 2010) in connection with muscle-stretching exercises (Dunteman and Swarm 1995; Sarlani et al. 2005/a; Fabian and Fejerdy 2010). Since too frequent injection can be injurious to the muscle, local application of local anesthetics can be repeated several times within a week if effective but not thereafter (Laskin and Block 1986; Fabian and Fejerdy 2010). Local anesthetics, when injected into a muscle, affect the hypertonus by preferential paralysis of both alpha and gamma motoneurons (fusimotor fibers) as well as the endings and afferent fibers leaving the muscle spindles (Mathews and Rushworth 1957; Harris and Griffin 1975); therefore, there is no need to infiltrate muscle tissues directly when the innervating nerve is available for block anesthesia (conduction anesthesia) (Mathews and Rushworth 1957). If block anesthesia is unaccomplishable, 0.5 ml anesthetics should be injected into the painful muscle area (Laskin and Block 1986; Fabian and Fejerdy 2010). Importantly, local anesthetics should be used *without any vasoconstrictor* (Bell 1969; Clark 1981; Laskin and Block 1986; Dunteman and Swarm 1995) to promote the infiltration of the tissues, to decrease the time span of the treatment, and especially to prevent the decrease of *blood flow* in the muscle (Fabian and Fejerdy 2010). Following an application of local anesthetics, relief from pain and a decrease of muscle spasms occur, which may be utilized for gentle muscle-stretching exercises (Laskin and Block 1986; Fabian and Fejerdy 2010). Importantly, *muscular exercises should be carried out very carefully during the period of anesthesia* because the protective reflexes of the muscles are inhibited (Fabian and Fejerdy 2010).

13.6. Management of Anaphylactic Reactions

Although allergic reactions in dentistry are fortunately rare and primarily belong to the delayed type (type IV) reactions appearing in relation to dentures (Hansen and West 1997; Garhammer et al. 2001; Fabian and Fejerdy 2010), occasionally rather severe and dangerous local anesthetic-related or denture-related allergic reactions may occur (Hansen and West 1997; Fabian and Fejerdy 2010). Therefore, great care should be taken with patients with a history of *urticaria, allergic type asthma bronchiale, angiooedema, anaphylactic shock, or any other IgE mediated (type I) reactions* (Fabian and Fejerdy 2010; Rasmussen et al. 2013) because patients with these premised pathologies are at *higher risk* of a *life-threatening* IgE-mediated (type I) *allergic reaction* (Fabian and Fejerdy 2010; Rasmussen et al. 2013). Dentists should be prepared for first aid interventions against severe anaphylactic reactions, especially if dealing with such patients (Fabian and Fejerdy 2010; Rasmussen et al. 2013). Mild symptoms such as pruritus or urticaria can be controlled through the administration of 0.2 to 0.5 mL of 1:1000 epinephrine (equivalent to 0.2 to 0.5 mg epinephrine) intramuscularly, with repeated doses as required at three minute intervals for severe reactions (Austen 1991; Fabian and Fejerdy 2010; Rasmussen et al. 2013) up to a total of 0.8 mg (Rasmussen et al. 2013). An intravenous infusion should be initiated to provide a route for the administration of epinephrine (diluted 1:50.000) and volume expanders if intractable hypotension occurs (Austen 1991; Fabian and Fejerdy 2010). Intubation or laryngotomy (i.e. incision of the cricothyroid membrane) may also be needed if laryngeal angioedema appears (Fabian and Fejerdy 2010; Rasmussen et al. 2013).

13.7. Contraindications

There are various medical (and/or dental) contraindications, possible side effects, and adverse effects, as well as possible dangerous interactions that should be considered very carefully before the initiation of medicamentous therapy (Bell 1969; Laskin and Block 1986; Friedlander et al. 2004; Pedersen and Bjerrum 2013). Utilizing pharmacological databases and *up-to-date* pharmacological knowledge, dentists should be familiar with the potential hazards before prescribing a medication (Bell 1969; Laskin and Block 1986; Friedlander et al. 2004). Considering the premised precautions, *short-term* (1 to 2 weeks, or a maximum of 3 to 4 weeks) administration of several medicaments can be carried out by the dentist (Bell 1969; Miyamoto and Ziccardi 1998; Laskin and Block 1986; Toyofuku and Kikuta 2006).

Nevertheless, long-term medicamentous treatment of long-standing symptoms (if any) is clearly within the scope of medical professionals (Fabian and Fejerdy 2010; Beck et al. 2012). Therefore, *if long-term medication is needed for any reason, it is necessary to place the patient under physician care* (Laskin and Block 1986; Fabian and Fejerdy 2010). In the case of pregnancy, lactation, any serious systemic disease, or strongly compromised health, referral to medical professionals responsible for the treatment of the systemic disease at issue and/or management of strongly compromised health is highly recommended before starting any medicamentous therapy (Fabian and Fejerdy 2010), even short-term therapy.

It should also be considered that not only the administration, but also the removal of a medication, may be contraindicated (Fabian and Fejerdy 2010). In the case of medication abuse, the removal of a medication should be carried out by the professional who is regularly responsible for the administration of the medication at issue (Fabian and Fejerdy 2010).

Conclusion

Medication is an important supplementary modality of implant dentistry, even if there are various medical (and/or dental) contraindications, possible side effects, and adverse effects, as well as possible dangerous interactions that should be considered (Bell 1969; Laskin and Block 1986; Friedlander et al. 2004; Pedersen and Bjerrum 2013). Utilizing pharmacological databases and *up-to-date* pharmacological and clinical knowledge, dentists should be familiar with both the benefits and potential hazards before prescribing a medication (Bell 1969; Laskin and Block 1986; Friedlander et al. 2004).

References

AAOS; ADA (American Academy of Orthopaedic Surgeons; American Dental Association). American Academy of Orthopaedic Surgeons and the American Dental Association Prevention of Orthopaedic Implant Infection in Patients Undergoing Dental Procedures Guideline. Rosemont, IL: American Academy of Orthopaedic Surgeons; 2012.

Austen, KF. Diseases of immediate type hypersensitivity. In: Wilson JD, Braunwald E, Isselbacher KJ, Petersdorf RG, Martin JB, Fauci AS, Root RK, editors. Harrison's Principles of Internal Medicine Vol. 2. (Twelfth Edition). New York: McGraw-Hill, 1991, 1422–1428.

Bakke, M; Bjorndal, L; Dolleris, SH; Nygaard, BU; Marcusen, M. Analgesic and anti-inflammatory drugs in general dental practice in Denmark. Danish Dent J, 2013, 117, 812–820.

Beck, A; Varga, G; Hermann, P; Fabian, G; Fejerdy, P; Fabian, TK. Methods for the treatment of denture induced psychogenic symptoms. In: Fabian TK, Fejerdy P, Hermann P, editors. Dentures. Types, benefits and potential complications. New York: Nova Science Publishers, 2012, 165–197.

Bell, WH. Nonsurgical management of the pain-dysfunction syndrome. J Am Dent Assoc, 1969, 79, 161–170.

Benoliel, R; Elishoov, H; Sharav, Y. Orofacial pain with vascular-type features. Oral Surg Oral Med Oral Pathol Oral Radiol Endod. 1997, 84, 506–512.

Bowen-Antolin, A; Pascua-Garcia, MT; Nasimi, A. Infections in implantology: From prophylaxis to treatment. Med Oral Patol Oral Cir Bucal, 2007, 12, E323–E330.

Chaco, J. Electromyography of the masseter muscles in Costen's syndrome. J Oral Med, 1973, 28, 45–46.

Clark, GT. Management of muscular hyperactivity. Int Dent J, 1981, 31, 216–225.

Dahlstrom, L. Electromyographic studies of craniomandibular disorders: a review of the literature. J Oral Rehabil, 1989 16, 1–20.

Dahlstrom, L. Conservative treatment methods in craniomandibular disorder. Swed Dent J, 1992, 16, 217–230.

Derra C; Egle, UT. Psychopharmaka in der Schmerztherapie. In: Egle UT, Hoffmann SO, Lehmann KA, Nix WA editors. Handbuch Chronischer Schmerz. Grundlagen, Pathogenese, Klinik und Therapie aus bio-psycho-sozialer Sicht. Stuttgart - New York: Schattauer GmbH, 2003, 352–359.

Dunteman, E; Swarm, R. Atypical facial "neuralgia". (Case reports). Anesth Analg, 1995, 80, 188–190.

Fabian, TK; Fabian, G. Dental stress. In: Fink G, editor in chief. Encyclopedia of stress. (vol. 1.). San Diego: Academic Press; 2000; 567–659.

Fabian, TK; Fabian, G; Fejerdy, P. Dental stress. In: Fink G, editor in chief. Encyclopedia of stress. Second edition. (vol. 1.) .Oxford: Academic Press, 2007, 733–736.

Fabian, TK; Fejerdy P. Psychogenic denture intolerance. Theoretical background, prevention and treatment possibilities. New York: Nova Science Publishers, 2010.

Friedlander, AH; Marder, SR; Sung, EC. Panic disorder. Psychopathology, medical management and dental implications. J Am Dent Assoc, 2004, 135, 771–778.

Garhammer, P; Schmalz, G; Hiller, KA; Reitinger, T; Stolz, W. Patients with local adverse effects from dental alloys: frequency, complaints, symptoms, allergy. Clin Oral Invest, 2001, 5, 240–249.

Gonzalez-Lemonnier, S; Bovaira-Forner, M; Penarrocha-Diago, MA; Penarrocha-Oltra, D. Relationship between preoperative anxiety and postope-rative satisfaction in dental implant surgery with intravenous conscious sedation. Med Oral Patol Oral Cir Bucal, 2010, 15, e379–e382.

Gonzalez-Lemonnier, S; Bovaira-Forner, M; Penarrocha-Diago, D; Penarrocha-Diago, MA. Hemodynamic and ventilatory changes during implant surgery with intravenous conscious sedation. Med Oral Patol Oral Cir Bucal, 2011, 16, e541–e545.

Grond, S; Lehmann, KA. Analgetika: Anwendung, Nutzen und Probleme. In: Egle UT, Hoffmann SO, Lehmann KA, Nix WA editors. Handbuch Chronischer Schmerz. Grundlagen, Pathogenese, Klinik und Therapie aus bio-psycho-sozialer Sicht. Stuttgart - New York: Schattauer GmbH, 2003, 334–345.

Hansen, PA; West, LA. Allergic reaction following insertion of a Pd-Cu-Au fixed partial denture: a clinical report. J Prosthodont, 1997, 6, 144–148.

Harris, R; Griffin, CJ. Neuromuscular mechanisms and the masticatory apparatus. In: Griffin CJ, Harris R editors. The temporomandibular joint syndrome. The masticatory apparatus of man in normal and abnormal function. (Monographs in oral science, Vol. 4.) Basel - Munchen - Paris - London - New York - Sydney: Karger, 1975, 45–64.

Hillerup, S; Risby, C. Lokal anaesthesia and sedation. Danish Dent J, 2013, 117, 822–826.

Hong, SB; Kim, JS; Shin, SI; Han, JY; Herr, Y; Chung, JH. Clinical treatment of postoperative infection following sinus augmentation. J Periodontal Implant Sci, 2010, 40, 144–149.

Kalyvas, DG; Tarenidou, M. Influence of nonsteroidal anti-inflammatory drugs on osseointegration. J Oral Sci, 2008, 50, 239–246.

Khoury, SB; Thomas, L; Walters, JD; Sheridan, JF; Leblebicioglu, B. Early wound healing following one-stage dental implant placement with and without antibiotic prophylaxis: A pilot study. J Periodontol, 2008, 79, 1904–1912.

Kuong, EE; Ng, FY; Yan, CH; Fang, CXS; Chiu, PKY. Antibiotic prophylaxis after total joint replacements. Hong Kong Med J, 2009, 15, 458–462.

Larsen, T; Ciofu, O; Moesby, L; Kirkevang, LL, Poulsen, AH. Antibiotics in dental practice. Danish Dent J, 2013, 117, 718–729.

Laskin, DM; Block, S. Diagnosis and treatment of myofacial pain-dysfunction (MPD) syndrome. J Prosthet Dent, 1986, 56, 75–84.

Lockhart, PB; Brennan, MT; Fox, PC; Norton, J; Jernigan, DB; Strausbaugh, LJ; Infectious Disease Society of America Emerging Infections Network. Decision-making on the use of antimicrobial prophylaxis for dental procedures: A survey of infectious disease consultants and review. Clin Infect Dis, 2002, 34, 1621–1626.

Lu, DP. The use of hypnosis for smooth sedation induction and reduction of postoperative violent emergencies from anesthesia in pediatric dental patients. J Dentistry Children, 1994, 182–185.

Mathews, PBC; Rushworth G. The selective effect of procaine on the stretch reflex and tendon jerk of soleus muscle when applied to its nerve. J Physiol Lond, 1957, 135, 245–262.

Miyamoto, SA; Ziccardi, VB. Burning mouth syndrome. Mt Sinai J Med, 1998, 65, 343–347.

Pedersen, AML; Bjerrum, L. Polypharmacy and odontological practice. Danish Dent J, 916–920.

Rasmussen, EHR; Fast, S; Tagesen, J; Bygum, A. Angioedema with and without urticaria – a dental perspective. Danish Dent J, 2013, 117, 474–480.

Rethman, MP; Watters III, W; Abt, E; Anderson, PA; Boyer, K; Carroll, KC; Evans, RP; Futrell, HC; Garvin, K; Glenn, SO; Goldberg, MJ; Hanson, NB; Hellstein, J; Hewlett, A; Kolessar, D; Moucha, C; O'Donnell, RJ; Osmon, DR; O'Toole, JE; Rinella, A; Steinberg, MJ. Prevention of Orthopaedic Implant Infection in Patients Undergoing Dental Procedures Executive Summary on the AAOS/ADA Clinical Practice Guideline. AAOS/ADA; 2012.

Sarlani, E; Balciunas, BA; Grace, EG. Orofacial pain - Part I. Assessment and management of musculoskeletal and neuropathic causes. AACN Clin Issues, 2005/a, 16, 333–346.

Sarlani, E; Balciunas, BA; Grace, EG. Orofacial pain - Part II. Assessment and management of vascular, neurovascular, idiopathic, secondary, and psychogenic causes. AACN Clin Issues, 2005/b, 16, 347–358.

Toyofuku, A; Kikuta, T. Treatment of phantom bite syndrome with milnacipran - a case series. Neuropsych Dis Treatment, 2006, 2, 387–390.

Wakita, R; Kohase, H; Fukayama, H. A Comparison of Dexmedetomidine Sedation With and Without Midazolam for Dental Implant Surgery. Anesth Prog, 2012, 59, 62–68.

Wilson, W; Taubert, KA; Gewitz, M; Lockhart, PB; Baddour, LM; Levison, M; Bolger, A; Cabell, CH; Takahashi, M; Baltimore, RS; Newburger, JW; Strom, BL; Tani, LY; Gerber, M; Bonow, RO; Pallasch, T; Shulman, ST; Rowley, AH; Burns, JC; Ferrieri, P; Gardner, T; Goff, D; Durack, DT. Prevention of infective endocarditis: Guidelines from the American Heart Association - A guideline from the American Heart Association Rheumatic Fever, Endocarditis and Kawasaki Disease Committee, Council on Cardiovascular Disease in the Young, and the Council on Clinical Cardiology, Council on Cardiovascular Surgery and Anesthesia, and the Quality of Care and Outcomes Research Interdisciplinary Working Group. J Am Dent Assoc, 2008, 139, 3S–24S.

CHAPTER 14

IMPLANT FAILURE, COMPLICATIONS, AND ADVERSE EFFECTS

Abstract

Implant failure can be considered the status of an implant performance that falls below an acceptable level. The distinction between a failed implant and a failing implant is clinically important because the failure process might be slow, even if continual. In general, there are three major etiologic factors behind implant failure: bacterial infection, impaired healing, and overload. *Complications* are all the locally appearing conditions that appear postoperatively; thus, complications may or may not lead to implant failure. Complications should be distinguished from surgical accidents. Complications may be divided into two subclasses: early stage and late stage. Although various mechanisms are expectable, not all the mechanisms responsible for the appearance of complications are known, and the causative mechanisms often remain obscure. The most common causes are poor surgical technique (and/or an excessively traumatic surgical approach), bacterial contamination of the host site, decreased bone density, the presence of a bone dehiscence, a thin alveolar crest, wound dehiscence during healing, postoperative infection, excessive loading, the fabrication of an inadequate denture, and bad oral hygiene. *Adverse effects* are considered conditions of general health significance appearing in relation to the oral implant treatment. The appearance of adverse effects in relation to oral implants is rare. Despite the high success rate of oral implants, implant failures, complications, or adverse effects may occur. It should be emphasized that not only early diagnosis and adequate treatment, but also prevention seem to be crucial for all three conditions. In this respect, proper oral hygiene, the prevention of bacterial infection during and following surgery, the prevention of overload of the implant system, the avoidance of poor and/or excessively traumatic surgical techniques (including avoidance of overheating of the bone), and the fabrication of a proper denture seem to be the most important.

14.1. Introduction

Implant failure can be considered the status of an implant performance that falls below an acceptable level (Sakka and Coulthard 2011). Despite the high success rate of oral implants, implant failures may occur (Schwartz-Arad et al. 2008; Sakka and Coulthard 2011). The distinction between a failed implant and a failing implant is clinically important because the failure process might be slow, even if continual (Isidor 1998; Sakka and Coulthard 2011). In general, there are three major etiologic factors behind an implant failure: bacterial infection, impaired healing, and overload (Esposito et al. 1999; Sakka and Coulthard 2011).

Complications are all the locally appearing conditions that appear postoperatively (Annibali et al. 2008); thus, complications may or may not lead to implant failure. Complications should be distinguished from surgical accidents (Annibali et al. 2008). Complications may be divided into two subclasses: early stage and late stage (Annibali et al. 2008). Although various mechanisms are expectable, not all the mechanisms responsible for these complications are known, and the causative mechanisms often remain obscure. The most common causes are poor surgical technique (and/or an excessively traumatic surgical approach), bacterial contamination of the host site, decreased bone density, the presence of a bone dehiscence, a thin alveolar crest, wound dehiscence during healing, postoperative infection, excessive loading, the fabrication of an inadequate denture, and bad oral hygiene (Annibali et al. 2008; Lamas-Pelayo et al. 2008; Real-Osuna et al. 2012). Adverse effects are considered conditions of general health significance appearing in relation to oral implant treatment. The appearance of adverse effects in relation to oral implants is rare.

14.2. Implant Failure

14.2.1. General Considerations

Implant failure can be considered the status of an implant performance that falls below an acceptable level (Sakka and Coulthard 2011) (thus failed implants should certainly be removed). Despite the high success rate of oral implants, implant failures may occur (Schwartz-Arad et al. 2008; Sakka and Coulthard 2011). An implant failure encompasses clinical situations ranging from all symptomatic mobile implants to implants that show more than 0.2 mm of peri-implant bone loss after the first year of loading (Albrektsson et al. 1986; Sakka and Coulthard 2011) or show peri-implant bleeding and a probing depth exceeding 5 mm (Mombelli and Lang 2000; Sakka and Coulthard 2011). The distinction between a failed implant and a failing implant is clinically important because the failure process might be slow, even if continual (Isidor 1998; Sakka and Coulthard 2011). For example, a mobile implant, together with peri-fixtural radiolucency (referring to the lack of osseointegration), can be considered a “failed” implant (Esposito et al. 1998; Sakka and Coulthard 2011), while an implant with progressive marginal bone loss without marked mobility can be considered a “failing” implant (Esposito et al. 1998; Sakka and Coulthard 2011). In general, there are three major etiologic factors behind implant failure: bacterial infection, impaired healing, and overload (Esposito et al. 1999; Sakka and Coulthard 2011).

14.2.2. Clinical Signs of Failure

Major clinical manifestations of peri-implant disease include general signs of inflammation like gingival bleeding, pus secretion, swelling, and bone loss (Schmidlin et al.

2012), but pain, fistulas, soft tissue hyperplasias, color changes of the marginal peri-implant tissues, and early/late mucosal dehiscences may also appear (Sakka and Coulthard 2011). Although all of these symptoms may point to implant failure, early mucosal (wound) dehiscences can also be present in relation to retained sutures, an inadequate flap design, or premature wearing of a denture (Sakka and Coulthard 2011). Peri-implant disease may appear at any time after implant placement. In general, an early appearance may be more serious than if the same complications occur later because of the disturbance of the bone healing and osseointegration process (Sakka and Coulthard 2011).

Another important clinical sign of implant failure is the clinically marked mobility of the fixture. The mobility of the fixture may be horizontal, vertical, or rotational and is the key sign of a failed implant (Sakka and Coulthard 2011). Although clinically noticeable mobility can occasionally be present without distinct radiographic signs of bone changes (Grondahl and Lekholm 1997; Sakka and Coulthard 2011), in most cases, peri-fixture radiolucency, suggesting the absence of direct bone-implant contact, also appears (Grondahl and Lekholm 1997; Sakka and Coulthard 2011). Mobility may also appear in the case of a fracture of the fixture (or other parts of the implant system, including the denture). In this case, a fracture line and radiolucency around the coronal part of the fractured fixture may appear on the radiograph, whereas the apical part of the fractured fixture usually remains osseointegrated (Gargallo-Albiol et al. 2008).

Importantly, clinical signs of inflammation in the absence of mobility and peri-implant radiolucency may point more to a failing implant than a failed one (Sakka and Coulthard 2011). Thus, a failing implant with peri-implantitis and signs of peri-implant inflammation and increased marginal bone loss may still be stable clinically. Therefore, signs of inflammation in relation to peri-implant disease cannot be used alone to determine the fate of an implant (Sakka and Coulthard 2011; Schmidlin et al. 2012) but should be evaluated in relation to other parameters such as mobility and radiographic changes (Sakka and Coulthard 2011; Schmidlin et al. 2012).

14.2.3. Peri-Implantitis and Other Infections

Peri-implant disease can be classified into two major groups: peri-implant mucositis and peri-implantitis (Lindhe et al. 2008). Both are of infectious origin caused by the development of a bacterial biofilm (Mombelli et al. 1987; Leonhardt et al. 1999; Lindhe et al. 2008; Unursaikhan et al. 2012) with a spectrum of pathogens similar to that of periodontal inflammation (Mombelli et al. 1987; Schmidlin et al. 2012; Sakka and Coulthard 2011). Peri-implant mucositis may be reversible and cured/managed by nonsurgical therapy (Lang at al. 2011; Sakka and Coulthard 2011), whereas the management of peri-implantitis is rather problematic, and roughly every fourth implant with peri-implantitis may be lost despite repeated treatment (Leonhardt et al. 2003). For both the prevention and treatment of peri-implantitis, the principal objective is the complete removal of the bacterial biofilm, including calcified plaque, from implant surfaces (Unursaikhan et al. 2012).

Similar to peri-implant disease, most soft tissue complications other than peri-implant mucositis (hyperplastic mucositis, fistulations, and mucosal abscess) also seem mainly to have an infectious etiology (Sanchez-Garces and Gay-Escoda 2004; Sakka and Coulthard 2011). Fistulations and hyperplastic mucositis are often found in relation to loose prosthetic components (Zarb and Schmitt 1990; Sakka and Coulthard 2011), whereas abscesses can occasionally be seen in relation to food particles trapped in the peri-implant crevice (Ibbott et al. 1993; Sakka and Coulthard 2011).

In rare cases, a unique *periapical form* of peri-implantitis (also referred to as "retrograde peri-implantitis" or an "implant periapical lesion") may also appear (Silva et al. 2010). This involves the periapical area of the fixture where there is normal bone around the coronal portion of the fixture (Silva et al. 2010). This kind of implant failure is normally accompanied by pain, swelling, tenderness, and fistulation, and its progression may lead to a failed implant (Silva et al. 2010). This unique lesion is also of bacterial origin in most cases, although, in certain cases, overheating during surgery, excessive implant tightening, and implant overload may also play a role in its etiology (Silva et al. 2010).

14.2.4. Impaired Osseointegration

There are various factors that may lead to impaired healing (osseointegration) and consequent implant failure (Annibali et al. 2008; Sakka and Coulthard 2011). Poor surgical technique and lack of irrigation leading to overheating (Annibali et al. 2008; Sakka and Coulthard 2011), as well as an excessively traumatic surgical approach (Annibali et al. 2008), may be considered the most important reasons. Micromotions during the healing phase (i.e. in the case of one-stage surgery and immediate load) surely play a significant role as well (Annibali et al. 2008; Sakka and Coulthard 2011). Several local factors like compromised bone quality and a bacterially infected implant site (i.e. because of pre-existing periodontal and/or periapical pathologies in the case of immediate implant placement) should also be considered as major reasons for impaired healing (Sakka and Coulthard 2011; Todescan et al. 2012). Certain systemic characteristics of the patient, for example diabetes mellitus if the patient has poor metabolic control (Elsubeihi and Zarb 2002; Todescan et al. 2012), may also play a major role in an implant failure with regard to impaired healing (Sakka and Coulthard 2011). Although each of the above factors may lead to impaired healing and consequent implant failure by itself, the risk of implant failure may be especially high if more than one of these factors appear at the same time.

14.2.5. Overload of the Bone

Implant failures related to the mechanical overload of the bone include those situations in which the functional load applied to the implants exceeds the capacity of the fixture attached to the bone to withstand it (Sakka and Coulthard 2011). Overload because of the strength and/or direction of masticatory forces (including cases of poor denture design) may be considered a major reason for this kind of implant failure (Sakka and Coulthard 2011). Besides these possibilities, a *very high* ratio of the length of the *osseointegrated* part of the fixture and the height of all other parts (*not*-osseointegrated part of fixture + abutment + denture) of the implant system, referred to as the "crown-to-implant" ratio (Lee et al. 2012), may also lead to the overload of the bone, even if recent data indicate that implants with a *moderately* higher crown-to-implant ratio show *less* peri-implant marginal bone loss than implants with a low ($x \leq 1$) C/I ratio (Lee et al. 2012).

14.2.6. Overload of the Implant System (Fracture)

Mechanical overload of an implant system may lead to implant failure if a fracture of the implant fixture occurs (Rangert et al. 1995; Balshi 1996; Gargallo-Albiol et al. 2008). In this case, metal fatigue appears, which leads to a fracture, most typically in the third or fourth year of loading (Gargallo-Albiol et al. 2008). Major causes of mechanical overload include inadequate size (especially a diameter below 3.75 mm) of the implant, anatomical determinations (i.e. strong masticatory muscles, molar region), bruxism or other parafunctional activity, inadequate prosthesis (i.e. inadequate occlusion, cantilever structures, high span bridges), and excessive peri-implant vertical bone loss (Rangert et al. 1995; Balshi 1996; Gargallo-Albiol et al. 2008). Fluoride corrosion of titanium implants may also play a role (Roselino Riberio et al. 2007).

In a fracture of the fixture, the apical part of the fixture at issue usually remains osseointegrated (Gargallo-Albiol et al. 2008). This apical part may be utilized for prosthetic purposes following certain corrections if the fracture line appears coronal near the fixture-abutment interface. If the fracture line appears more apically, the fractured fixture may either be removed by means of explantation trephine or the remnant apical fragment can be left integrated in the bone (Petropoulos et al. 2004; Gargallo-Albiol et al. 2008). Not only fixtures, but also other parts of the implant system, like the abutment and the denture, may also be fractured; however, these cases are not considered as an implant failure but rather as a "simple" complication.

14.3. Complications

14.3.1. General Considerations

Complications are all the locally appearing conditions that appear postoperatively (Annibali et al. 2008); thus, complications may or may not lead to implant failure. Complications should be distinguished from surgical accidents (Annibali et al. 2008) (which are *not* discussed in this chapter) and also from adverse effects that are considered conditions of general health significance appearing in relation to the oral implant treatment. Complications may be divided into two subclasses: early stage and late stage (Annibali et al. 2008).

Although various mechanisms are expectable, not all the mechanisms responsible for the appearance of complications are known, and the causative mechanisms often remain obscure. The most common causes are poor surgical technique (and/or an excessively traumatic surgical approach), bacterial contamination of the host site, decreased bone density, the presence of a bone dehiscence, a thin alveolar crest, wound dehiscence during healing, postoperative infection, excessive loading, the fabrication of an inadequate denture, and bad oral hygiene (Annibali et al. 2008; Lamas-Pelayo et al. 2008; Real-Osuna et al. 2012). Some of the most important complications were already introduced above in relation to implant failure, while others will be introduced below.

14.3.2. Early-Stage Complications

Early-stage complications may include infection, edema, hematomas, bleeding, flap dehiscence, and temporary or permanent sensory disorders (Abarca et al. 2006; Annibali et al. 2008; Lamas-Pelayo et al. 2008). In very rare cases, emphysema may also appear, resulting from a sudden rise of intraoral pressure (i.e. the patient sneezes) if air is forced (through the mucoperiosteal tissue of an imperfectly approximated flap) in between the tissues (Lauc and Kobler 1998; Annibali et al. 2008). With the exception of sensory disorders, early-stage complications are usually easy to handle based on general surgical after-care principles.

In the case of sensory disorders, a radiographic investigation should be performed first to identify any pathological changes (e.g. penetration of an implant into the mandibular canal) that may be associated with the injury (Annibali et al. 2008; Fukuda et al. 2012). If such changes are not radiographically visible, and the symptoms of the patient are mild, a "wait-and-see attitude" and administration of NSAIDs, antibiotics, and vitamins (B, C, D, E) are advisable (Annibali et al. 2008; Fabian and Fejerdy 2010; Beck et al. 2012), followed by administration of physical therapy like PEMF, transcutaneous electric nerve stimulation (TENS) or low-level laser therapy (Annibali et al. 2008; Fabian and Fejerdy 2010; Beck et al. 2012). In contrast, if nerve injury is observed radiologically (or intraoperatively) and/or the symptoms are serious and/or persist or worsen, the patient should be referred (as soon as possible, but *at the latest* within a month after exposure) to an expert team familiar with the treatment of such conditions (Fabian and Fejerdy 2010; Fukuda et al. 2012). Treatment may be medicamentous or surgical depending on the extent of the pathological alterations and the neurological symptoms reported by the patient (Annibali et al. 2008; Fabian and Fejerdy 2010; Beck et al. 2012; Fukuda et al. 2012).

14.3.3. Late-Stage Complications

The most important late-stage complications are exposure of the cover screw because of perforation of the mucoperiosteum, maxillary sinusitis, the appearance of peri-implant bony defects, and very rarely, a mandibular fracture (Annibali et al. 2008; Lamas-Pelayo et al. 2008; Hong et al. 2010; Lee and Lee 2010; Raffoul and Kofod 2013).

Spontaneous exposure of the cover screw is a frequent complication (Annibali et al. 2008), which may occur because of extremely thin tissue surrounding the implant, acute mechanical trauma, pressure from an inadequate removable denture, or loosening of the cover screw (Annibali et al. 2008). This condition usually does not require treatment, but to facilitate oral hygiene, the area of exposure may be extended and the cover screw replaced with a healing abutment (Annibali et al. 2008).

Sinusitis is a complication resulting from bacterial contamination of the maxillary sinus during surgery performed under non-aseptic conditions (Annibali et al. 2008; Hong et al. 2010; Lee and Lee 2010). Bacterial contamination may also occur during healing because of wound dehiscence or because of implant displacement into the sinus causing a foreign body reaction and chronic infection (Annibali et al. 2008; Hong et al. 2010; Lee and Lee 2010). Sinusitis may present either in acute form or in chronic form from its offset (Annibali et al. 2008; Hong et al. 2010; Lee and Lee 2010). Treatment may be medicamentous and/or surgical depending on the clinical situation (Annibali et al. 2008; Hong et al. 2010; Lee and

Lee 2010). If surgical treatment is needed, the patient should be referred to an oral/maxillofacial surgeon familiar with surgical interventions of the maxillary sinus.

A horizontal or vertical bony defect around the implant is a complication that may be observed by assessing the bone-implant interface at the time of second-phase surgery (Annibali et al. 2008). There may be various causes for such defects; however, the causative mechanism often remains obscure (Annibali et al. 2008). The treatment of these conditions is similar to the treatment of other bony defects, which is discussed in detail elsewhere.

A mandibular fracture is a rare complication. There are only a few cases reported in the literature, and most of them are in relation with severely resorbed jaws (Annibali et al. 2008; Lamas-Pelayo et al. 2008; Raffoul and Kofod 2013). In the case of a fracture, the patient should be referred to an oral/maxillofacial surgeon familiar with the treatment of jaw fractures.

14.4. Adverse Effects

Adverse effects are considered conditions of general health significance appearing in relation to oral implant treatment. The appearance of adverse effects in relation to oral implants is rare. Allergic reactions do not seem to play any significant role concerning the dental applications of titanium alloys (Neumann and Kevenhoerster 2009). Sensitization through titanium is rare. Although a few individual cases have been described for orthopedic or cardiologic (pacemaker implant) applications, no type IV allergic reactions have been described for oral applications of titanium alloys to date (Neumann and Kevenhoerster 2009).

Similarly, overall both titanium oxide and pure titanium (both ionic or particle) show very low toxicity (Neumann and Kevenhoerster 2009), even if, in rare cases, both titanium oxide and titanium itself may cause certain toxic effects and disorders like yellow nail syndrome (Berglund and Carlmark 2011). Somewhat higher toxicity potential may also arise from titanium alloy additives like aluminum and vanadium, as well as from several titanium corrosion products (Letic-Gavrilovic et al. 2000; Neumann and Kevenhoerster 2009; Tomsia et al. 2011); however, it should be emphasized that there is currently no indication of clinically relevant systemic toxicity caused by oral titanium alloy implants (Neumann and Kevenhoerster 2009).

Rare cases of certain other disorders like orbital cellulitis (Wilk et al. 2012), exfoliative cheilitis (Pigatto et al. 2011), and benign paroxysmal positional vertigo (BPPV) (Rodriguez-Gutierrez and Rodriguez-Gomez 2007; Chiarella et al. 2007) were also reported in relation to dental implants; however, pathogenically, these cases remain speculations. There are also a few reports of individual cases of malignant tumors in the tissue surrounding titanium alloys (Friedman and Vernon 1983; Eguia del Valle et al. 2008), but pathogenically these cases also remain speculations (Neumann and Kevenhoerster 2009). Given the great number of titanium alloy dental implants used throughout the world, tumorigenicity is practically ruled out (Neumann and Kevenhoerster 2009).

Conclusion

Despite a high success rate of oral implants, implant failures (Sakka and Coulthard 2011), other complications (Annibali et al. 2008; Lamas-Pelayo et al. 2008; Real-Osuna et al. 2012), or adverse effects (Letic-Gavrilovic et al. 2000; Neumann and Kevenhoerster 2009; Tomsia et al. 2011) may occur. It should be emphasized that not only early diagnosis and adequate treatment, but also prevention, seem to be crucial for all three conditions (Annibali et al. 2008; Lamas-Pelayo et al. 2008; Sakka and Coulthard 2011; Real-Osuna et al. 2012). In this respect, proper oral hygiene, prevention of bacterial infection during and following surgery, prevention of overload of the implant system, avoidance of poor and/or excessively traumatic surgical techniques (including avoidance of overheating of the bone), and fabrication of proper dentures seem to be the most important preventative actions to take (Annibali et al. 2008; Lamas-Pelayo et al. 2008; Sakka and Coulthard 2011; Real-Osuna et al. 2012).

References

Abarca, M; van Steenberghe, D; Malevez, C; De Ridder, J; Jacobs, R. Neurosensory disturbances after immediate loading of implants in the anterior mandible: an initial questionnaire approach followed by a psychophysiological assessment. *Clin Oral Invest*, 2006, 10, 269–277.

Albrektsson, T; Zarb, G; Worthington, P; Ericsson, AR. The long-term efficacy of currently used dental implants: a review and proposed criteria of success. *Int J Oral Maxillofac Implants*, 1986, 1, 11–25.

Annibali, S; Ripari, M; La Monaca, G; Tonoli, F; Cristalli, MP. Local complications in dental implant surgery: Prevention and treatment. *ORAL & Implantology*, 2008, 1, 21–33.

Balshi TJ. An analysis and management of fractured implants: a clinical report. *Int J Oral Maxillofac Implants*, 1996, 11, 660–666.

Beck, A; Varga, G; Hermann, P; Fabian, G; Fejerdy, P; Fabian, TK. Methods for the treatment of denture induced psychogenic symptoms. In: Fabian TK, Fejerdy P, Hermann P, editors. *Dentures. Types, benefits and potential complications.* New York: Nova Science Publishers, 2012, 165–197.

Berglund, F; Carlmark, B. Titanium, sinusitis and the yellow nail syndrome. *Biol Trace Elem Res*, 2011, 143, 1–7.

Chiarella, G; Leopardi, G; De Fazio, L; Chiarella, R; Cassandro, C; Cassandro, E. Iatrogenic benign paroxysmal positional vertigo: review and personal experience in dental and maxillo-facial surgery. *Acta Otorhinolaryngol Ital*, 2007, 27, 126–128.

Eguia del Valle, A; Martinez-Conde Llamosas, R; Lopez Vicente, J; Uribarri Etxebarria, A; Aguirre Urizar, JM. Primary oral squamous cell carcinoma arising around dental osseointegrated implants mimicking peri-implantitis. *Med Oral Patol Oral Cir Bucal*, 2008, 13, E489–E491.

Elsubeihi, ES; Zarb, GA. Implant prosthodontics in medically challenged patients: The University of Toronto experience. *J Can Dent Assoc*, 2002, 68, 103–108.

Esposito, M; Hirsch, JM; Lekholm, U; Thomsen, P. Biological factors contributing to the failures of osseointegrated oral implants (I). Success criteria and epidemiology. *Eur J Oral Sci*, 1998, 106, 527–551.

Esposito, M; Hirsch, J; Lekholm, U; Thomsen P. Differential diagnosis and treatment strategies for biologic complications and failing oral implants: a review of the literature. *Int J Oral Maxillofac Implants*, 1999, 14, 473–90.

Fabian, TK; Fejerdy P. *Psychogenic denture intolerance. Theoretical background, prevention and treatment possibilities*. New York: Nova Science Publishers; 2010.

Friedman, KE; Vernon, SE. Squamous cell carcinoma developing in conjunction with a mandibular staple bone plate. *J Oral Maxillofac Surg*, 1983, 41, 265–266.

Fukuda, KI; Ichinohe, T; Kaneko, Y. Pain management for nerve injury following dental implant surgery at Tokyo Dental College Hospital. *Int J Dentistry*, 2012, Article ID: 209474. DOI: 10.1155/2012/209474.

Gargallo-Albiol, J; Satorres-Nieto, M; Puyuelo-Capablo, JL; Sanchez-Garces, MA, Pi-Urgell, J; Gay-Escoda, C. Endosseous dental implant fractures an analysis of 21 cases. *Med Oral Patol Oral Cir Bucal*, 2008, 13, E124–E128.

Grondahl, K; Lekholm, U. The predictive value of radiographic diagnosis of implant instability. *Int J Oral Maxillofac Implants*, 1997, 12, 59–64.

Hong, SB; Kim, JS; Shin, SI; Han, JY; Herr, Y; Chung, JH. Clinical treatment of postoperative infection following sinus augmentation. *J Periodontal Implant Sci*, 2010, 40, 144–149.

Ibbott, CG; Kovach, RJ; Carlson-Mann, LD. Acute periodontal abscess associated with an immediate implant site in the maintenance phase: a case report. *Int J Oral Maxillofac Implants*, 1993, 8, 699–702.

Isidor, F. Mobility assessment with the Periotest system in relation to histologic findings of oral implants. *Int J Oral Maxillofac Implants* 1998, 13, 377–383.

Lamas-Pelayo, J; Penarrocha-Diago, M; Marti-Bowen, E; Penarrocha-Diago, M. Intraoperative complications during oral implantology. *Med Oral Patol Oral Cir Bucal*, 2008, 13, E239–E243.

Lang, NP; Berglundh, T. Group 4 of the Seventh European Workshop on Periodontology. Periimplant diseases: where are we now? Consensus of the Seventh European Workshop on Periodontology. *J Clin Periodontol*, 2011, 38, (Suppl. 11) 178–181.

Lauc, T; Kobler, P. Early post-operative complications in oral implantology. *Coll Antropol*, 1998, 22, 251–257.

Lee, KC; Lee, SJ. Clinical features and treatments of odontogenic sinusitis. *Yonsei Med J*, 2010, 51, 932–937.

Lee, KJ; Kim, YG; Park, JW; Lee, JM; Suh, JY. Influence of crown-to-implant ratio on periimplant marginal bone loss in the posterior region: a five-year retrospective study. *J Periodontal Implant Sci*, 2012, 42, 231–236.

Leonhardt, A; Renvert, S; Dahlen, G. Microbial findings at failing implants. *Clin Oral Implants Res*, 1999, 10, 339–345.

Leonhardt, A; Dahlen, G; Renvert, S. Five-year clinical, microbiological, and radiological outcome following treatment of peri-implantitis in man. *J Periodontol*, 2003, 74, 1415–22.

Letic-Gavrilovic, A; Scandurra, R; Abe, K. Genetic potential of interfacial guided osteogenesis in implant devices. *Dental Materials J*, 2000, 19, 99–132.

Lindhe, J; Meyle, J; Group D of the Sixth European Workshop on Periodontology. Peri-implant diseases: Consensus report of the Sixth European Workshop on Periodontology. *J Clin Periodontol*, 2008, 35 (Suppl. 8), 282–5.

Mombelli, A; van Oosten, MA; Schurch Jr., E; Land, NP. The microbiota associated with successful or failing osseointegrated titanium implants. *Oral Microbiol Immunol*, 1987, 2, 145–151.

Mombelli, A; Lang, NP. Clinical parameters for the evaluation of dental implants. *Periodontol*, 2000, 1994, 81–86.

Neumann, A; Kevenhoerster, K. Biomaterials for craniofacial reconstruction. *GMS Curr Top Otorhinolaryngol Head Neck Surg*, 2009, 8, Doc08. DOI: 10.3205/ cto000060.

Petropoulos, VC; Wolfinger, GJ; Balshi, TJ. Complications of mandibular molar replacement with a single implant: A case report. *J Can Dent Assoc*, 2004, 70, 238-242.

Pigatto, PD; Berti, E; Spadari, F; Bombeccari, GP; Guzzi, G. Exfoliative cheilitis associated with titanium dental implants and mercury amalgam. *J Dermatol Case Rep*, 2011, 5, 89–90.

Raffoul, L; Kofod, T. Fracture of the atrophic mandible associated with implant treatment. *Danish Dent J*, 2013, 117, 396–399.

Rangert, B; Krogh, PH; Langer, B; Van Roekel, N. Bending overload and implant fracture: a retrospective clinical analysis. *Int J Oral Maxillofac Implants*, 1995, 10, 326–34.

Real-Osuna, J; Almendros-Marques, N; Gay-Escoda, C. Prevalence of complications after the oral rehabilitation with implant-supported hybrid prostheses. *Med Oral Patol Oral Cir Bucal*, 2012, 17, e116–e121.

Rodriguez-Gutierrez, C; Rodriguez-Gomez, E. Positional vertigo afterwards maxillary dental implant surgery with bone regeneration. *Med Oral Patol Oral Cir Bucal*, 2007, 12, E151–153.

Roselino Riberio, AL; Noreiga, JR; Dametto, FR; Vaz, LG. Compressive fatigue in titanium dental implants submitted to fluoride ions action. *J Appl Oral Sci*, 2007, 15, 299–304.

Sakka, S; Coulthard, P. Implant failure: Etiology and complications. *Med Oral Patol Oral Cir Bucal*, 2011, 16, e42–e44.

Sanchez-Garces, MA; Gay-Escoda, C. Periimplantitis. *Med Oral Patol Oral Cir Bucal*, 2004, 9, (Suppl.) 63–74.

Schmidlin, PR; Sahrmann, P; Ramel, C; Imfeld, T; Müller, J; Roos, M; Jung, RE. Peri-implantitis prevalence and treatment in implant-oriented private practices: A cross-sectional postal and internet survey. *Schweiz Monatsschr Zahnmed*, 2012, 122, 1136–1144.

Schwartz-Arad, D; Laviv, A; Levin, L. Failure causes, timing and cluster behavior: an 8-year study of dental implants. *Implant Dent*, 2008, 17, 200–207.

Silva, GC; Oliveira, DRF; Vieira, TC; Magalhaes, CS; Moreira, AN. Unusual presentation of active implant periapical lesions: a report of two cases. *J Oral Sci*, 2010, 52, 491–494.

Todescan, S; Lavigne, S; Kelekis-Cholakis, A. Guidance for the maintenance care of dental implants: Clinical review. *J Can Dent Assoc*, 2012, 78, c107.

Tomsia, AP; Launey, ME; Lee, JS; Mankani, MH; Wegst, UGK; Saiz, E. Nanotechnology approaches to improve dental implants. *Int J Maxillofac Implants*, 2011, 26(Suppl), 25–49.

Unursaikhan, O; Lee, JS; Cha, JK; Park, JC; Jung, UW; Kim, CS; Cho, KS; Choi, SH. Comparative evaluation of roughness of titanium surfaces treated by different hygiene instruments. *J Periodont Implant Sci*, 2012, 42, 88–94.

Wilk, G; Modrzejewska, M; Lachowicz, E; Lisiecka-Opalko, K; Mysliwiec, L; Rutkowski, D. Kotrych, K; Burzynska, K; Golubinska, E. From ophthalmologist to dentist via radiology. *Pol J Radiol*, 2012, 77, 21–27.

Zarb, GA; Schmitt, A. The longitudinal clinical effectiveness of osseointegrated dental implants: the Toronto study. Part III: Problems and complications encountered. *J Prosthet Dent*, 1990, 64, 185–94.

CHAPTER 15

GENERAL HEALTH CONSIDERATIONS

Abstract

There are only a few conditions that can be considered absolute contraindications with respect to dental implant rehabilitation, such as disease processes like recent myocardial infarction, recent cerebrovascular stroke, recent heart surgery, immune suppression, blood dyscrasias, *active* neoplastic disease undergoing treatment, drug abuse, certain psychiatric disorders, and more recently, *intravenous* bisphosphonate treatment. Accordingly, data suggest that patients with osteoporosis, cardiovascular diseases, and hypothyroidism are not at greater risk of implant failure. On the other hand, there are certain conditions that may negatively influence or jeopardize the implant treatment outcome. The most important such conditions, like the age of the patient, smoking habits, poorly controlled diabetes mellitus, *orally* administered bisphosphonate treatment, and certain conditions in relation to tumor disorders, will be discussed in this chapter.

15.1. Introduction

There are only a few conditions that can be considered absolute contraindications with respect to dental implant rehabilitation, such as disease processes like recent myocardial infarction, recent cerebrovascular stroke, recent heart surgery, immune suppression, blood dyscrasias, *active* neoplastic disease undergoing treatment, drug abuse, certain psychiatric disorders, and more recently, intravenous bisphosphonate treatment (Hwang and Wang 2006; Minguez-Serra et al. 2008; Schropp and Storsken 2013). Accordingly, data suggest that patients with osteoporosis, cardiovascular diseases, and hypothyroidism are not at greater risk of implant failure (Elsubeihi and Zarb 2002; Mellado-Valero et al. 2010). On the other hand, there are certain conditions that may negatively influence or jeopardize the implant treatment outcome (Stanford 2007). The most important of these conditions will be discussed in greater detail below in this chapter.

15.2. Age of the Patient

Osseointegrated dental implants were designed for the mature jaws of adults (Branemark 1977); however, they may also be needed for the treatment of children and adolescents (Thilander et al. 2001) because of various conditions such as congenital absence (aplasia, hypodontia) of teeth (Thilander et al. 2001; Richardson and Russell 2001; Nishimura et al. 2006), trauma (Thilander et al. 2001), ectodermal dysplasia (Bergendal et al. 1991; Oesterle et al. 1993; Bergendal et al. 1996; Gjorup et al. 2013), and several hereditary disorders like dentinogenesis imperfecta (DGI), dentine dysplasia (DD) (Barron et al. 2008; Depprich et al. 2007; Gjorup et al. 2013), or others.

Experimental and clinical studies have indicated that osseointegrated dental implants do not behave like normally erupting teeth during the dento-alveolar development and growth of the jaws; and this difference between natural teeth and implants frequently results in the infraocclusion of the osseointegrated implants (Odman et al. 1991; Thilander et al. 1992; Thilander et al. 1994; Thilander et al. 2001). Further, disturbances of the natural developmental processes may also occur due to the insertion of osseointegrated implants and complications like the appearance of tooth-implant contact because of tooth-implant collision caused by the eruptive (or other) movement of the teeth (Thilander et al. 2001). Although in rare cases of total aplasia (as in ectodermal dysplasia), treatment with implants could be advocated in childhood (Bergendal et al. 1991; Oesterle et al. 1993; Bergendal et al. 1996; Gjorup et al. 2013); a general conclusion from the above considerations may be that dental implants should not be inserted into young individuals until permanent dentition is fully erupted and skeletal growth is completed or almost completed (Thilander et al. 1994; Bergendal et al. 1996; Richardson and Russell 2001). Though 18 years of age may be considered as a guide for implant placement in this respect (Barron et al. 2008), it should be emphasized that a fixed chronological age is not the best guide because there is a great deal of individual variation (Thilander et al. 2001; Richardson and Russell 2001) ranging between 15 and 21 years of age (Richardson and Russell 2001).

However, it should also be emphasized that a stage of fully erupted permanent teeth and skeletal maturation (completed or almost completed) is not sufficient to avoid *all kinds of* infraocclusion (Thilander et al. 2001; Schropp and Storsken 2013) because there is a "continuous tendency of infraocclusion" with osseointegrated implants due to the slight continuous eruption of the adjacent teeth occurring in post-adolescence (Thilander et al. 2001; Schropp and Storsken 2013). Further, several studies have also demonstrated that significant changes in craniofacial dimensions occur even during adulthood (Sarnas and Solow 1980; Bjork and Skiller 1983; Behrents 1985; Thilander et al. 2001), including changes of the dento-alveolar height, indicating eruptive movement of the natural teeth in adults as well (Forsberg et al. 1991; Tallgren and Solow 1991; Thilander et al. 2001). Thus, a slight continuous eruption of teeth can be observed even after established occlusion in post-adolescence (Ainamo and Talari 1976; Iseri and Solow 1996; Thilander et al. 1999; Thilander et al. 2001); and there are physiological occlusal changes not only from adolescence into young adulthood, but also into old age (Thilander et al. 2001).

It should also be emphasized with respect to the age of the patient that despite age-related tendencies toward systemic illness among older adults, there are no general limitations in relation to implant placement in older adults or the elderly (Bryant and Zarb 2002; Elsubeihi and Zarb 2002). In general, it can be considered that the outcomes of oral implant therapy are comparable among older and younger adults (Bryant and Zarb 2002; Elsubeihi and Zarb 2002), and old age itself will not influence the outcome of oral implant therapy involving either partial or complete prostheses (Bryant and Zarb 2002). The insertion of oral implants (followed by established prosthodontic protocols) will meet routinely with predictable outcomes if the patient is able to undergo minor oral surgery (Bryant and Zarb 2002), and the osseointegrated oral implants can be maintained with either fixed or removable prostheses regardless of age (Bryant and Zarb 2002). On the other hand, it should also be noted that the frequency of occurrence of those compromised general health conditions that may jeopardize a treatment outcome can be higher in the elderly (Stanford 2007). But in these cases, the disorder/condition itself, not the greater age of the patient, is the limiting factor.

15.3. Smoking

Smoking addiction is directly related to dental implant failure, and there is a general consensus regarding the negative effect of smoking on long-term implant survival (Sham et al. 2003). It is very likely that smokers have a somewhat higher rate of early implant failure and a significantly higher prevalence of late implant failure than nonsmokers (Elsubeihi and Zarb 2002; Stanford 2007), in part (but not exclusively) because patients who smoke are also considered at high risk of peri-implantitis (Elsubeihi and Zarb 2002; Todescan et al. 2012; Sham et al. 2003). The exact mechanism by which smoking exerts its negative effect on the healing and maintenance of peri-implant tissues is not yet fully understood (Elsubeihi and Zarb 2002). However, it may be considered that cigarette smoking impairs peri-implant healing and osseointegration by affecting the circulatory and immune systems and by impairing normal cellular function (Elsubeihi and Zarb 2002). Furthermore, it appears that cigarette smoking during adulthood is associated with decreased bone density later in life (Elsubeihi and Zarb 2002).

Smoking cessation protocols offered and initiated by dental professionals (Bain 1996; Sandhu 2001) show considerable promise in improving the success rate of osseointegration in smokers (Sham et al. 2003) There are significant differences between failure rates between non-smokers and smokers and between smokers who have adopted the smoking cessation protocol and those who continue smoking (Bain 1996; Sham et al. 2003).

15.4. Diabetes Mellitus

The placement of dental implants in patients with metabolically controlled diabetes appears to be just as successful as in the general population (Elsubeihi and Zarb 2002; Beikler and Flemming 2003; Todescan et al. 2012; Inbarajan et al. 2012), whereas poorly controlled diabetic patients are more difficult to manage, and a delay in surgery is recommended until better control is achieved (Elsubeihi and Zarb 2002; Beikler and Flemming 2003; Todescan et al. 2012). Therefore, screening for diabetes and ensuring that implant patients are under good metabolic control are recommended to increase the chances of successful treatment (Beikler and Flemming 2003; Mellado-Valero et al. 2007). Patients who do not demonstrate strict metabolic control should be examined for the causative mechanism, and glycemic control should be re-assessed and optimized prior to implant surgery (Beikler and Flemming 2003), in part (but not exclusively) because diabetes mellitus patients, if they have poor metabolic control, are potentially at high risk of peri-implantitis (Elsubeihi and Zarb 2002; Todescan et al. 2012).

Although the importance of metabolic control of diabetic patients is emphasized in the scientific literature in relation to the success of implant therapy (Oates et al. 2009, 2013), it should be noted that there are no clear (evidence-based, unambiguous) clinical data supporting a significantly increased number of implant failures for diabetic patients lacking good glycemic control (Dowell et al. 2007; Oates et al. 2013), even if there are clear alterations (some "delay") of the osseointegration processes under hyperglycemic conditions (Oates et al. 2009). Accordingly, more recent studies seem to support the use of dental implant therapy for patients also in the absence of good glycemic control, with appropriate accommodation for the premised delay in implant osseointegration (Oates et al. 2013), even if this represents a clear shift in attitude toward diabetic patient care when compared to previous protocols (Oates et al. 2013).

15.5. Bisphosphonate Treatment

Bisphosphonates are widely used for the treatment of diseases such as multiple myeloma, bone metastases, and malignant hypercalcemia, as well as for the prevention and treatment of osteoporosis and other skeletal diseases such as Paget's disease (Fleisch 1998; Minguez-Serra et al. 2008; Blazsek et al. 2009; Johansen et al. 2013). Recent data show that the administration of bisphosphonates (in certain concentrations and durations) may induce bone formation around titanium implants due to their osteoclast inhibitory (and possibly also osteoblast stimulating) activity (Aspenberg 2009; Blazsek et al. 2009). On the other hand, if the bone surrounding the implant fixture presents a medium to high concentration of bisphosphonates, turnover and remodeling processes may be hindered or prevented—with the risk of necrosis of the surrounding bone (Minguez-Serra et al. 2008).

Clinical observations have revealed that bisphosphonates may cause bisphosphonate-related osteonecrosis of the jaws (BRONJ) in certain cases (Blazsek et al. 2009; Wood 2010; Minguez-Serra et al. 2008; Shin et al. 2010; Masroori and Schiodt 2013). Therefore, clinicians must be aware of the potential risk of osteonecrosis in patients treated with bisphosphonates via either the oral or intravenous route (Minguez-Serra et al. 2008; Shin et al. 2010; Masroori and Schiodt 2013), and all patients considered for implant surgery should be asked if they have ever received bisphosphonates intravenously (Minguez-Serra et al. 2008; Wood 2010; Schropp and Storsken 2013). Implant placement can be initiated only if the patient does not receive (and has not previously received) these drugs (Wood 2010; Minguez-Serra et al. 2008). In patients treated with intravenous bisphosphonates, it is necessary to avoid any kind of invasive oral procedure unless they are considered absolutely necessary (Minguez-Serra et al. 2008; Wood 2010; Masroori and Schiodt 2013). Thus, a dental implant is absolutely contraindicated for any patient who is receiving (and strongly contraindicated if they have previously received) bisphosphonates intravenously (Minguez-Serra et al. 2008; Wood 2010).

The principal discussion arises when bisphosphonate treatment is administered via the oral route (Minguez-Serra et al. 2008; Masroori and Schiodt 2013). In the case of administration via the oral route, caution is required, and it is advisable to avoid surgical procedures or to indicate them only when truly necessary (Minguez-Serra et al. 2008; Masroori and Schiodt 2013). Special care should be taken if there are other risk factors such as the prolonged use of bisphosphonates, concomitant estrogen or corticoid treatment, and advanced age (Minguez-Serra et al. 2008). If surgical treatment should be done, the patient must be informed of the potential complications (Minguez-Serra et al. 2008). Accordingly, if the patient is programmed to receive bisphosphonate therapy, the dental professional must carry out an accurate oral exploration to ensure that all teeth amenable to extraction are dealt with before the start of bisphosphonate therapy (Minguez-Serra et al. 2008), and the patient should be informed that there may be a higher risk of osteonecrosis around existing oral implants (Shin et al. 2010; Junquera et al. 2011).

Bisphosphonate-induced osteonecrosis of the jaw has been widely reported (Minguez-Serra et al. 2008; Wood 2010), which has resulted in altered dosing regimens, including shorter courses of intravenous bisphosphonates for many disease sites (Wood 2010). The reduced dosing regimens may allow for the placement of dental implants in the future (Wood 2010); however, the risk of postoperative osteonecrosis following the cessation of intravenous therapy with bisphosphonates remains uncertain (Minguez-Serra et al. 2008).

15.6. Tumor Disorders

Patients with tumor disorders can be treated successfully with oral implants, and there is no limitations on implant treatment because of the tumor disorder itself (Wood 2010; Sailer et al. 2010; Infante-Cossio et al. 2011; Korfage et al. 2011; Carini et al. 2012/a, b). However, certain information is needed before a decision is made about an implant, such as (Wood 2010): the type of chemotherapy drugs used, the timing of the implant in relation to the last chemotherapy treatment, and the anticipated interval before the next (if any) chemotherapy treatment (Wood 2010). It should also be kept in mind that chemotherapy combined with radiation treatment may cause necrosis of the jaw bones (Wood 2010; Korfage et al. 2011) and/or other orofacial complications (Korfage et al. 2011; Schropp and Storsken 2013). Irradiation of the orofacial region itself (without being combined with chemotherapy) may also cause serious complications certainly (Schropp and Storsken 2013). It should also be emphasized that surgery is absolutely contraindicated for tumor disorder patients receiving (and strongly contraindicated if they have previously received) bisphosphonates intravenously (Wood 2010).

A large number of chemotherapy agents are currently used. Some of them are relatively innocuous (Wood 2010), while others are highly toxic (Wood 2010; Korfage et al. 2011), and as such, may prevent wounds from healing, may interfere with osseointegration, and may cause a reduction in hemoglobin, platelets, and white blood cells due to their toxic effect on bone marrow (Wood 2010; Johansen et al. 2013). Recovery from chemotherapy may take up to 28 days (or even longer) from the date of the drug delivery; therefore, the patient should wait a minimum of one month (preferably 60 days) after the final chemotherapy treatment before undergoing implant surgery (Wood 2010). Further, any mouth sores (possibly caused by the chemotherapy) should be resolved and blood cell counts should be within normal ranges before implant placement (Wood 2010). If repeated chemotherapy treatments are needed (and the placement of the implant is urgent for whatever reason), it is advisable to have a window of at least 60 days after the completion of the last chemotherapy and a further 60 days (preferably longer) following the placement of the implant.

Conclusion

There are only a few conditions that can be considered absolute contraindications with respect to dental implant rehabilitation, and the number of those conditions that may negatively influence or jeopardize the treatment outcome of dental implant therapy is not very high. Nevertheless, dentists must not underestimate the importance of various general health conditions of their patients. All patients considered for implant surgery should be evaluated carefully in this respect. It should be also emphasized that this chapter is dedicated to only the most important aspects of this issue, but dentists are responsible for all conditions of their patients, including those that were not discussed in this chapter.

References

Ainamo, J; Talari, A. Eruptive movements of teeth in human adults. In: Poole DFG, Stack MV, editors. *The eruption and occlusion of teeth*. London: Butterworths, 1976, 97–107.

Aspenberg, P. Bisphosphonates and implants. An overview. *Acta Orthopedica*, 2009, 80, 119–123.

Bain, CA. Smoking and implant failure-benefits of a smoking cessation protocol. *Int J Oral Maxillofac Implants*, 1996, 11, 756–9.

Barron, MJ; McDonnell, ST; MacKie, I; Dixon, MJ. Hereditary dentine disorders: dentinogenesis imperfecta and dentine dysplasia. *Orphanet J Rare Diseases*, 2008, 3, 31.

Behrents, RG. *Growth in the aging craniofacial skeleton. (Monographs No 17. Craniofacial growth series).* Ann Arbor: University of Michigan, 1985, 1–145.

Beikler, T; Flemming, TF. Implants in the medically compromised patient. *Crit Rev Oral Biol Med*, 2003, 14, 305–316.

Bergendal, T; Eckerdal, O; Hallonsten, AL; Koch, G; Kurol, J; Kvint, S. Osseointegrated implants in the oral habilitation of a boy with ectodermal dysplasia: a case report. *Int Dent J*, 1991, 41, 149–156.

Bergendal, B; Bergendal, T; Hallonsten, AL; Koch, G; Kurol J; Kvint, S. A multidisciplinary approach to oral rehabilitation with osseointegrated implants in children and adolescents with multiple aplasia. *Eur J Orthodontics*, 1996, 18, 119–129.

Bjork, A; Skieller, V. Normal and abnormal growth of the mandible. A synthesis of longitudinal cephalometric implant studies over a period of 25 years. *Eur J Orthodontics*, 1983, 5, 1–46.

Blazsek, J; Dobo Nagy, C; Blazsek, I; Varga, R; Vecsei, B; Fejerdy, P; Varga, G. Aminobisphosphonate stimulates bone regeneration and enforces consolidation of titanium implant into a new rat caudal vertebrae model. *Pathol Oncol Res*, 2009, 15, 567–577.

Branemark, PI; Hansson, BO; Adell, R; Breine, U; Lindstrom, J; Hallen, O; Ohman, A. *Osseointegrated implants in the treatment of edentulous jaw. Experiences from a 10-year period.* Stockholm: Almquist and Wiksell International; 1977.

Bryant, SR; Zarb, GA. Outcomes of implant prosthodontic treatment in older adults. *J Can Dent Assoc*, 2002, 68, 97–102.

Carini, F; Bucalo, C; Saggese, V; Monai, D; Porcaro, G. Osteointegration in oncologic patients: a case report. *Annali di Stomatologia*, 2012/a, 3, (Suppl. 2) 37–40.

Carini, F; Francesconi, M; Saggese, V; Monai, D; Porcaro, G. Implant-supported rehabilitation of a patient with mandibular ameloblastoma. *Annali di Stomatologia*, 2012/b, 3, (Suppl. 2) 21–25.

Depprich, RA; Ommerborn, MA; Handschel, JGK; Naujoks, CD; Meyer, U; Keble, NR. Dentin dysplasia type I: a challenge for treatment with dental implants. *Head & Face Med*, 2007, 3, 31.

Dowell, S; Oates, TW; Robinson, M. A pilot study of implant success in individuals with type 2 diabetes mellitus with varying glycemic control. *J Am Dent Assoc*, 2007, 138, 355–361.

Elsubeihi, ES; Zarb, GA. Implant prosthodontics in medically challenged patients: The University of Toronto experience. *J Can Dent Assoc*, 2002, 68, 103–108.

Fleisch, H. Bisphosphonates: mechanisms of action. *Endocr Rev*, 1998, 19, 80–100.

Forsberg, CM; Eliasson, S; Westergren, H. Face height and tooth eruption in adults. A 20-year follow-up investigation. *Eur J Orthodontics*, 1991, 13, 249–254.

Gjorup, H; Daugaard-Jensen, J; Poulsen, S. Ten years with Danish centres of oral health in rare diseases. *Danish Dent J*, 2013, 117, 552–559.

Hwang, D; Wang, HL. Medical contraindications to implant therapy: part I: Absolute contraindications. *Implant Dent*. 2006, 15, 353–360.

Inbarajan, A; Veeravalli, PT; Vaidyanathan, AK; Grover, M. Short-term evaluation of dental implants in a diabetic population: an *in vivo* study. *J Adv Prosthodont*, 2012, 4, 134–138.

Infante-Cossio, P; Martinez-de-Fuentes, R; Garcia-Perla-Garcia, A; Jimenez-Castellanos, E; Gomez-Izquierdo, L. Myxofibroma of the maxilla. Reconstruction with iliac crest graft and dental implants after tumor resection. *Med Oral Patol Oral Cir Bucal*, 2011, 16, e532–e536.

Iseri, H; Solow, B. Continued eruption of maxillary incisors and first molars in girls from 9 to 25 years, studied by the implant method. *Eur J Orthodontics*, 1996, 18, 245–256.

Johansen, NB; Larsen, HL; Pedersen, AML. Treatment of patients with medical & psychiatric conditions, using medicines which are of interest to dentists. *Danish Dent J*, 2013, 117, 908–915.

Junquera, L; Gallego, L; Pelaz, A. Multiple myeloma and bisphosphonate-related osteonecrosis of the mandible associated with dental implants. *Case Report in Dentistry*, 2011, Article ID: 568246. DOI: 10.1155/2011/568246.

Korfage, A; Stellingsma, K; Jansma, J; Vissink, A; Raghoebar, GM. Oral rehabilitation with implant-based prostheses of two adult patients treated for childhood rhabdomyosarcoma. *Support Care Cancer*, 2011, 19, 1477–1480.

Masroori, P; Schiodt, M. Guidelines regarding tooth extractions on patients receiving bisphosphonate treatment. *Danish Dental J*, 2013, 117, 386–393.

Mellado-Valero, A; Ferrer-Garcia, JC; Herrera-Ballester, A; Labaig-Rueda, C. Effects of diabetes on the osseointegration of dental implants. *Med Oral Patol Oral Cir Bucal*, 2007, 12, E38–E43.

Mellado-Valero, A; Ferrer-Garcia, JC; Calvo-Catala, J; Labaig-Rueda, C. Implant treatment in patients with osteoporosis. *Med Oral Patol Oral Cir Bucal*, 2010, 15, e52–e57.

Minguez-Serra, MP; Salort-Llorca, C; Silvestre-Donat, FJ. Oral implants in patients receiving bisphosphonates: A review and update. *Med Oral Patol Oral Cir Bucal*, 2008, 13, E755–E760.

Nishimura, R; Nojima, K; Nishii, Y; Hanai, J; Arataki, T; Uchiyama, T; Yamaguchi, H. Multidisciplinary treatment of mandibular prognatism with multiple congenitally missing teeth. *Bull Tokyo Dent Coll*, 2006, 47, 25–31.

Oates, TW; Dowell, S; Robinson, M; McMahan, CA. Glycemic control and implant stabilization in type 2 diabetes mellitus. *J Dent Res*, 2009, 88, 367–371.

Oates, TW; Huynh-Ba, G; Vargas, A; Alexander, P; Feine, J. A critical review of diabetes, glycemic control and dental implant therapy. *Clin Oral Implants Res*, 2013, 24, 117–127.

Odman, J; Grondahl, K; Lekholm, U; Thilander, B. The effect of osseointegrated implants on the dento-alveolar development. A clinical and radiographic study in growing pigs. *Eur J Orthodontics*, 1991, 13, 279–286.

Oesterle, LJ; Cronin, RJ; Ranly, DM. Maxillary implants and the growing patient. *Int J Oral Maxillofac Implants*, 1993, 8, 377–38.

Richardson, G; Russell, KA. Congenitally missing maxillary lateral incisors and orthodontic treatment considerations for the single-tooth implant. *J Can Dent Assoc*, 2001, 67, 25–28.

Sailer, HF; Tarawneh, F; Fourkas, P; Antoniades, DZ; Athanasiou, AE. Surgical, orthodontic and prosthodontic rehabilitation of a patient with follicular ameloblastoma: A case report. *Eur J Dentistry*, 2010, 4, 192–196.

Sandhu, HS. A practical guide to tobacco cessation in dental offices. *J Can Dent Assoc*, 2001, 67, 153–157.

Schropp, L; Storsken, K. Implants versus conventional prosthetic rehabilitation. *Danish Dent J*, 2013, 117, 112–123.

Sham, ASK; Cheung, LK; Jin, LJ; Corbet, EF. The effects of tobacco use on oral health. *Hong Kong Med J*, 2003, 9, 271–277.

Sarnas, KV; Solow, B. Early adult changes in the skeletal and soft-tissue profile. *Eur J Orthodontics*, 1980, 2, 1–12.

Shin, EY; Kwon, YH; Herr, Y; Shin, SI; Chung, JH. Implant failure associated with oral bisphosphonate-related osteonecrosis of the jaw. *J Periodontal Implant Sci*, 2010, 40, 90–95.

Stanford, CM. Dental implants. A role in geriatric dentistry for the general practice? *J Am Dent Assoc*, 2007, 138, (Suppl. 9) 34S–40S.

Tallgren, A; Solow, B. Age differences in adult dentoalveolar heights. *Eur J Orthodontics*, 1991, 13, 149–156.

Thilander, B; Odman, J; Grondah, Lekholm, U. Aspects of osseointegrated implants inserted in growing jaws. A biometric and radiographic study in the young pig. *Eur J Orthodontics*, 1992, 14, 99–109.

Thilander, B; Odman, J; Grondahl, K; Friberg, B. Osseointegrated implants in adolescents. An alternative in replacing missing teeth? *Eur J Orthodontics*, 1994, 16, 84–95.

Thilander, B; Odman, J; Jemt, T. Single implants in the upper incisor region and their relationship to the adjacent teeth. An 8-year follow-up study. *Clin Oral Implants Res*, 1999, 10, 346–355.

Thilander, B; Odman, J; Lekholm, U. Orthodontic aspects of the use of oral implants in adolescents: a 10-year follow-up study. *Eur J Orthodontics*, 2001, 23, 715–731.

Todescan, S; Lavigne, S; Kelekis-Cholakis, A. Guidance for the maintenance care of dental implants: Clinical review. *J Can Dent Assoc* 2012, 78, c107.

Wood, B. A patient treated for lymphoma with chemotherapy is now interested in a dental implant. If her lymphoma recurs, will there be any ramifications for the implant? *J Can Dent Assoc*, 2010, 76, a91.

CHAPTER 16

FUTURE PERSPECTIVES

Abstract

Future implant dentistry will utilize the body's own healing and reconstructive mechanisms by means of materials and concepts that are not available for regular use now but can be readily extrapolated from current research efforts. Based on current developments, it is presumable that future implants will spontaneously heal and reconstruct surrounding tissues, which would revolutionize implant dentistry. It is also presumable that dental tissue engineering will provide an attractive alternative to traditional implantation therapies, with the hope that tissue-engineered teeth can be used to functionally replace missing teeth. However, tissue engineering-based therapies are in an early phase of development, and many issues need to be addressed before there are any clinical applications. Thus, it is likely that the classic approach of implant dentistry, based on the insertion and integration of non-vital alloplastic materials (primarily metals or ceramics) into the jaws, will continue to dominate implant dentistry. However, the implant systems used for this approach will undergo great development in upcoming years.

16.1. Introduction

Future implant dentistry will utilize the body's own healing and reconstructive mechanisms (Ratner 2001) by means of materials and concepts that are not available for regular use now, but can be extrapolated from current research efforts (Ratner 2001). Based on current developments, it is presumable that future implants will spontaneously heal and reconstruct surrounding tissues (Ratner 2001), which would revolutionize implant dentistry (Ratner 2001). Dental tissue engineering will provide an attractive alternative to traditional implantation therapies (Yen and Yelick 2011), with the hope that tissue-engineered teeth can be used to functionally replace missing teeth (Yen and Yelick 2011). However, scientists working in the field are confronted daily with new challenges and limitations (Mitsiadis and Papagerakis 2011) that might postpone the generation and clinical use of tissue-engineered teeth for many years (Mitsiadis and Papagerakis 2011).

16.2. Future Implant Systems

The classical approach of implant dentistry is based on the insertion and integration of non-vital alloplastic materials (primarily metals or ceramics) into the jaws. The authors expect that this approach will continue to dominate implant dentistry, and also that implant systems used for this approach will undergo great development in the near future.

Fixtures with surfaces containing bone morphogenetic proteins (and/or other bioactive molecules) that are gradually released will be available for regular use in the near future (Albrektsson and Wennerberg 2005; Hanawa 2011). Similarly, titanium implants with precision-nanomachined surface textures and structure patterns that might couple into the spacing of mobile receptors on cell surfaces (and thus modulate healing) will also be available for clinical use soon (Ratner 2001). These improvements will surely improve the outcome of implants in grafted bone or where implants might otherwise be unstable (Albrektsson and Wennerberg 2005; Hanawa 2011; Ratner 2001). Based on the expectable improvement of the surface properties of fixtures, it is also likely that the fixtures will, in general, be shorter, and may also be thinner in the future.

It is also anticipated that the use of specific surface nanopatterns may lead to the development of fixtures able to induce the formation of periodontal ligament (PDL) or PDL-like structures surrounding their surface (Dangaria et al. 2011; Lin et al. 2011). Data indicate that periodontal ligament-derived dental progenitor cells (DPCs) can be used to induce the formation of periodontal ligament tissues on titanium implants, leading to organized PDL tissues surrounding titanium implant surfaces (Lin et al. 2011), especially because it is likely that DPCs of periodontal ligament origin exhibit the differentiative potential characteristics of stem cells (Lin et al. 2011) and are potentially also able to organize periodontal tissues around titanium fixtures placed in the jaw at the site of previously lost teeth (Lin et al. 2011). These data may hold the potential for the development of new implant insertion approaches aimed at the development of PLD around fixtures as alternatives to osseointegrated dental implants (Lin et al. 2011).

It is also very likely that the development of new ceramic materials (for example zirconia) will allow the manufacture of implant systems (i.e. fixtures and/or abutments and/or crowns) from ceramics, and this will lead to further enhanced esthetics (Albrektsson and Wennerberg 2005).

16.3. Tissue Engineering

Although there are various strategies for tissue engineering (Yen and Yelick 2011), the most promising studies usually utilize mesenchymal/ectomesenchimal stem cells, delivered or internally recruited, to generate orofacial structures in temporary (resorbable) scaffolding biomaterials (Mao et al. 2006; Duailibi et al. 2008). Many aspects of tissue engineering are likely to be realized in the foreseeable future and will represent an opportunity that dentistry cannot afford to miss (Mao et al. 2006). It is very likely that traditional bone grafts will be replaced by tissue-engineered bone tissue at first (Albrektsson and Wennerberg 2005; Pedersen et al. 2012). Later, it will also be possible to produce new, tissue-engineered teeth to replace missing teeth (Albrektsson and Wennerberg 2005).

The generation of a new whole tooth consists of recreating and mimicking the molecular and cellular events that occur during odontogenesis (Young et al. 2002; Duailibi et al. 2004, 2008; Mitsiadis and Papagerakis 2011; Yen and Yelick 2011). Thus, the process involves the initiation of growth and eruption of new teeth in the mouth of the patient (Mitsiadis and Papagerakis 2011) by means of manipulating and placing stem cells into biodegradable scaffolds in vitro (Young et al. 2002; Duailibi et al. 2004, 2008), and implanting these tissue-engineered systems into the bone of the jaws (Duailibi et al. 2008).

However, the use of tissue-engineered teeth poses several challenges that need to be solved prior to any clinical trial/application (Mitsiadis and Papagerakis 2011). The existing challenges include the need to determine consistent protocols to control the number, size, shape, and color of any newly developing teeth (Young et al. 2002; Duailibi et al. 2004, 2008; Mitsiadis and Papagerakis 2011; Yen and Yelick 2011), as well as to considerably shorten the time of enamel and root formation and tooth eruption (Mitsiadis and Papagerakis 2011; Yen and Yelick 2011), and to create suitable jaw implantation site environments that enable tooth development (Yen and Yelick 2011). Despite these premised challenges, we can hope that rapid scientific and technological advancement will provide solutions that will allow tissue-engineered teeth to become a routine treatment for individuals with missing teeth (Mitsiadis and Papagerakis 2011) in time.

16.4. Diagnostic and Surgical Tools

It is presumable that improved three-dimensional diagnostic tools (e.g. CBCT) will be available for general use, leading to improved treatment planning and a more general use of surgical guides (Albrektsson and Wennerberg 2005). Proper computerized monitoring of chewing patterns, leading to more accurate adjustment of occlusion of implant-supported prostheses, will also be available (Albrektsson and Wennerberg 2005). It is also likely that more advanced techniques for the assessment of bone quality will be available based on new methods of analysis, for example Raman-spectroscopy (Morris and Mandair 2011).

It is also predictable that the possibility to virtually visualize the drill in the bone and the adjacent anatomical structures in real time by means of computer-assisted navigational surgery will be used more widely, especially in patients with challenging surgical anatomy (Ng et al. 2005). It is also likely that the premised computer-assisted navigational surgery will be supplemented with telerobotic-assisted drilling systems (Kasahara et al. 2012) because these teleoperated surgery systems make it possible to perform precision drilling of bone that exceeds the capabilities of human dexterity (Kasahara et al. 2012). With the use of teleoperated robotic precision drilling combined with real-time direct virtual vision, both surgeons and patients are assured of greater surgical safety (Ng et al. 2005; Kasahara et al. 2012), which will increase the confidence and reduce the surgical stress in both the patient and the clinician (Ng et al. 2005; Kasahara et al. 2012).

It is also very likely that a better understanding of the importance of surgical and prosthodontic skills will arise gradually from newly designed quality-control tests in the near future (Albrektsson and Wennerberg 2005).

16.5. Other Perspectives

The development of new methods to treat peri-implantitis is predictable. A future approach may be based on implant disinfection by means of electrolysis utilizing the electrical conductivity of titanium implant systems (Mohn et al. 2011). In this promising approach, alkalinity (i.e. the anode) or active oxidants (i.e. the cathode) can be generated via electrolysis in the body fluids surrounding the fixture and/or abutment, which can reduce viable counts of adhering bacteria, especially if the implants are used as cathodes and oxidative species are generated (Mohn et al. 2011).

It is also very likely that the use of several physiotherapies, especially electrical and electromagnetic treatments, will see a revival based on a better understanding of the relation between such externally applied signals and cellular functions (Albrektsson and Wennerberg 2005; Beck et al. 2012; Fabian et al. 2012/a). Further, it is also presumable that psychological and psychosomatic aspects of dental implant therapy will be an emerging issue in the near future (Beck et al. 2012; Fabian and Fejerdy 2010; Fabian et al. 2012/b)

Conclusion

The classical approach of implant dentistry based on the insertion and integration of non-vital alloplastic materials (primarily metals and ceramics) into jaws will continue to dominate implant dentistry. However, the implant systems used for this approach will undergo great development. Although the prospect of tissue-engineered teeth is also very attractive, it is unlikely that they will replace routine clinical dental practices in the near future (Mitsiadis and Papagerakis 2011). Tissue engineering-based therapies are in an early phase of development, and many issues need to be addressed before there is any clinical application (Mitsiadis and Papagerakis 2011).

References

Albrektsson, T; Wennerberg, A. The impact of oral implants – Past and future, 1966-2042. *J Can Dent Assoc*, 2005, 71, 327–327d.

Beck, A; Varga, G; Hermann, P; Fabian, G; Fejerdy, P; Fabian, TK. Methods for the treatment of denture induced psychogenic symptoms. In: Fabian TK, Fejerdy P, Hermann P, editors. *Dentures. Types, benefits and potential complications.* New York: Nova Science Publishers, 2012, 165–197.

Dangaria, SJ; Ito, Y; Yin, LL; Valdre, G; Luan, X; Diekwisch, TGH. Apatite microtopographies instruct signaling tapestries for progenitor-driven new attachment of teeth. *Tissue Engineering (Part A)*, 2011, 17, 279–290.

Duailibi MT, Duailibi SE, Young CS, Vacanti JP, Bartlett JD, Yelick PC. Bioengineered teeth from cultured rat tooth bud cells. *J Dent Res*, 2004, 83, 523–528.

Duailibi, SE; Duailibi, MT; Zhang, W; Asrican, R; Vacanti, JP; Yelick, PC. Bioengineered dental tissues grown in the rat jaw. *J Dent Res*, 2008, 87, 745–750.

Fabian, TK; Fejerdy P. *Psychogenic denture intolerance. Theoretical background, prevention and treatment possibilities.* New York: Nova Science Publishers; 2010, 162–170.

Fabian, TK; Beck, A; Fabian, G; Fejerdy, P; Hermann, P. Pulsed electromagnetic field (PEMF) therapy for peri-implant healing and bone remodeling. In: Fabian TK, Fejerdy P, Hermann P, editors. *Dentures. Types, benefits and potential complications.* New York: Nova Science Publishers, 2012/a, 243–254.

Fabian, TK; Beck, A; Gotai, L; Hermann, P; Fejerdy, P. Psychogenic complications of making dentures. Theoretical background, prevention and treatment possibilities. In: Fabian TK, Fejerdy P, Hermann P, editors. *Dentures. Types, benefits and potential complications.* New York: Nova Science Publishers, 2012/b, 199–241.

Hanawa, T. A comprehensive review of techniques for biofunctionalization of titanium. *J Periodontal Implant Sci*, 2011, 41, 263–272.

Kasahara, Y; Kawana, H; Usuda, S; Ohnishi, K. Telerobotic-assisted bone-drilling system using bilateral control with feed operation scaling and cutting force scaling. *Int J Med Robotics Comput Assist Surg*, 2012, 8, 221–229.

Lin, Y; Gallucci, GO; Buser, D; Bosshardt, D; Belser, UC; Yelick, PC. Bioengineered periodontal tissue formed on titanium dental implants. *J Dent Res*, 2011, 90, 251–256.

Mohn, D; Zehnder, M; Stark, WJ; Imfeld, T. Electrochemical disinfection of dental implants – a proof of concept. *PLoS One*, 2011, 6, e16157.

Mao, JJ; Giannobile, WV; Helms, JA; Hollister, SJ; Krebsbach, PH; Longaker, MT; Shi, S. Craniofacial tissue engineering by stem cells. *J Dent Res*, 2006, 85, 966–979.

Mitsiadis, TA; Papagerakis, P. Regenerated teeth: the future of tooth replacement? *Regen Med*, 2011, 6, 135–139.

Morris, MD; Mandair, GS. Raman assessment of bone quality. *Clin Orthop Relat Res*, 2011, 469, 2160–2169.

Ng, FC; Ho, KH; Wexler, A. Computer-assisted navigational surgery enhances safety in dental implantology. *Ann Acad Med Singapore*, 2005, 34, 383–388.

Pedersen, TO; Blois, AL; Xue, Y; Xing, Z; Cottler-Fox, M; Fristad, I; Leknes, KN; Lorens, JB; Mustafa, K. Osteogenic stimulatory conditions enhance growth and maturation of endothelial cell microvascular networks in culture with mesenchimal stem cells. *J Tissue Engineering*, 2012, 3, Article ID: 2041731412443236. DOI: 10.1177 /2041731412443236.

Ratner, BD. Replacing and renewing: Synthetic materials, biomimetics, and tissue engineering in implant dentistry. *J Dent Education*, 2001, 65, 1340–1347.

Yen, AH; Yelick, PC. Dental tissue regeneration – A mini-review. *Gerodontology*, 2011, 57, 85–94.

Young CS, Honda M, Terada S, Vacanti JP, Bartlett JD, Yelick PC. Tissue engineering of complex tooth structures on biodegradable polymer scaffolds. *J Dent Res*, 2002, 81, 695–700.

CONCLUSION

The applied anatomy of orofacial tissues is very important for dentists practicing implant dentistry. In the relevant chapter, the "hottest topics" of applied maxillary and mandibular anatomy were discussed to help the reader avoid unsuccessful surgical interventions due to misunderstanding practical morphological details of high clinical importance and to help implant planning from both the surgical and prosthodontic viewpoint.

The major diagnostic tool for implant dentistry is X-ray diagnostics, which usually includes the evaluation of several two-dimensional images, like intraoral radiographs and images of orthopantomography, as well as three-dimensional images, such as cone-beam computed tomography. *Intraoral radiographs* are primarily used for follow up, including the examination of the bone-implant interface for signs of failure, such as a radiolucent rim around the implant body and loss of crestal bone and augmented/grafted bone. *Orthopantomography* (also referred to as *panoramic radiography*) is one of the most frequently used modalities for presurgical planning, including both finding an appropriate location for an implant and measuring the available bone. *Cone-beam computed tomography* systems belong to the highest level of computed tomography systems. These systems were designed specifically for visualization of the maxillofacial region and offer both two- and three-dimensional images with high spatial resolution. CBCT offers a great advantage when compared to medical CT in terms of accuracy, scan time reduction, dose reduction, and its lower number of artifacts.

A large number of various biomaterials may be used for implant surgery, and their number is increasing continuously. It is rather difficult for researchers and clinicians to keep up in this field. Therefore, there is a need for general reviews on available current scientific data to keep related knowledge up-to-date and functional. In the relevant chapter, the most important current knowledge related to biomaterials used for implant surgery was summarized.

Although the success rate of implant treatments is high, achieving osseointegration is still a challenging task for clinicians. Understanding the basic phenomena behind osseointegration may help a clinician solve more complex cases appearing in praxis. It may also help to be up-to-date on the rather complex market of various implant products and treatment trends and their related protocols. Although contact osteogenesis is considered as optimum currently, it is very likely that proper osseointegration may also occur via distance osteogenesis. The latter may gain more theoretical and clinical importance in the future if developments in relation to resorbable or partially resorbable coatings lead to a breakthrough.

The surface roughness properties of implants strongly influence peri-implant gingival healing processes; and it is also obvious that the properties of surface morphology are equally important at both the microscale and nanoscale level. Although smooth titanium surfaces are used conventionally in the trans-gingival region, it seems to be rather difficult to find out which surface properties should be considered as optimal for gingival closure, especially because not only surface roughness, but also chemical composition and physical properties like hydrophilicity and others affect the behavior of peri-implant gingival tissues. Since the proper healing and attachment of peri-implant gingival tissues is crucial for the success of implant placement, future research should focus on improving connective tissue and epithelial attachment on implant fixtures and also on abutments in the case of two-piece implant systems.

The preservation of the alveolar ridge may be crucial for successful implant placement in many cases. For the preservation of the alveolar bone following tooth extraction, the use of common preservation techniques like "socket grafting," guided bone regeneration, immediate implant placement, and (in certain cases) forced eruption of compromised teeth may be used. Invasive techniques should be used very carefully, as the advancement of flaps may result in an increased inflammatory response, in a decrease in vestibular dimension and in the creation of unesthetic scars. Therefore guided bone regeneration and immediate implant placement should be used only if indicated. Reducing extraction trauma and limiting flap elevation (if any) are essentials for each of these procedures.

Physiotherapies were found to be beneficial for a wide variety of therapeutic processes over the last few decades. Data in the literature has revealed that bone formation and soft tissue healing around dental implants can also be significantly promoted by physiotherapeutic treatment. Although various modalities of physiotherapy have been found to be beneficial to a wide variety of therapeutic processes in implant dentistry, the exact mechanisms by which they affect alveolar bone and other peri-implant tissues is far from fully understood. However, certain mechanisms are already recognized, and the increased amount of knowledge may be utilized in clinical practice. Although physiotherapies in general can be seen as noninvasive tools, the few contraindications related to their use should be considered carefully for safe and successful application.

The most important surgical aspects dentists should consider in relation to implant dentistry include principles of implant site preparation and implant placement, the timing of implant site preparation (immediate, early, and delayed implant placement), the timing of loading (immediate, early, and delayed loading), the type of loading (functional, nonfunctional, and progressive), surgical management of various implant failures (peri-implantitis, fracture), several forms of bone augmentation, the major techniques of sinus floor elevation (including the management of sinus membrane perforation), and soft tissue surgery, as well as certain important related topics like the assessment of bone quality and primary stability. Besides these, several more advanced surgical techniques, like alveolar distraction osteogenesis, alveolar nerve lateralization, alveolar nerve transposition, and the use of tilted, zygomatic, and tuberal implantation, as well as principles of virtual implant placement and navigational surgery may also be considered.

The abutment is a highly important part of most implant systems. Positioned between the fixture and the denture, the abutment makes it possible to connect dentures to fixtures and to modify the long axis of the implant-abutment-denture complex if needed. The disadvantage of the use of an abutment is the appearance of two (i.e. the fixture-abutment and the abutment-denture) interfaces, from which at least one could be discounted if the abutment is not used. On the other hand, the use of an abutment clearly increases the plasticity and adaptability of the whole implant system. Further, creative use of the abutment, together with provisional restoration, is a rather efficient tool for soft tissue modeling (contouring, profiling), which is crucial for obtaining the proper soft tissue esthetic in many cases.

Besides available bone, surgical technique, bone quality, and osseointegration processes, the outcome of dental implant therapy also strongly depends on factors like surgical technique, the vertical positioning of the fixture, the shape and surface properties of the neck of the fixture, and the fixture-abutment interface, as well as the "crown-to-implant" ratio and the mechanical stress exposure of the peri-implant bone during mastication. Besides these, patients who have undergone implant therapy should also receive adequate maintenance care, including regular recalls and proper personal and professional oral hygiene (avoiding fluoride corrosion), as well as immediate and adequate therapeutic interventions (if needed), to reach a favorable outcome. With optimal maintenance care, a marginal bone loss of roughly 1.1 mm during the first year and 0.1 mm per year thereafter may be considered a satisfactory outcome.

The survival rate and marginal bone loss values of short implants are comparable to (or may be even better than) those of longer implants. Similarly, results in relation to narrow implants are also rather good and comparable to those of regular diameter implants. Orthodontic mini-implants serve as temporary skeletal anchorage devices and are excellent alternatives to conventional orthodontic intraoral or extraoral (headgear) anchorages. All these data clearly indicate that special-sized implants are qualified for regular use in dentistry.

Even though a dental treatment may have been carried out properly, there is no assurance that the patient will be satisfied with the therapy. A normative evaluation by a dentist and a subjective evaluation by the patient related to the dental treatment may be rather different. Therefore the factors unrelated to operative/technological dental skills but that contribute to the success of dental treatments are becoming more and more important in the field of implant dentistry.

Medication is an important supplementary modality of implant dentistry, even if there are various medical (and/or dental) contraindications, possible side effects, and adverse effects, as well as possible dangerous interactions that should be considered. Utilizing pharmacological databases and *up-to-date* pharmacological and clinical knowledge, dentists should be familiar with both the benefits and potential hazards before prescribing a medication.

Despite the high success rate of oral implants, implant failure, other complications, or adverse effects may occur. It should be emphasized that not only early diagnosis and adequate treatment, but also prevention, seem to be crucial in the case of all these conditions. In this respect, proper oral hygiene, prevention of bacterial infection during and following surgery, prevention of the overload of the implant system, avoidance of poor and/or excessively traumatic surgical techniques (including avoidance of overheating of the bone), and fabrication of proper dentures seem to be the most important.

There are only a few conditions that can be considered absolute contraindications with respect to dental implant rehabilitation, and the number of those conditions that may negatively influence or jeopardize the treatment outcome of dental implant therapy is not very high. Nevertheless, dentists must not underestimate the importance of various general health conditions of their patients. All patients considered for implant surgery should be evaluated carefully in this respect. It should be also emphasized that the relevant chapter is dedicated to the most important aspects of this issue only, but dentists are responsible for all conditions involving their patients, including those that were not discussed in the chapter.

The classic approach to implant dentistry, based on the insertion and integration of non-vital alloplastic materials (primarily metals or ceramics) into the jaw, will continue to dominate implant dentistry. However, the implant systems used for this approach will undergo great development. Although the prospect of tissue-engineered teeth is also very attractive, it is unlikely that they will replace routine clinical dental practices in the near future. Tissue engineering-based therapies are in an early phase of development and many issues need to be addressed before any clinical application occurs.

AUTHORS' CONTACT INFORMATION

Dr. Tibor Károly Fábián,
Kattesundet 8, 2.tv
5700 Svendborg
Denmark/EU
Tel:+ 45-22-87-81-98
Email: fabiantiborkaroly@gmaii.com

Hans Christian Hidalgo Wulff,
Tandklinikken Sydfyn,
Egevaenget 8.
5771 Stenstrup
Denmark/EU
Tel: +45- 6226-2233
Email: tandklinikken-stenstrup@mail.dk

INDEX

#

A

B

C

D

E

F

G

H

I

M

N

O

P

Q

R

S

U

V